ESTHETIC
COMPOSITE BONDING

TECHNIQUES AND MATERIALS

Revised Reprint

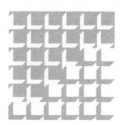

ESTHETIC
COMPOSITE BONDING

TECHNIQUES AND MATERIALS

Revised Reprint

RONALD E. JORDAN, D.D.S., M.S.D., F.I.C.D., F.R.C.D.(C)

Professor
Department of Restorative Dentistry

Associate Dean
Clinical Affairs
Faculty of Dentistry
University of Western Ontario
London, Ontario

BOKSMAN · COMFORTES · FEIGENBAUM · FRIEDMAN
GRATTON · GWINNETT · JORDAN · MOPPER · SUZUKI

1988 B.C. Decker Inc. · Toronto · Philadelphia

Publisher

B.C. Decker Inc.
3228 South Service Road
Burlington, Ontario   L7N 3H8

B.C. Decker Inc.
320 Walnut Street, Suite 400
Philadelphia, Pennsylvania   19106

Sales and Distribution

United States and Possessions	**The C.V. Mosby Company** 11830 Westline Industrial Drive Saint Louis, Missouri 63146
Canada	**The C.V. Mosby Company, Ltd.** 5240 Finch Avenue East, Unit No. 1 Scarborough, Ontario M1S 4P2
United Kingdom, Europe and the Middle East	**Blackwell Scientific Publications, Ltd.** Osney Mead, Oxford OX2 OEL, England
Australia	**Holt-Saunders Pty. Limited** 9 Waltham Street Artarmon, N.S.W. 2064 Australia
Japan	**Igaku-Shoin Ltd.** Tokyo International P.O. Box 5063 1-28-36 Hongo, Bunkyo-ku, Tokyo 113, Japan
Asia	**Holt-Saunders Asia Limited** 10/F, Inter-Continental Plaza Tsim Sha Tsui East Kowloon, Hong Kong

Esthetic Composite Bonding - Techniques and Materials (Revised Reprint)   ISBN 1-55664-039-0

Library of Congress catalog card number: 87-70934

Printed in Hong Kong   10   9   8   7   6   5   4   3   2   1

To my wife Wilona, daughters Anne, Jane, and Sally, and sons John, David, and Peter,
without whose patience, understanding, and support
this book could not have been written.

CONTRIBUTORS

LEENDERT BOKSMAN, D.D.S., B.Sc., F.A.D.I.
Associate Professor
Division of Operative Dentistry
Faculty of Dentistry
University of Western Ontario
London, Ontario

ISAAC COMFORTES, D.D.S.
Assistant Clinical Professor of Restorative Dentistry

Special Lecturer in Esthetic Dentistry
University of Southern California
School of Dentistry
Los Angeles, California

NORMAN L. FEIGENBAUM, D.D.S.
Private Practitioner
New York, New York

Editor
The Forum of Esthetic Dentistry

MARK J. FRIEDMAN, D.D.S.
Assistant Clinical Professor of Restorative Dentistry

Special Lecturer in Esthetic Dentistry
University of Southern California
Los Angeles, California

DONALD R. GRATTON, D.D.S., M.S.
Associate Professor and Coordinator
Clinical Fixed Prosthodontics
Faculty of Dentistry
University of Western Ontario
London, Ontario

A. JOHN GWINNETT, B.D.S., L.D.S.R.C.S., Ph.D.
Professor
Department of Oral Biology and Pathology
School of Dental Medicine
State University of New York at Stony Brook
Stony Brook, New York

DAVID R. JORDAN, M.D.
Department of Ophthalmology
Ottawa General Hospital
Ottawa, Ontario

**RONALD E. JORDAN, D.D.S.,
M.S.D., F.I.C.D., F.R.C.D.(C)**
Professor
Department of Restorative Dentistry

Associate Dean
Clinical Affairs
Faculty of Dentistry
University of Western Ontario
London, Ontario

K. WILLIAM MOPPER, B.A., D.D.S., M.S.
Private Practitioner
Winnetka, Illinois

Diplomat of the American Board of Pedodontics

MAKOTO SUZUKI, D.D.S., M.S., F.I.C.D.
Associate Professor and Chairman
Division of Fixed Prosthodontics
Faculty of Dentistry
University of Western Ontario
London, Ontario

PREFACE

The purpose of *Esthetic Composite Bonding* is to provide clinical information on composite resin bonding techniques and materials as they relate to a wide variety of applications. The book is oriented primarily to the practitioner of general dentistry and to undergraduate dental students. The data presented are the direct result of approximately 10 years of clinical research activity that was sponsored primarily by Ontario Provincial Health grants.

It is a well known fact that the practice of general dentistry has recently undergone significant change. Primarily as a result of the effectiveness of patient education and preventive programs, the incidence of dental caries is currently very low. Accordingly, the profile of general dental practice has changed from the conventional restorative approach to include a much greater emphasis on esthetic dentistry. Composite bonding techniques are therefore of fundamental importance to the practitioner. A working knowledge of the composite materials used in crown restoration, treatment of the discolored dentition, dentin bonding, posterior restorations, resin-bonded retainers, and fissure sealants constitutes the "bread and butter" of general practice dentistry.

No individual can possibly claim expertise in all phases of composite restorative dentistry. Thus, contributors who have demonstrated special talents in specific areas have been selected to enrich this publication. Doctors Norman Feigenbaum and J. William Mopper are internationally recognized experts in bonding techniques, particularly as they relate to direct veneers. Doctors Mark Friedman and Isaac Comfortes, both well known in the field of esthetic dentistry, present some interesting and innovative ideas on the subject. My colleagues, Doctors Makoto Suzuki, Donald Gratton, and Len Boksman who have been extensively involved for 12 years in clinical research related to composite materials and techniques, provide a wealth of information based on clinical observations of long-term standing. Dr. A. J. Gwinnett, a widely recognized pioneer in the vast area of bonding, provides a highly valuable scientific approach to the subject.

Although visible-light-cured composite materials are excellent for esthetic bonding techniques, it is now known that particular caution must be exercised in using light-cure units, since long-term exposure to visible light prematurely ages the retinal tissues. Dr. David R. Jordan presents valuable information in this important area.

To all of my contributors I offer my most sincere thanks; it is an honor to "have you aboard".

Ronald E. Jordan

CONTENTS

1

R O N A L D   E.   J O R D A N
A.   J O H N   G W I N N E T T

METHODS AND MATERIALS

There is nothing more gratifying than the sight of an intact young anterior dentition in an adolescent or preadolescent patient (Fig. 1-1), particularly the healthy, natural gingival-enamel relationship that is characteristically observed in young dentitions (Fig. 1-2). The natural gingival-enamel relationship in the young patient is tenuous (Dello-Russo, 1984) and usually is disrupted by operative procedures (Fig. 1-3). This is not meant to imply that a negative gingival response routinely follows full-coverage restorations. However, when a negative response does occur, it is extremely difficult to reverse by conservative means. For this reason, everything possible must be done to maintain the natural gingival-enamel relationship in its intact form. The major role of composite resin materials is that of "buying time" during the adolescent and early adult periods to attain this goal. In order to illustrate the concept of buying time and its clinical significance, two patients are presented for consideration.

A 14-year-old female was treated conservatively with ultraviolet-light-cured composite (Nuvafil[4]) for the restoration of two fractured maxillary central incisor crowns (Figs. 1-4 and 1-5). The restorations are shown at 7-year recall (Fig. 1-6). The right central incisor restoration was highly acceptable at this time, having no discoloration or fracture. The left central incisor (Fig. 1-7) showed marked discoloration within the immediately adjacent tooth structure, the result of dentin cracking (Jordan et al, 1977) with associated microleakage caused by placement of a single self-threading pin. The restoration was removed and replaced with a visible-light-cured composite material (Prismafil[18]) (Fig. 1-8); the result, 2 years later, is shown in Figure 1-9. Nine years after the original treatment, the natural gingival-enamel relationship is maintained, and it may remain that way for a lifetime as a result of conservative treatment with composite materials.

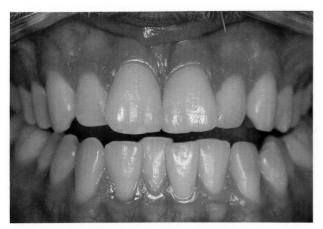

Figure 1-1 Anterior dentition of a 20-year-old patient.

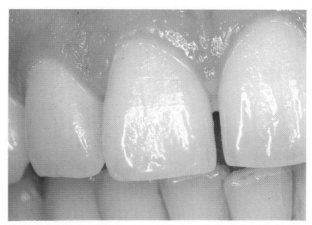

Figure 1-2 The healthy, natural gingival-enamel relationship in a young patient.

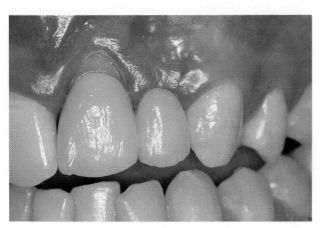

Figure 1-3 Gingival recession in association with a full-crown restoration on the maxillary left centralincisor.

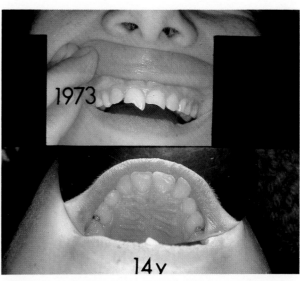

Figure 1-4 Fractured maxillary central incisors in a 14-year-old patient as seen preoperatively.

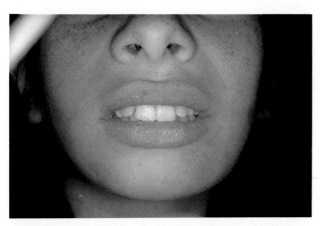

Figure 1-5 Composite restorations in the maxillary central incisors.

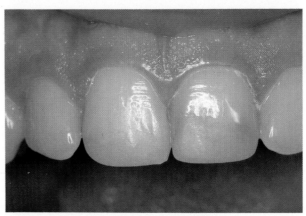

Figure 1-6 Seven-year recall appearance of the maxillary incisor composite restorations.

A 17-year-old patient with an extensively discolored large composite restoration in a nonvital right central incisor (Fig. 1-10) was treated by means of a full-coverage porcelain fused to metal crown. The result, at 4-year recall, is shown in Figure 1-11. The gingival inflammation associated with the restoration is self-evident.

Principle: The results of a failed composite restoration are easily reversed by conservative means, whereas failure of a full-coverage restoration is difficult, if not impossible, to reverse by conservative treatment procedures.

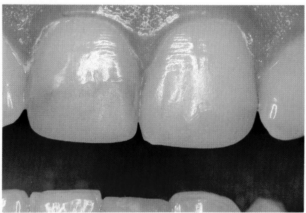

Figure 1–7 Close-up view of the pin-retained maxillary left central incisor restoration showing discoloration surrounding the pin.

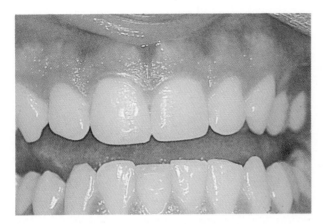

Figure 1-8 Maxillary left central incisor after restoration with light-cured composite material.

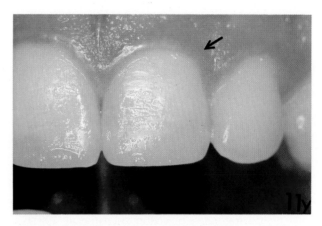

Figure 1-9 Restored maxillary incisors of the patient shown in Figures 1-5 through 1-8 at 9-year recall. The patient is 23 years of age and the intact gingival-enamel relationship is maintained.

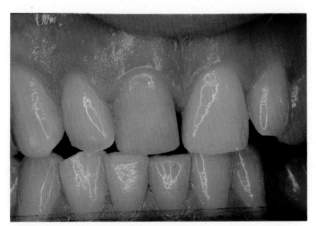

Figure 1-10 A large discolored composite restoration in the maxillary right central incisor prior to full coverage.

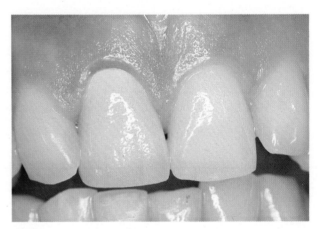

Figure 1-11 The central incisor shown in Figure 1-10 at 4-year recall.

The major reason that composite materials are so useful in terms of conservative operative dentistry is that, unlike other restorative materials, they are directly bondable to tooth structure (Gwinnett and Matsui, 1967) (Figs. 1-12 and 1-13). There are four basic types of bonding methods, all of which are extremely significant clinically:

1. Resin-enamel bonding (Fig. 1-14)
2. Resin-dentin bonding (Fig. 1-15)
3. Resin-resin bonding (Fig. 1-16)
4. Resin-metal bonding (Fig. 1-17)

Clinical success relative to each bonding method is clearly dependent on the choice of appropriate resin material and on the proper manipulative technique involved in the clinical restorative procedure (Jordan et al, 1981). The material-technique interaction is all-important in confirming the reliability of the clinical result. Accordingly, the dual material technique approach will be presented throughout this book.

There are many different materials that may be successfully used for conservative bonding procedures, and it is important that the practitioner choose the appropriate material for the purpose at hand. It may be hazardous to base this choice on physical properties alone because few, if any, such properties, by themselves, can reliably predict the clinical performance of a composite material in a given situation (Dennison, 1982). Clinical observations carried out for at least 2 years in controlled trials have proved to be a much more reliable predictor of performance. Unfortunately, few new materials are subjected to controlled long-term clinical performance trials before their introduction to dental practitioners.

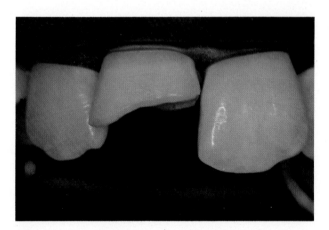

Figure 1-12   An extensively fractured maxillary right central incisor.

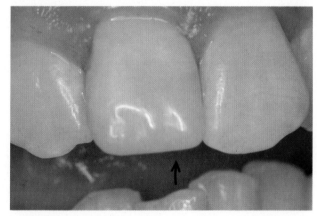

Figure 1-13   The incisor shown in Figure 1-12 after direct bonding with composite material.

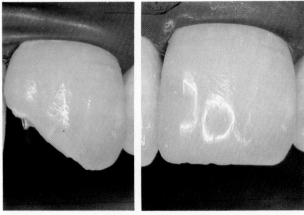

Figure 1–14   Incisal fracture, right central incisor and discolored class III restorations, maxillary lateral incisors prior to restoration.

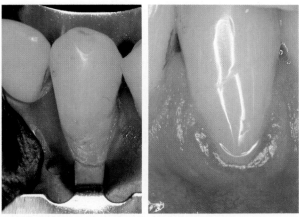

Figure 1–15   Typical example of resin-dentin bonding; preoperative (*left*) and postoperative (*right*).

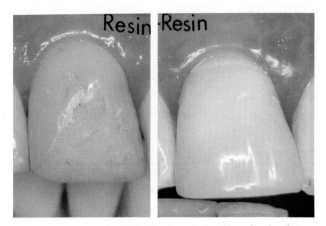

Figure 1–16   Typical example of resin-resin bonding; discolored composite restoration (*left*), veneered with new composite (*right*).

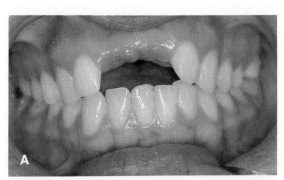

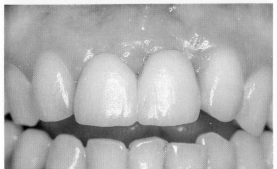

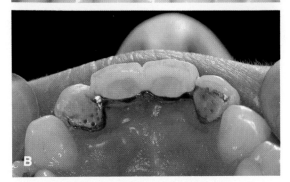

Figure 1–17   *A*, Missing maxillary central incisors (*top*) restored with metal resin-bonded fixed prosthesis (*bottom*). *B*, Lingual view of the resin-bonded fixed prosthesis.

Composite materials consist of two major components, namely, the resin binding matrix and the inorganic filler phases (Fig. 1-18). The resin binding matrix is not highly variable among composite materials; Bowen's resin bisphenol A-glycidyl methacrylate (Bis-GMA) constitutes the resin matrix of most composite materials, and urethane dimethacrylate is occasionally used as the matrix in some composite materials. However, no significant differences in clinical performance between Bis-GMA and urethane dimethacrylate have thus far been demonstrated. Composite materials differ mainly relative to their inorganic filler component. The type of inorganic filler, the size of the particles, and the extent of inorganic loading, all of which vary widely among composite materials, may be used by the operator to predict the clinical performance of a particular composite material. In initially assessing a new composite material, the practitioner should determine not only the size of the inorganic filler particle, but also the extent of inorganic loading by weight within the material, for both provide extremely valuable clinical information relative to the polishability of the material and to its degree of fracture resistance when placed in stress-bearing situations.

Size of the Inorganic Filler Particle

The inorganic filler particle may be as small in diameter as 0.04 microns or it may be as large as 15 to 30 microns. The polishability of the composite material varies over a wide range dependent on filler particle size. Composite materials in which the inorganic filler is submicron in size normally demonstrate superpolishable clinical characteristics (Fig. 1-19). That is, after proper finish, they present a smooth, highly reflective, glass-like surface similar to intact enamel surfaces.

Composite materials in which the inorganic filler particle size is between 1 and 8 microns are only semipolishable (Fig. 1-20). They present a duller, less reflective surface after finishing.

Materials in which the inorganic filler particle size is greater than 10 microns are considered to be nonpolishable (Fig. 1-21) since they present a dull, nonreflective surface after finishing. Caution should be exercised in using such materials in patients whose oral hygiene is not strictly controlled; the rough surfaces associated with such materials are plaque-retentive and prone to discoloration.

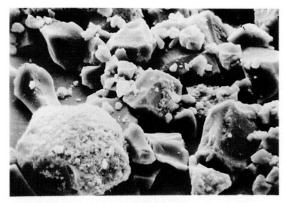

Figure 1–18   Scanning electron micrograph (500 ×) of inorganic filler particles in a composite material.

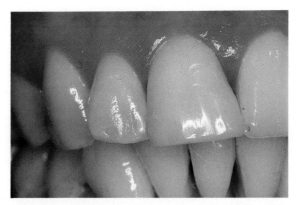

Figure 1-19   A large composite restoration in the maxillary right central incisor. The inorganic filler particle size in the composite material is submicron (.04 microns).

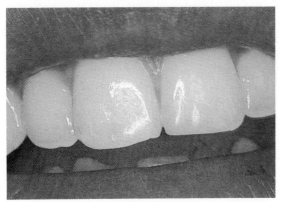

Figure 1–20   Mesioincisal composite restoration maxillary left central incisor. The inorganic filler particle size in the composite material is 5 microns.

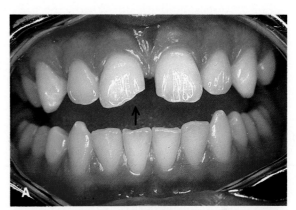

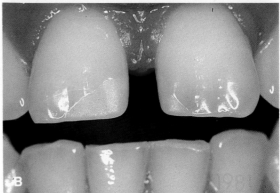

Figure 1-21   Fractured maxillary central incisors. *A*, Nine years after restoration. *B*, With a composite material in which the inorganic filler particle size is 15 microns.

Extent of Inorganic Loading

The amount of inorganic filler content by weight in a composite material is an important clinical consideration that can be used to predict the fracture resistance of a material placed in stress-bearing class IV situations (Lambrechts et al, 1982). A composite material that is inorganically loaded by weight 75 percent or more is termed a ''heavy-filled'' or ''macrofilled'' material. On the other hand, a composite material loaded inorganically by weight 66 percent or less is referred to as a ''lightly filled'' or ''microfilled'' material. The difference between lightly filled and heavy-filled composite materials is a most important clinical consideration since the latter are known to be highly resistant to fracture in stress-bearing situations, whereas the former are considerably less fracture-resistant (Fig. 1-22).

The size of the inorganic filler particle and the extent of inorganic loading by weight are interrelated variables. Thus far, it has not been possible to ''heavy load'' a composite material in which the inorganic filler particle size is submicron. On the other hand, if the inorganic filler particle size is 1 micron or greater, heavy inorganic loading is possible.

When a practitioner is confronted with a new composite material, therefore, the questions he should ask are: What is the size of the inorganic filler particle in microns, and what is the extent of inorganic loading by weight? Having determined the answers to these questions, he can easily categorize the composite material into microfilled, macrofilled, or hybrid (Lutz and Phillips, 1983). On the basis of this categorization, the clinician may reliably predict the clinical performance of a particular composite material.

Microfilled Composites

Microfilled materials[5-15] (Table 1-1) are by far the most polishable and esthetically acceptable of all composite systems. The inorganic filler in most microfilled composite materials is colloidal silica, which is a fine white powder with a particle size of approximately 0.04 microns. The submicron inorganic filler particle automatically yields a high degree of smooth surface polishability. Microfilled materials subjected to a carefully controlled finishing technique characteristically demonstrate a glossy, highly reflective surface not unlike that of glazed porcelain (Fig. 1-23). Unfortunately, the use of a submicron filler particle in a composite material precludes heavy inorganic loading, since the base resin (Bis-GMA or urethane dimethacrylate) is capable of accepting only a relatively limited amount of the microparticle inorganic filler. Indeed, the maximum inorganic loading with a microfilled material is usually in the vicinity of 51 to 52 percent and can be as little as 36 to 37 percent. This is in stark contrast to the inorganic loading level of other composite systems, which varies between 75 and 80 percent.

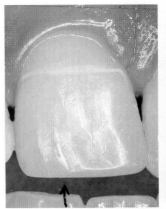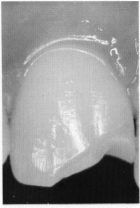

Figure 1-22 A lightly filled mesioincisal composite restoration in the maxillary left central incisor at time of insertion *(left)* and at 18-month recall *(right)* showing cohesive fracture.

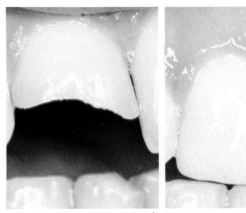

Figure 1-23 An extensively fractured right central incisor *(left)* restored with microfilled composite *(right)*.

TABLE 1-1   Composite Materials

	Large-Particle Macrofilled	Microfilled	Small-Particle Macrofilled	Hybrids
Particle size in microns	> 10	0.04	1 to 5	0.04+ < 5
Self-cured	Adaptic[1] Concise[2]	Phaseafill[5] Estic Microfil[6] Silar[7] Isopast[8] Superfil[9]	Profile[16] Simulate[17]	Miradapt[21] Finesse[22] P–10[23] Conclude[24]
Light-cured	Visiofil[3] Nuvafil[4]	Certain[10] Durafill[11] Silux[12] Heliosit[13] Rembrandt[14] Paste laminate[14a] Extra smooth[14b] Visiodispers[15]	Prismafil[18] Estilux[19] Command[20] Aurafil[27] Valux[32]	Brilliant Lux[25] Command Ultrafine[26] Herculite XR[31] P–30[28] Visarfil[29] Profile TLC[30]
Clinical features	High fracture resistance Nonpolishable Discoloration† Plucking	Less fracture resistance Superpolishable Color stable* No plucking	Fracture-resistant Semipolishable Color stable* No plucking	Fracture-resistant Polishable Color stable* No plucking
Indications	Large Class IV "Light on heavy" technique	"Protected" Class III and V Small Class IV labial veneers	Large Class IV Crown build-up Posterior restorations	Large Class IV Crown build-up Posterior restorations

*Light-cured
†Self-cured

The base or binding resin in most microfilled materials is Bis-GMA. The Bis-GMA resin accepts only a limited quantity of colloidal silica before it becomes extremely viscous and difficult to handle. In an effort to attain maximum inorganic loading, manufacturers pulverize a heat-polymerized ''prepolymer'' made up of an admixture of colloidal silica and Bis-GMA (Fig. 1-24). The resultant mistermed ''organic'' filler particles (i.e., colloidal silica-loaded Bis-GMA) are then incorporated into additional Bis-GMA, thus producing the microfilled composite material (Figs. 1-25 and 1-26). The so-called ''organic'' filler particles, usually large in diameter, can range in size between 20 and 100 microns and are the primary reason for the high viscosity of microfilled composite materials.

The microfilled materials are highly polishable, but lightly filled inorganically in comparison to other materials. What is the clinical significance of this difference? In general, the less the inorganic loading, the lower the fracture resistance of the material when placed in stress-bearing situations. This should not be interpreted as meaning that microfilled composites are contraindicated as class IV restoratives. The practitioner, however, in utilizing these materials in stress-bearing areas, must be extremely careful to adjust the occlusion not only in centric relation, but also in protrusive and lateral protrusive excursions. Should this not be done, a cohesive fracture of the microfilled composite material is likely (see Fig. 1-22).

The ideal composite material would surely demonstrate a unique combination of smooth surface polishability together with heavy inorganic loading and thus maximum durability in stress-bearing areas. The ultimate in anterior composite materials has not yet been developed; generally, in a particular system, what is gained in one important feature (polishability) almost automatically involves sacrifice of another (fracture resistance). Thus, a ''trade-off'' situation exists relative to differential clinical choice.

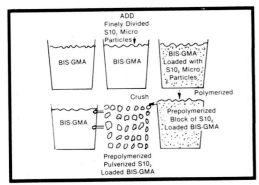

Figure 1-24 Diagrammatic illustration of the manufacturing process of a microfilled composite. The resin Bis-GMA is loaded with colloidal silica microfiller (*top*). The mixture is heat-polymerized to produce the prepolymer which is pulverized to form colloidal silica-loaded Bis-GMA particles (*bottom*).

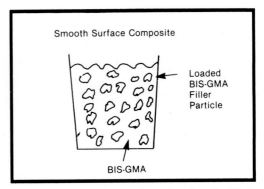

Figure 1-25 Diagrammatic illustration of a microfilled composite. It is made up of a Bis-GMA resin matrix with colloidal silica-loaded Bis-GMA filler particles.

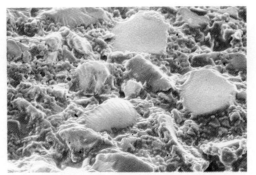

Figure 1-26 Scanning electron micrograph (300 ×) of a fracture specimen of microfilled composite material (Silar[7]). The large colloidal silica-loaded "filler" particles are irregular in shape and measure several microns. (Courtesy of Dr. A. J. Gwinnett, State University of New York at Stony Brook.)

Macrofilled Composites

A large number of macrofilled composite materials are available for clinical use (see Table 1–1). Such materials are characterized by a large inorganic filler particle, ranging in diameter between 1 micron and 15 microns (see Fig. 1-18). Because of their large particle size, these materials are not so ''high-gloss'' polishable as the microfilled systems. They present a duller, lusterless finished surface after polishing (see Fig. 1-21). The macrofiller particle size may be small or large. Composite materials in which the size of the inorganic filler particles is between 1 and 8 microns are referred to as *small-particle macrofilled systems*.[16-20] Such materials may be finished to a smooth topography, but the surface is duller and less reflective than is observed with microfilled materials (see Fig. 1-20). The small-particle macrofilled material therefore may be regarded as being semipolishable.

If the inorganic filler particle in a composite material is larger than 10 microns, such a material is essentially nonpolishable since it presents a dull, lusterless surface after finishing (Fig. 1-27). Composite materials with inorganic filler particles greater than 10 microns in size are known as *large-particle macrofilled systems*.[1-4]

The macrofilled composite materials differ significantly from the microfilled systems in that they invariably contain much more inorganic filler. The inorganic filler content of the macrofilled materials usually ranges between 75 and 80 percent or greater by weight. Clinical observations carried out on such materials during the past few years indicate that they are more resistant to fracture than are the microfilled materials when placed in class IV situations exposed to heavy occlusal loads (Figs. 1-28 through 1-31). What is sacrificed, therefore, in terms of polishability in the macrofilled materials is more than compensated for in terms of increased fracture resistance.

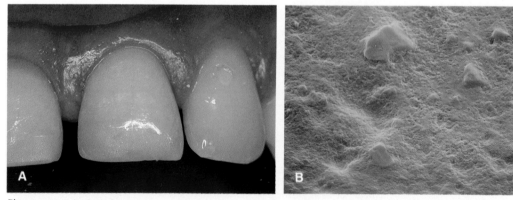

Figure 1-27 *A,* Incisal restoration of a composite material containing 15-micron inorganic filler particles. *B,* Scanning electron micrograph (300 ×) of the same composite surface.

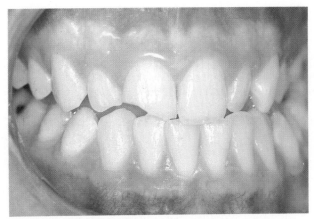

Figure 1-28 Fractured maxillary right central incisor before restoration with microfilled composite.

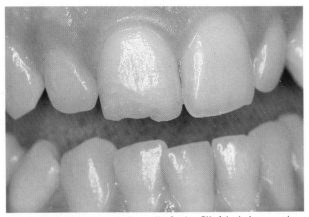

Figure 1-29 Eighteen-month recall of microfilled incisal restoration showing cohesive fracture.

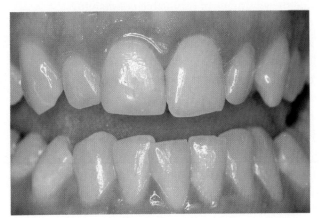

Figure 1-30 The maxillary right central incisor shown in Figures 1-28 and 1-29 after restoration with macrofilled composite (Prismafil[18]).

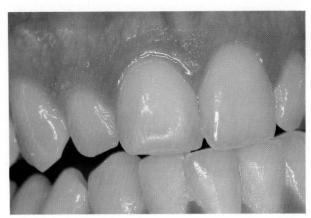

Figure 1-31 Three-year recall appearance of macrofilled composite restoration, maxillary right central incisor.

Typical clinical situations in which the macrofilled materials are preferable to the microfilled systems are as follows:

1. Very large coronal restorations exposed to heavy occlusal stress, particularly where "light group contact" cannot be equitably spread over adjacent enamel surfaces, especially during protrusive and lateral protrusive function (Fig. 1-32).
2. Large incisal restorations on mandibular anterior teeth (Fig. 1-33).
3. In posterior class II situations where esthetics are a major consideration (Fig. 1-34).

Hybrid Composites

The newest of the composite materials are the "hybrid" systems[21-30] (see Table 1–1), so called because they are bimodally filled. They contain two different types of inorganic filler particles, namely, microparticles (0.04 micron) in combination with macroparticles (1 to 15 microns). The hybrid materials are generally more polishable than the macrofilled, but less so than the microfilled systems (Fig. 1-35). Since they are generally heavy-loaded inorganically (i.e., 76% to 80% or more by weight), they combine the advantage of reasonable polishability with a high degree of fracture resistance when placed in stress-bearing situations.

A large number of microfilled, macrofilled, and hybrid composite materials have already been introduced, and probably many more will follow in each category as the result of a highly competitive market situation. Unfortunately, long-term clinical observations have not been carried out on the vast majority of materials currently available to the profession. The wise practitioner should be highly selective in his use of the available materials.

The microfilled materials are especially indicated for protected clinical situations such as class III and class V labial veneer restorations, and small class IV situations in which the occlusion can be carefully adjusted. The macrofilled and hybrid materials, on the other hand, are primarily indicated in more highly demanding stress-bearing class IV situations. The careful practitioner will accordingly keep one acceptable microfilled material and one good macrofilled or hybrid material available for routine use in situations in which each is indicated.

In the event that the practitioner requires the best of two worlds, the microfilled-macrofilled combination can be used in the form of a "laminating" technique. For example, given a large class IV situation, the main body of the restoration may be built up by means of a macrofilled composite, and a microfilled material may be used as a labial veneer. Such a laminated restoration demonstrates the ideal combination of fracture resistance and high-gloss polishability (see Chapter 9).

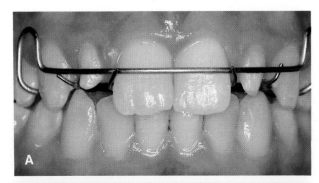

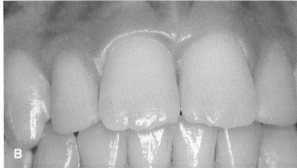

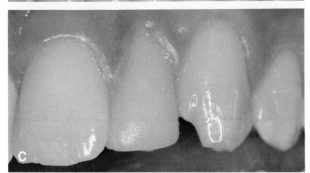

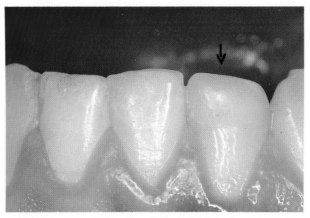

Figure 1-33 Large incisal macrofilled composite (Prismafil[18]) restoration of mandibular left lateral incisor at 2-year recall.

Figure 1-32 *A,* Peg lateral incisors in a young patient. *B,* After crown build-up with macrofilled composite (Nuvafil[4]), and *C,* At 5-year recall.

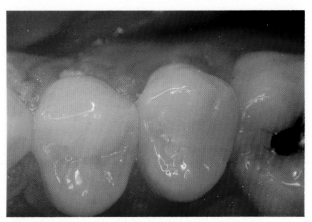

Figure 1-34 Disto-occlusal macrofilled composite restoration (Prismafil[18]) of maxillary second premolar at 3-year recall.

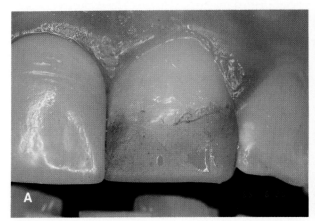

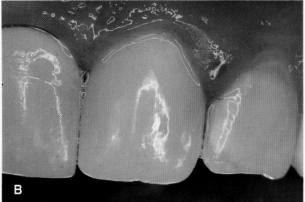

Figure 1-35 *A,* A worn discolored distoincisal restoration, maxillary left central incisor. *B,* After restoration with hybrid composite material (Command Ultrafine[26]).

Self-Cured Versus Light-Cured Composite Materials

The microfilled, macrofilled, and hybrid composite materials may be either autopolymerized (self-cured) or light-cured.

The self-curing mechanism involves the interaction between a catalyst paste (benzoyl peroxide) and an accelerator paste (tertiary aromatic amine) in order to create free radicals. The latter open up the unsaturated carbon bonds in the methacrylate grouping to provide an activated or receptive site for bonding with other activated groups. Polymerization into molecular chains continues until termination of the reaction. At the end point, the catalytic constituents remain and are a potential source of problems for the restoration. In the oral environment, the tertiary aromatic amines may undergo chemical change that results in a color shift in the restoration (Pollack and Blitzer, 1984). The latter is seen clinically as a darkening known as "amine discoloration" (Fig. 1-36).

Another clinical problem that has been commonly observed, particularly with the self-cured macrofilled composite materials, is often referred to as "plucking". When such materials are placed in stress-bearing class IV, I or II situations, the inorganic filler particles progressively and cumulatively separate from the surrounding resin matrix, and the end result after 2 or 3 years is observed as severe wear and loss of contour (Fig. 1-37).

The introduction of light-cured composite materials resulted in a marked improvement in both color stability and resistance to plucking. In the early 1970s, the first light curing was introduced as an option for the clinician in the form of ultraviolet-light-cured composite materials. The mechanism still involves the generation of free radicals, but instead of a chemical source of energy, the new systems use photon energy from lamps. The action of ultraviolet light in the long-wavelength range on a photosensitive ether chemical formed the basis of the first light-activated resins. These developed in tandem with the rapidly evolving acid-etch technique. Restorative systems catered to the needs of this new technique in which free-flowing resin formulations were used as bonding agents for the relatively more viscous composites, which contained very little free monomer. The bonding agents are primarily made up of Bis-GMA resin to which other diluent resins are added to enhance the rheologic properties of the resin formulations. These free-flowing monomers readily penetrate the enhanced enamel porosity (Gwinnett, 1982) created by phosphoric acid conditioning (Fig. 1-38). Following their polymerization in situ, the resin and enamel composite serves to anchor or bond the bulk of the composite restoration, which sits on the tissue (Fig. 1-39).

Long-term clinical observations on ultraviolet-light-cured materials (Nuvafil[4]) have clearly shown that they are more color-stable than self-cured systems and they more readily resist loss of contour when placed in stress-bearing situations (Fig. 1-40).

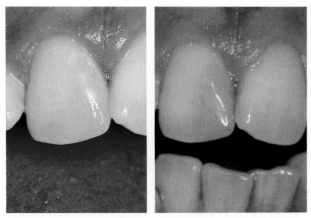

Figure 1-36 A mesioincisal self-cured composite restoration, maxillary right central incisor, at time of placement *(left)* and at 1-year recall *(right)* showing "amine" discoloration.

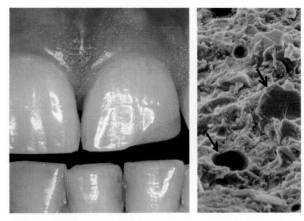

Figure 1-37 A class IV distoincisal composite restoration at 4-year recall *(left)*. Scanning electron micrograph (400 ×) of composite surface *(right)*.

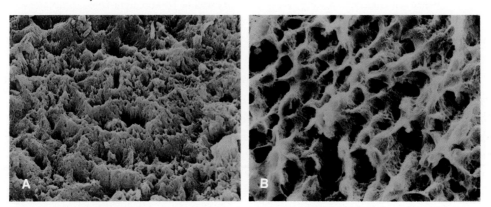

Figure 1-38 *A,* Scanning electron micrograph of microporous phosphoric acid-etched enamel surface (300 ×). *B,* Scanning electron micrograph of resin tags (300 ×). (Courtesy of Dr. A. J. Gwinnett, State University of New York at Stony Brook.)

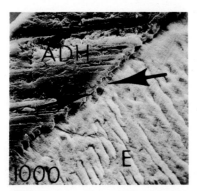

Figure 1-39 Scanning electron micrograph (1,000 ×) of resin-enamel interface. (Courtesy of Dr. A. J. Gwinnett, State University of New York at Stony Brook.)

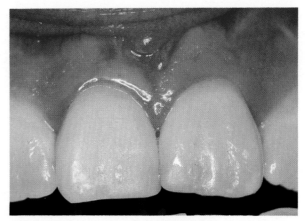

Figure 1-40 Mesioincisal ultraviolet light-cured composite (Nuvafil[4]) restorations in the maxillary central incisors at 10-year recall.

Ultraviolet-light-cured composite materials, however, despite their proven usefulness, demonstrate a major limitation. They are, for the most part, unreliable when placed in thick, confined, proximal situations, particularly where there exists a labial or lingual plate of enamel overlying the composite material (Figs. 1-41 to 1-43). The major limitation of ultraviolet light as a polymerization mechanism is that it is not capable of curing composite materials to clinically acceptable depths of thickness or of curing composite materials effectively through calcified tissues.

The advent of visible-light cure constitutes a major advance in composite resin restorative dentistry because three clinical advantages are associated with visible-light-cured composite systems:

1. "Command" cure. The curing time of visible-light-cured composite materials is, to a much greater extent, under the control of the operator.
2. Fast, deep, reliable cure. Within 40-second period, a minimum of 2.5 to 3.0 mm of composite thickness may be reliably cured even through overlying labial or lingual enamel.
3. Enhanced color stability. Light-cured material is demonstrably more color-stable than self-cured systems (Fig. 1-44). This may well be because light-cured composite materials contain no tertiary amine accelerator, the presence of which, in self-cured materials, is regarded as being a causative factor in discoloration (Asmusen, 1983).

The clinical selection of a composite material must be carefully delineated between self- and light-cured on the one hand, and between microfilled, macrofilled, or hybrid on the other, depending on the particular clinical requirements facing the practitioner. There are some clinical situations in which self-cured materials are clearly indicated, whereas there are many in which light-cured materials constitute the best choice. In following chapters that deal with specific clinical situations, materials will be discussed in greater detail. In the meantime, Table 1–1 presents an overview of the various composite materials currently available, the categories into which they fall, and their clinical characteristics and indications.

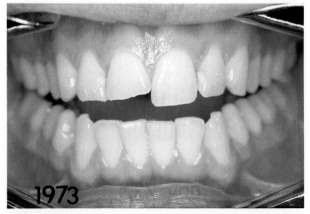

Figure 1–41 Incisal fracture, right central incisor and discolored class III restorations, maxillary lateral incisors prior to restoration.

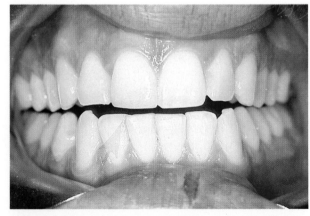

Figure 1–42 The anterior dentition shown in Figure 1-41 after restoration of maxillary left central incisor (class IV) and left and right lateral incisors (class III) with ultraviolet light-cured composite material (Nuvafil[4]).

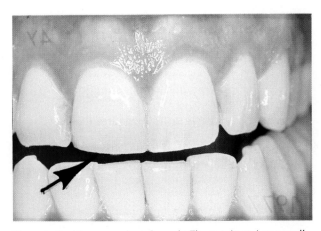

Figure 1–43 The restorations shown in Figure 1-42 at 4-year recall. Note the color stability of the incisal restoration on the right central incisor and the discoloration of the class III restorations on the mesial aspect of both lateral incisors.

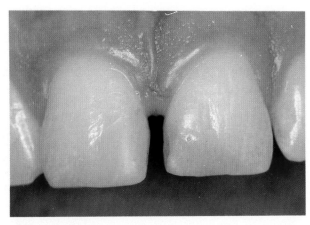

Figure 1–44 Mesioincisal light-cured composite (Prismafil[18]), right central incisor, and self-cured composite (Concise[2]), left central incisor, at 3-year recall.

References

Asmusen E. Factors affecting color stability of restorative resins. Acta Odontol Scand 1983; 41:11.

Dello-Russo NM. Placement of crown margins in patients with altered passive eruption. Int J Periodont Restor Dent 1984; 4:59.

Dennison JB. Status report on microfilled composite restorative resins. Council on dental materials, instruments and equipment. J Am Dent Assoc 1982; 105:488.

Gwinnett AJ, Matsui A. A study of enamel adhesives. The physical relationship between enamel and adhesive. Oral Biol 1967; 12:1615.

Gwinnett AJ. Bonding factors in technique which influences success. NY State Dent J 1982; 48:233.

Jordan RE, Suzuki M, Gwinnett AJ. Conservative applications of acid etch resin techniques. Dent Clin North Am 1981; 25:307.

Jordan RE, Suzuki M, Gwinnett AJ, Hunter JK. Restoration of fractured and hypoplastic incisors by the acid etch resin technique: a three year report. J Am Dent Assoc 1977; 95:795.

Lambrechts P, Ameye G, Vanherle G. Conventional and microfilled composite resins: II chip fractures. J Prosthet Dent 1982; 48:527.

Lutz F, Phillips RW. A classification and evaluation of composite resin systems. J Prosthet Dent 1983; 50:480.

Pollack BF, Blitzer MH. Discoloration in composite and microfill resins. Gen Dent 1984; 2:130.

Product Information

Product	Manufacturer/Distributor	Purpose
1. Adaptic	Johnson and Johnson 20 Lake Drive, CN7060 East Windsor, NJ 08520	Large-particle, macrofilled, self-cured composite
2. Concise	Dental Products/3M Company 3M Center 270–5N–02 St. Paul, MN 55144	Large-particle, macrofilled, self-cured composite
3. Visiofil	ESPE-Premier Sales Corp. Romano Dr., P.O. Box 111 Norristown, PA 19401	Large-particle, macrofilled, visible-light-cured composite
4. Nuvafil	L. D. Caulk Co. P.O. Box 359 Milford, DE 19963	Large-particle, macrofilled, ultraviolet-light-cured composite
5. Phaseafill	Phasealloy Co. 1050 Greenfield Drive El Cajon, CA 92021	Self-cured, microfilled composite
6. Estic microfil	Wright Dental Ltd. 257 Centre E. Richmond Hill, Ontario L4C 1A7	Self-cured, microfilled composite
7. Silar	Dental Products/3M Company 3M Center 270–5N–02 St. Paul, MN 55144	Self-cured, microfilled composite
8. Isopast	Vivadent USA Inc. P.O. Box 304 Tonawanda, NY 14150	Self-cured, microfilled composite
9. Superfil	Harry J. Bosworth Co. 7227 North Hamlin Ave. Skokie, IL 60076	Self-cured, microfilled composite
10. Certain	Johnson and Johnson 20 Lake Drive, CN7060 East Windsor, NJ 08520	Visible-light-cured, microfilled composite 52% filled by weight
11. Durafill	Kulzer Inc. 10015 Muirlands Blvd., Unit G Irvine, CA 92714	Visible-light-cured, microfilled composite 52% filled by weight
12. Silux	Dental Products/3M Company 3M Center 270–5N–02 St. Paul, MN 55144	Visible-light-cured, microfilled composite 52% filled by weight
13. Heliosit	Vivadent USA Inc. P.O. Box 304 Tonawanda, NY 14150	Visible-light-cured, microfilled composite 52% filled by weight
14. Rembrandt	DenMat Inc. 3130 Skyway Dr., Unit 501 Santa Maria, CA 93456	Visible-light-cured, microfilled composite 18% filled by weight
14a. Paste Laminate 14b. Extra Smooth	DenMat Inc. 3130 Skyway Dr., Unit 501 Santa Maria, CA 93456	A 52% filled, light-cured microfill
15. Visiodispers	ESPE-Premier Sales Corp. Romano Dr., P.O. Box 111 Norristown, PA 19401	Visible-light-cured, microfilled composite
16. Profile	S. S. White Co. Three Parkway Philadelphia, PA 19102	Self-cured, small-particle, macrofilled composite
17. Simulate	Kerr-Sybron Co. P.O. Box 455 Romulus, MI 48174	Self-cured, small-particle, macrofilled, composite

Product Information

Product	Manufacturer/Distributor	Purpose
18. Prismafil	L. D. Caulk Co. P.O. Box 359 Milford, DE 19963	Visible-light-cured, small-particle, macrofilled composite
19. Estilux	Kulzer Inc. 10015 Muirlands Blvd., Unit G Irvine, CA 92714	Visible-light-cured, small-particle, macrofilled composite
20. Command	Kerr-Sybron Co. P.O. Box 455 Romulus, MI 48174	Visible-light-cured, small-particle, macrofilled composite
21. Miradapt	Johnson and Johnson 20 Lake Drive, CN7060 East Windsor, NJ 08520	Heavy-filled, self-cured, hybrid composite
22. Finesse	L. D. Caulk Co. P.O. Box 359 Milford, DE 19963	Lightly-filled, self-cured, hybrid composite
23. P–10 24. Conclude	Dental Products/3M Company 3M Center 270–5N–02 St. Paul, MN 55144	Heavy-filled, self-cured, hybrid composite
25. Brilliant Lux	Coltene Co. Feldwiesen Strasse 20, CH-9450 Altstatten, Switzerland	Heavy-filled, visible-light-cured, hybrid composite
26. Command Ultrafine	Kerr-Sybron Co. P.O. Box 455 Romulus, MI 48174	Heavy-filled, visible-light-cured, hybrid composite
27. Aurafil	Johnson and Johnson 20 Lake Drive, CN7060 East Windsor, NJ 08520	Heavy-filled, visible-light-cured, small-particle, macrofilled composite
28. P–30	Dental Products/3M Company 3M Center 270–5N–02 St. Paul, MN 55144	Heavy-filled, visible-light-cured, hybrid composite
29. Visarfil	DenMat Inc. 3130 Skyway Dr., Unit 501 Santa Maria, CA 93456	Heavy-filled, visible-light-cured, hybrid composite
30. Profile TLC	S. S. White Co. Three Parkway Philadelphia, PA 19102	Heavy-filled, visible-light-cured, hybrid composite
31. Herculite XR	Kerr-Sybron Co. P.O. Box 455 Romulus, MI 48174	Heavy-filled, visible-light-cured, hybrid composite
32. Valux	Dental Products/3M Company 3M Center 270-5N-02 St. Paul, MN 55144	Visible-light-cured, small-particle, macrofilled composite material

2

RONALD E. JORDAN

R E S I N - E N A M E L   B O N D I N G

Resin-enamel bonding is by far the most frequently utilized, most reliable, and most predictable of all bonding procedures involving composite resin materials (Jordan et al, 1981). The basis for enamel bonding involves the use of phosphoric acid etching (Buonocore, 1955). The application of phosphoric acid to an enamel surface renders it self-retentive (Silverstone, 1975) owing to the fact that microporosities are thereby formed which extend between 25 and 50 microns deep (Gwinnett, 1976) into the subsurface enamel (Fig. 2-1). Should a free-flow bonding resin be placed on such an enamel surface, the resin enters the enamel micro-porosities in the form of long projecting tags, thereby forming a deeply penetrative interlocking relationship at the resin-enamel boundary (Fig. 2-2) which is unique in operative dentistry. The most intimate marginal relationship attainable with restorative materials such as silver amalgam, gold foil, cast gold, and fused porcelain consists at best of a butt-type joint at the material-enamel interface (Fig. 2-3). Using resin materials with an acid-etch technique, the clinician may attain a more intimate marginal relationship consisting of resin tags inter-locking deeply with enamel microporosities (Fig. 2-4). Such a relationship provides not only a conservative means of securing *retention* of resin materials to tooth structure (Fig. 2-5), but also a reliable method of eliminating the marginal leakage (Hembree and Andrew, 1976) for which resin materials have been notorious (Fig. 2-6). Discoloration and leakage around the marginal periphery of a resin restoration are primarily due to a contraction gap at the enamel interface resulting from polymerization shrinkage (Fig. 2-7). Phosphoric acid etching of enamel surfaces prior to the introduction of resin materials eliminates the contraction gap at the enamel boundary and thereby enhances the marginal seal of the material on a long-term basis (Fig. 2-8).

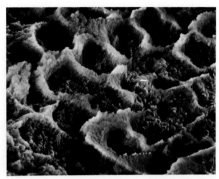

Figure 2-1 Scanning electron micrograph (5,000 ×) of phosphoric acid-etched enamel surface. (Courtesy of Dr. A. J. Gwinnett, State University of New York at Stony Brook.)

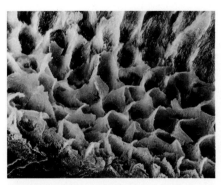

Figure 2-2 Scanning electron micrograph (1,800 ×) of resin tags. (Courtesy of Dr. A. J. Gwinnett, State University of New York at Stony Brook.)

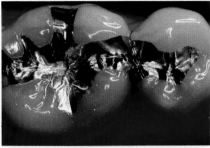

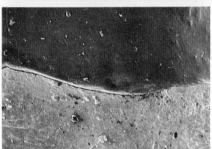

Figure 2-3 Butt-type joint at amalgam-enamel interface clinically (*top*) and scanning electron micrograph (20 ×) (*bottom*).

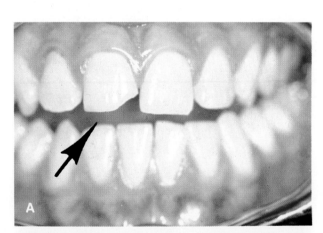

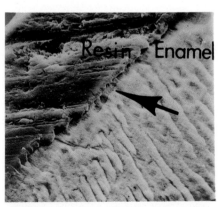

Figure 2-4 Scanning electron micrograph (1,000 ×) of interlocking relationship at resin-enamel interface. (Courtesy of Dr. A. J. Gwinnett, State University of New York at Stony Brook.)

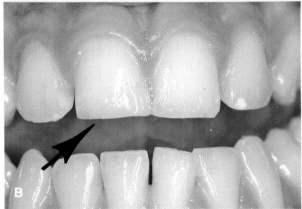

Figure 2-5 *A*, Mesioincisal fracture, maxillary right central incisor (*top*), *B*, after restoration (*bottom*).

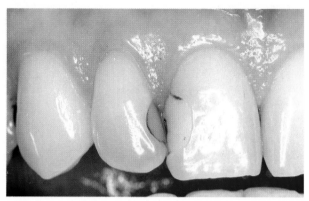

Figure 2–6 Class III resin restoration in non-etched preparations at 5-year recall.

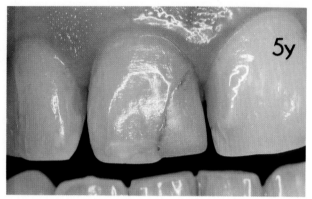

Figure 2–7 Class IV resin restoration in non-etched preparation.

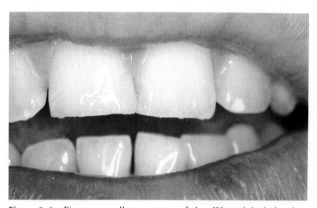

Figure 2–8 Five-year recall appearance of class IV mesioincisal resin restoration on a phosphoric acid-etched enamel surface.

The innumerable clinical applications of resin-enamel bonding are based on what is termed the *one millimeter circumferential principle*:

> If the area to be restored or recontoured is surrounded by one millimeter of circumferential peripheral enamel, mechanical retention in the form of pins, slots, grooves, or undercuts is usually unnecessary since phosphoric acid etching of the enamel periphery provides the sole basis for reliable long-term resin retention. (Jordan et al, 1977).

The "one millimeter" principle can be applied reliably in the conservative long-term treatment of a wide variety of clinical problems including:

1. Incisal fractures
2. Labial veneers
3. Extensive crown restoration in nonvital teeth
4. Mandibular incisal restorations
5. Diastema closure
6. Peg lateral build-up
7. Hypoplastic defects
8. White spot lesions
9. Cervical demineralized lesions

In each of these procedures, the clinician's choice of an appropriate composite *material* combined with a carefully controlled *clinical technique* are all-important factors.

RESTORATION OF INCISAL FRACTURE

Materials. Conservative restoration of an extensively fractured young incisor crown (Fig. 2-9) may be an exceedingly demanding procedure since the primary requisites for the material of choice involve a combination of esthetic acceptability, resistance to fracture and abrasive wear, and biological acceptability. Full coverage, in the form of a porcelain jacket or porcelain fused to metal crowns are options which should be carefully considered. There is no question as to their esthetic acceptability and resistance to fracture and abrasive wear; these are the major advantages of full-coverage restorations. However, full coverage should be avoided in the young adolescent or early adult dentition because the pulp chambers are usually large, and accordingly, the pulp response to the combined irritants of trauma, extensive preparation, temporization, and cementation is unpredictable. Further, since the young anterior teeth have not reached the state of full eruption, the gingival response to placement of full crown margins beneath the free gingival crest is often less than positive (Dello Russo, 1984).

Composite crown build-up should be seriously considered as an alternative in the young patient, since esthetics, biological acceptability, and resistance to abrasive wear are all excellent (Jordan et al, 1977). Fracture resistance varies with the material selected. However, should fracture of the composite restoration occur, it is easily and reliably repaired (Chan and Boyer, 1983).

Composite crown build-up may be done with microfilled, macrofilled, or hybrid materials. The microfilled materials should be used to restore incisal fractures only when the maxillo-mandibular relationship is normal and when the remaining natural teeth can serve as the primary support for centric, protrusive, and protrusive lateral functions. When the occlusion is heavy and the incisal composite restoration is expected to bear most of the "occlusal load", particularly in protrusive and protrusive lateral function, macrofilled or hybrid types of "heavy-filled" composite materials are specifically indicated because of their greater fracture resistance in stress-bearing situations.

Regarding the clinical situation under consideration, a hybrid material such as Herculite XR[1] or a macrofilled material such as Valux[45], may be selected for the restoration primarily because of the polishability and fracture resistance of the materials. The following technique may be used successfully for the crown build-up irrespective of the materials utilized.

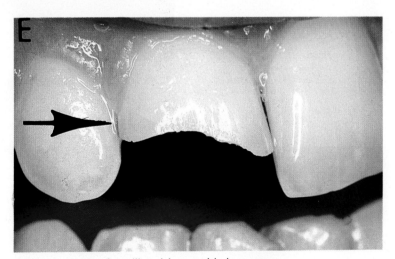

Figure 2-9 Fractured maxillary right central incisor crown.

Shade Selection. The proper shade should be selected before the field is isolated since dehydrated enamel "whitens" considerably, thus negating the possibility of a proper shade match after rehydration. Multiple shades are an important requirement with composite materials, and it is essential that at least four shades be available: light, light yellow, light gray, and dark yellow. Unfortunately, few shade guides provided by manufacturers accurately indicate the shade of the composite material. To further complicate the problem of shade selection, light-cured composite materials undergo a shade transformation on being subjected to light (Fig. 2-10). Accordingly, before a new composite material is used clinically, fabrication of a "customized" shade guide is recommended. The base shades (light, light yellow, light gray, and dark yellow) are placed in four different transparent crown forms and cured. Subsequently, "half-to-half" mixtures of the base shades are placed in another four different crown forms and cured. (Half light yellow and half light gray is a commonly used admixture.) An accurate custom shade guide is thus provided (Fig. 2-11) which greatly simplifies precise shade matching clinically, particularly with light-cured composite materials.

Preparation. A bullet-nosed diamond (Fig. 2-12) is used to prepare a "chamfer-shoulder" around the entire enamel periphery. The preparation should extend cervically approximately 1 mm beyond the edge of the fractured enamel and, in depth, should involve at least half of the enamel thickness (Fig. 2-13). Ideally, the chamfer should be cut as far through the enamel thickness as possible without exposing dentin in order to allow a maximal bulk of composite material to overlie cut tooth structure. Particular care should be taken to ensure that the chamfer preparation is not too shallow, or a "halo" effect will occur in the final restoration (Fig. 2-14).

Proper instrumentation involves the use of a bullet-nosed diamond carbide pair of points (RCBIIK 4–5 Duet²) (Fig. 2-15) together with a thin tapering diamond point (201.3F Tapering Diamond³) in order to prepare the interproximal regions of the chamfer.

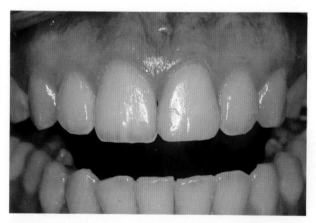

Figure 2–10 Labial veneer restoration, maxillary left central incisor 4 weeks after placement.

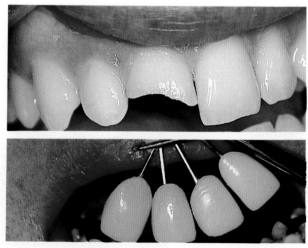

Figure 2–11 Custom shade guide (*bottom*) used to determine shade preoperatively (*top*).

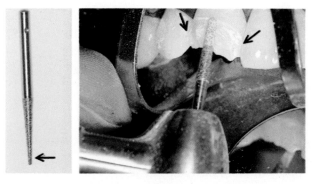

Figure 2-12 A bullet-nosed diamond (*left*) used to prepare peripheral chamfer-shoulder (*right*).

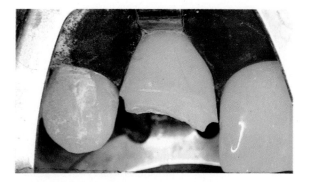

Figure 2-13 Completed chamfer preparation.

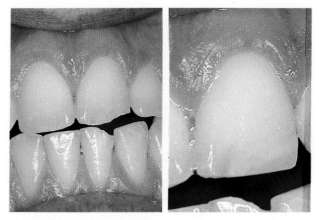

Figure 2-14 Fractured maxillary left central incisor (*left*); after restoration (*right*) showing "halo".

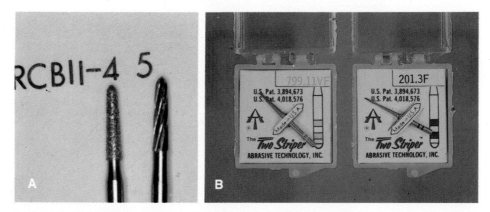

Figure 2-15 *A*, Diamond carbide pair of "duet" points (RCBIIK 4–5 Duet²) used for chamfer preparation. *B*, Thin-tapering diamond point (201.3F³) (*right*) for interproximal preparation.

The chamfer preparation may be extended cervically beyond 1 mm if indicated by such clinical circumstances as demineralized or hypoplastic enamel in the cervical or middle thirds and the requirement for increased retention and full labial veneers. In any event, the chamfer preparation must extend around the entire labial, lingual, mesial, and distal circumferential periphery of the crown in incisal fracture restorations.

The chamfer-shoulder preparation has several advantages:

1. It enhances the *retention* of the restoration by exposing the subsurface enamel to the effects of the phosphoric acid conditioning solution (Fig. 2-16).
2. It provides a *clearly defined marginal periphery* to which the composite resin material may be finished precisely.
3. It allows for *bulk marginal finish* of the composite material. Bevels should be avoided since the inevitable result is a thin fin of marginal composite material, which is not only highly friable but difficult to finish (Fig. 2-17). Bulk marginal finish is recommended in order to minimize the problem of "white line margin" (Fig. 2-18), which is frequently encountered when composite materials are used.
4. It provides a gradual *resin-lap joint* which results in a masking effect at the resin-enamel interface, thereby improving esthetic results (Fig. 2-19).

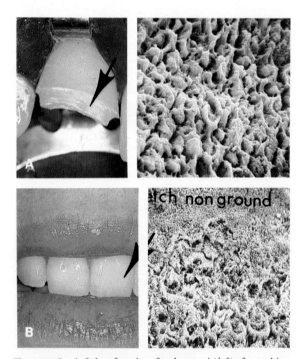

Figure 2-16 *A,* Subsurface chamfered enamel (*left*) after etching (*right*) shows highly porous surface under scanning electron micrograph (2,000 ×). *B,* Intact enamel surface (*left*) after etching shows shallow microporosity distribution (*right*) under scanning electron micrograph (2,000 ×).

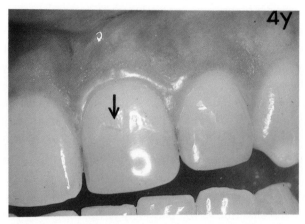

Figure 2-17   Class IV composite restoration, maxillary left central incisor at 4-year recall showing marginal ''ledge'' with associated discoloration.

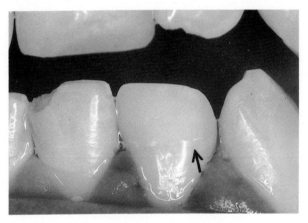

Figure 2–18   Typical ''white line'' margin in a composite restoration.

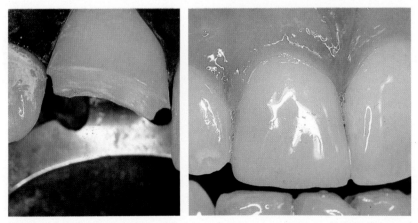

Figure 2–19   Chamfer preparation (*left*) allows a resin lap joint which masks the resin-enamel interface (*right*).

The chamfer-shoulder preparation, properly etched, forms the sole basis for reliable long-term retention of the incisal restoration (Fig. 2-20). Pins, particularly self-threading pins, are not indicated for accessory retention. Self-threading pins are neither necessary nor desirable for long-term retention (Jordan et al, 1977) and, in fact, may be directly associated with esthetic failure of the restoration (Fig. 2-21). When a self-threading pin, even of small diameter, is inserted into the restricted dentin thickness in the incisal region of an anterior tooth, cracking of the dentin (Suzuki et al, 1973) at the pin periphery frequently occurs (Fig. 2-22). The dentin cracking is often accompanied by cracking or checking of the overlying enamel. Subsequent to insertion of the composite material, microleakage occurs through the enamel, and dentin cracks are accompanied by corrosion of the pin periphery. As a result, a dark gray or blue sulfide-type deposit occurs in the dentin surrounding the buried pin, almost invariably causing a discoloration at the periphery of the composite restoration (Fig. 2-23). In a recently completed long-term clinical research project at The University of Western Ontario (Jordan et al, 1977), such discoloration was observed in 30 percent of cases in which self-threading pins were utilized (Fig. 2-24).

Self-threading pins also result in clinically undetectable pulp exposures (Fig. 2-25). Although pins are rarely indicated in the anterior region, they are frequently required posteriorly in order to retain large amalgam or composite restorations. In such instances, in order to minimize the problems associated with dentin cracking, the pin should be made self-tapping by means of a simple modification (Baum, 1982), and before placement the end should be coated with a small amount of calcium hydroxide (Hydroxyline[4]) (Fig. 2-26).

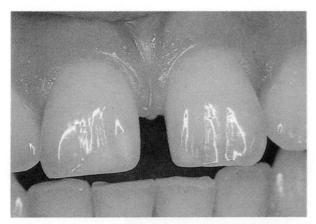

Figure 2-20 Mesioincisal composite restoration in the maxillary central incisors at 7-year recall.

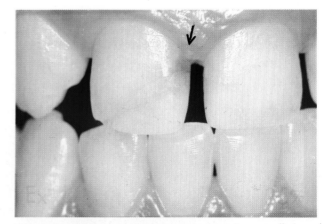

Figure 2-21 Pin-retained composite restoration at 3-year recall. Arrow indicates a crack in the enamel and discoloration.

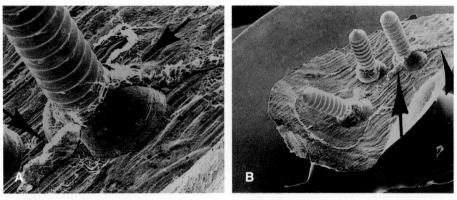

Figure 2-22   *A*, Scanning electron micrograph (40 ×) of pin periphery showing dentin cracking. (Courtesy of Dr. A. J. Gwinnett, State University of New York at Stony Brook.) *B*, Scanning electron micrograph (10 ×) of a pin-retained composite restoration. Arrows indicate dentin cracking at pin periphery. (Courtesy of Dr. A. J. Gwinnett, State University of New York at Stony Brook.)

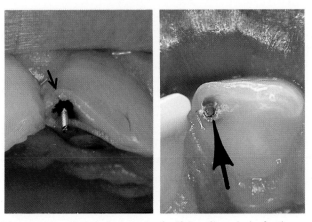

Figure 2-23   Clinical photograph of self-threading pin in dentin showing cracking of enamel (*left*) and discoloration around pin periphery (*right*).

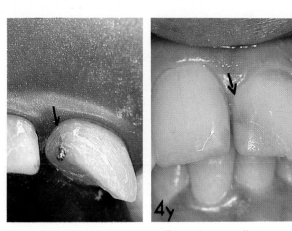

Figure 2-24   Typical pin-cracking effect at 4-year recall.

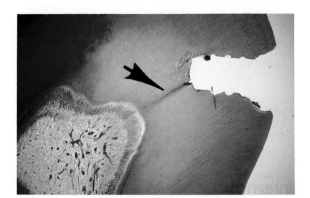

Figure 2-25   Photomicrograph showing dentin cracking at periphery of self-threading pin. Hematoxylin and eosin stain (20 ×).

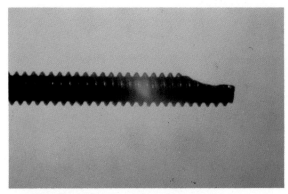

Figure 2-26   Cutting a small portion off the end diameter of a self-threading pin renders it self-tapping, thereby minimizing dentin-enamel cracking.

Pulp Protection. Pulp studies and clinical experience both clearly indicate that among the most toxic materials in operative dentistry are those used in composite restorative techniques (Goto and Jordan, 1972). Accordingly, *thermal sensitivity* subsequent to placement of a composite restoration is pathognomonic of pulp irritation (Figs. 2-27 and 2-28).

> Principle: Under no circumstances should phosphoric acid or resin materials* be placed in contact with freshly cut or accidentally exposed dentin.

Phosphoric acid may be placed on an enamel surface with impunity. However, when phosphoric acid is inadvertently applied to a freshly cut dentin surface (Fig. 2-29), the peritubular dentin is destroyed (Gwinnett, 1982) and the dentin tubules are widened (Fig. 2-30), thus providing a dual source of cumulative irritation to pulp tissues, namely, (1) the direct toxic effect of phosphoric acid entering the widenend tubules, and (2) the superimposed irritation from the resin material entering the tubules. The histologic result is shown in Figure 2-31.

Pulp protection must accordingly be carefully *controlled.* Three precautions are recommended in the controlled pulp protection technique, namely:

1. An **acid-resistant** pulp protective should be utilized.
2. The pulp protective should be applied to all exposed dentin, particularly the dentin on the gingival floor of a class II or class III cavity preparation.
3. A controlled technique of phosphoric acid etching should be utilized in order to minimize dissolution of the pulp protective.

Calcium hydroxide materials probably offer the best pulp protection under composite systems (Goto and Jordan, 1972). Unfortunately, many calcium hydroxide materials undergo dissolution and ''washout'' during phosphoric acid etching (Fig. 2-32). Accordingly, an acid-resistant pulp protective (Hwas and Sandrik, 1984) should be utilized (Table 2-1).

(*Exception: certain dentin bonding agents; see Chapter 4.)

TABLE 2–1   Acid-resistant Pulp Protective Materials for Composite Restorations

Material	Manufacturer	Type	Effectiveness
Advanced Formula Dycal[40]	L.D. Caulk	Calcium hydroxide	++
Ketac-Cem[28]	ESPE-Premier	Glass ionomer	++++
Life[42]	Kerr-Sybron	Calcium hydroxide	+++
Poly-F-Plus[32]	DeTreys/AD	Polycarboxylate	++++
Reolit[43]	Vivadent	Calcium hydroxide	++
G-C Lining Cement[44]	GC Intl. Corp.	Glass ionomer	+ + + +
VLC Dycal[46]	L.D. Caulk Co.	Calcium Hydroxide	+ + + +

++   Highly acid-resistant
+++   Very highly acid-resistant
++++ Totally acid-resistant

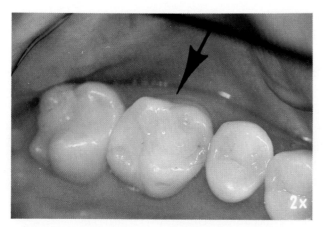

Figure 2-27 Maxillary left first molar restored with class II composite. Patient experienced thermal sensitivity postoperatively.

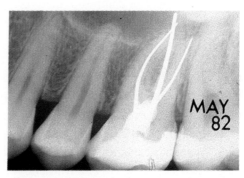

Figure 2-28 Radiograph of the same molar (as shown in Fig. 2-27) 6 months later.

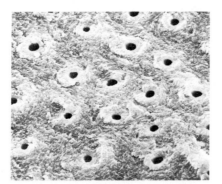

Figure 2-29 Scanning electron micrograph (3,000 ×) of cut dentin surface showing tubular morphology. (Courtesy of Dr. A. J. Gwinnett, State University of New York at Stony Brook.)

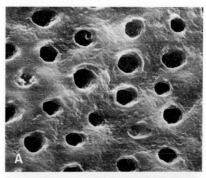

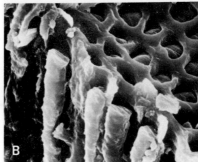

Figure 2-30 Scanning electron micrograph (3,000 ×) of phosphoric acid-etched dentin, *A,* Note wide opening to dentin tubules filled with columns of resin, *B,* (Courtesy of Dr. A. J. Gwinnett, State University of New York at Stony Brook.)

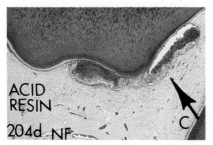

Figure 2-31 Photomicrograph of pulp subjacent to a composite restoration 204 days postoperatively. Arrow indicates pulp abscess, Hematoxylin and eosin stain (40 ×).

The acid-resistant pulp protective should be carefully applied to the axial wall, pulpal floor, and as much dentin as possible on the gingival wall of a class II or III cavity preparation before placement of composite materials. Since the *gingival dentin tubules* are usually in relatively close approximation to the underlying pulp (Fig. 2-33), direct acid application should be carefully avoided.

A controlled phosphoric acid-etching technique, which is carefully carried out in order to avoid "washout" of the pulp protective, will be discussed subsequently. Unfortunately, in certain clinical circumstances calcium hydroxide and other opaque materials cannot be used for pulp protection because of a "shine-through" problem (Fig. 2-34). Accordingly, when shallow labial dentin is exposed in an anterior tooth (i.e., in a class V situation or a labial hypoplastic defect), the dentin should be covered either by a light-cured dentin bonding resin (see Chapter 6) or a synthetic (Caviline[5]) or nitrocellulose (Universal[6]) varnish (Fig. 2-35). Such materials seal the dentin tubules and are completely compatible with composite materials placed over them (Fig. 2-36). Copal-type varnishes have been shown to be somewhat incompatible with composite materials placed in contact with them (Jendresen and Stanley, 1981).

Acid Etching

There is overwhelming clinical evidence that all composite resin restorations (class III, IV, or V) are greatly enhanced by the routine utilization of enamel acid-etching techniques (Jordan et al, 1977). There are four important considerations in acid etching, namely, *method, time, concentration*, and *type of acid* utilized (Gwinnett, 1982). All may significantly affect the longevity of the restoration.

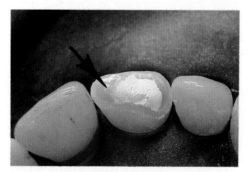

Figure 2-32 Incisal fracture after all dentin was covered with calcium hydroxide and the enamel subsequently phosphoric acid-etched. Note "washout" of pulp protective.

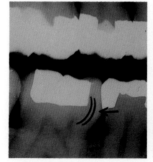 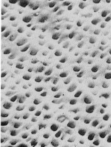

Figure 2-33 Bite-wing radiograph (*left*) and diagrammatic illustration of the continuity of open dentin tubules (*right*) with pulp chamber.

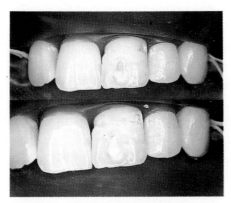

Figure 2-34 Labial composite restoration showing "shine-through" of subajacent calcium hydroxide.

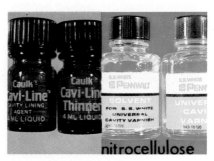

Figure 2-35 Synthetic varnishes.

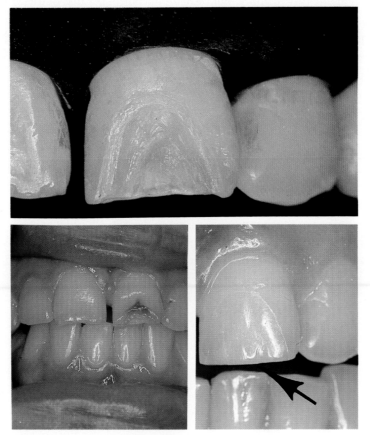

Figure 2-36 Shallow labial dentin (*top*) covered with synthetic varnish. After placement of composite veneer restoration (*bottom*).

Method. With a fine-tipped, soft-bristle brush[7], acid is applied to the enamel in a dabbing motion (Fig. 2-37). Such a brush is recommended because (1) the fine tip confines the acid to the enamel periphery of the chamfer-shoulder preparation, thereby minimizing the acid dissolution of the calcium hydroxide liner (i.e., a controlled etching technique), and (2) the soft bristles prevent a heavy rubbing or scrubbing mode of acid application that would result in decreased retention due to the fracture of interstitial enamel surrounding the micropores (Gwinnett, 1976).

Time. The acid should be applied with a light stroking motion and constantly replenished with new acid for one full minute. The application time should be increased to 2 minutes for either fluorosed or deciduous enamel because both are relatively resistant to the etching procedure. During acid application, the brush should be repeatedly redipped to ensure the application of fresh acid to the enamel surface.

Acid Concentration. Although the subject is controversial, clinical as well as laboratory observations indicate that concentrations of 30 to 40 percent are the most reliably effective in creating microporous enamel surfaces (Rock, 1974).

Type of Acid. Either an *aqueous solution* or a *phosphoric acid gel* may be utilized. Aqueous solutions are easy to apply, but difficult to control because of their free-flow nature. Phosphoric acid gels (Scotchbond Etching Gel[39]), being highly viscous, are much more readily controlled clinically. In the treatment of cervical erosion lesions by means of dentin bonding materials (see Chapter 6) and in posterior composite restorations (see Chapter 7), the gel type phosphoric acid etchants are particularly indicated.

Post-Etch Cleaning. After acid etching the enamel surface should be thoroughly cleansed by means of a copious water lavage for at least 15 to 30 seconds (Fig. 2-38) and longer if possible (Soetopo et al, 1978). The prolonged water lavage is necessary to remove contaminant residues, consisting mainly of soluble calcium salts (Fig. 2-39), from the treated enamel surface prior to bonding. Failure to thoroughly do so may well inhibit effective resin bonding and constitutes a common reason for bond failure.

If an aqueous solution of phosphoric acid is used for etching, a 15-second period of water lavage is sufficient for thorough cleansing. However, should a gel etchant be utilized, a period of 30 to 45 seconds of water lavage is necessary (Gwinnett, 1982) since gels leave firmly adherent contaminant residues on enamel surfaces that are more difficult to remove (Fig. 2-40).

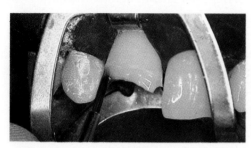

Figure 2-37   Use of fine-tipped brush for controlled application of phosphoric acid.

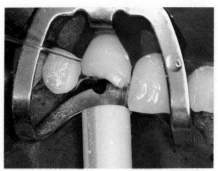

Figure 2-38   Thorough washing of the enamel surface by means of a copious water lavage.

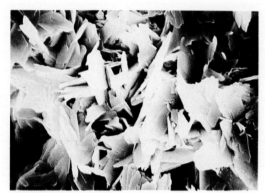

Figure 2-39   Scanning electron micrograph of crystalline reaction product remaining on enamel surface after phosphoric acid etching (400 ×).

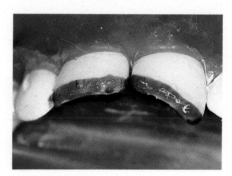

Figure 2-40   Firmly adherent gel etchant on enamel surfaces.

Drying the Enamel Surface. The enamel surface should be carefully dried after the water lavage is completed. Although chemical drying agents may be used, warm air drying is preferred. If the warm air from the syringe is contaminated with water droplets, a warm air dryer (Handi-Dry[8]) (Fig. 2-41) should be used. After drying, the enamel surface should present a chalky white opaque appearance (Fig. 2-42). At this point the enamel surface is said to be in a critical state for it is most sensitive to contamination (Fig. 2-43). Should even a small quantity of saliva come in contact with the etched enamel surface, within a short time the microporous surface becomes obliterated by a firmly adherent contaminant layer composed mainly of salivary proteins, i.e., pellicle (Fig. 2-44). Should this occur, the surface can only be effectively releatased by the application of phosphoric acid (Hormati et al, 1980) for a 15- to 20-second period (Fig. 2-45). The maintenance of strictly controlled dry conditions renders this measure unnecessary.

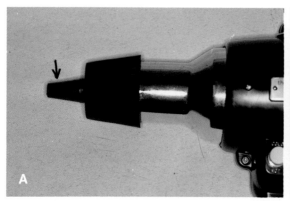
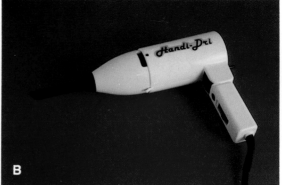

Figure 2–41 *A*, "Home-made" air dryer consisting of hair dryer with attached conical end. *B*, Commercially available warm air dryer (Handi-Dry[8]).

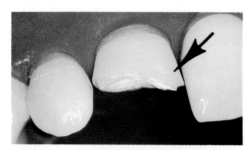

Figure 2–42 White opaque appearance of properly acid-etched enamel.

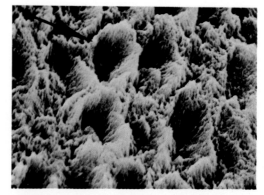

Figure 2–43 Scanning electron micrograph of microporous enamel surface after acid etching (2,000 ×). (Courtesy of Dr. A. J. Gwinnett, State University of New York at Stony Brook.)

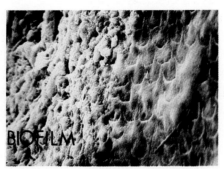

Figure 2-44 Scanning electron micrograph of salivary contaminated enamel surface (1,000 ×).

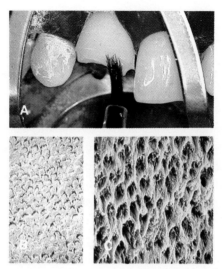

Figure 2-45 *A*, 15- to 20-second reapplication of phosphoric acid after salivary contamination "flows off" the salivary protein contaminant layer, *B*, thereby providing a clean enamel surface, *C*.

Bonding

Bonding resins have always been the source of a great deal of controversy. Some clinicians regard their use as a waste of time. Manufacturers, in their directions, often indicate that the use of a bonding resin is entirely optional. However, there is considerable evidence (Newman and Nevaste, 1975; Mitchem and Turner, 1974) both clinical and laboratory, attesting to the fact that the routine use of a bonding resin clearly enhances the composite resin restoration, particularly with regard to marginal integrity (Fig. 2-46). With few exceptions, composite materials are highly viscous in nature and thereby demonstrate limited penetrability into enamel microporosities. Being considerably less viscous, bonding resins flow more readily into the depths of the enamel microporosities, thereby ensuring full-length resin tags at the resin-enamel interface.

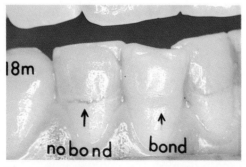

Figure 2-46 Labial composite restorations at 18-month recall. A bonding resin was not used on the lateral incisor (*left*), whereas an intermediary bonding resin was used on the central incisor (*right*).

The routine use of a bond resin, irrespective of the particular composite material utilized, is a necessary expedient since it ''buys the clinician time'' to effectively work with a composite material. Since most composite materials are highly viscous, they do not adapt well to acid-etched enamel surfaces. The problem is further complicated by the fact that the viscosity of a self-cured material rapidly increases with time after mixing, thereby compromising adaptation even further. Similarly, the viscosity of a light-cured composite material rapidly increases on extrusion from its container since room or operatory light begins the polymerization process. The use of a bonding resin buys the clinician time to properly manipulate the composite material irrespective of whether it is light- or self-cured. The mechanism by which this is brought about is the ''air-inhibited'' surface layer of the bond resin. Most bonding resins currently available consist of Bis-GMA with small quantities of dimethacrylate added as a diluent to lend fluidity to the material. These are known as ''unfilled'' bond resins (Fig. 2-47). Other bond resins, particularly the light-cured, may contain inorganic filler in the form of colloidal silica up to 50 percent by weight. These are called ''filled'' bond resins, and because of their inorganic filler content, they demonstrate better physical properties than the unfilled materials. The recently introduced phosphonate bond resins (Scotchbond;[30] Prisma Universal Bond;[47] and Bondlite[48]) are thought to result in an improved resin enamel bond.

The technique for applying the bonding resin should be carefully controlled, and so a fine-tipped, soft-bristle brush is used for this purpose (Fig. 2-48). Since they are relatively weak in comparison to composite materials, bonding resins should be placed in the form of a thin controlled film: a small bead of bonding resin is picked up on the end of the brush and applied carefully to the acid-etched enamel. Care must be taken to ensure that excess material is not applied beyond the margin of the preparation. After ''thin spreading'' with the fine-tipped brush, the bond resin surface should be carefully blown with an air syringe to further ensure the thin application of the material. Once the bond resin has been applied, the fine-tipped brush should be cleaned of all adherent resin material by dipping it into ethyl acetate or acetone solvent. The brush may then be used for successive applications.

Irrespective of whether a self-cured or a light-cured bond resin is utilized, it should be prepolymerized prior to the insertion of the composite material. This ensures a more easily controlled composite insertion technique. Accordingly, if a self-cured bond resin is utilized it should be allowed to set for a period of 90 seconds. In the event that a light-cured bond resin is utilized, it should be precured by means of the application of visible light for a 20-second period before composite insertion. After polymerization of the bond resin, a tacky, ''air-inhibited'' layer is observed on the surface (Fig. 2-49). This is a thin reactive surface layer of nonpolymerized bonding resin, which should neither be removed nor contaminated prior to the insertion of the composite material. It will not polymerize until it is covered with composite material. Thus the clinician has ample time to manipulate the composite material irrespective of whether it is self- or light-cured.

Manufacturers commonly recommend that the composite material be inserted over the bonding resin quickly, before the latter has set, to ensure maximum bonding between bonding and composite resin materials. This is not essential, however. If the bonding resin is allowed to set fully before placement of the composite resin and if the air-inhibited layer is left intact, there will be excellent bonding between composite and bonding resins because of the surface-reactive air-inhibited layer, which quickly polymerizes after the composite resin is placed, thereby ensuring a tight bond between the two materials.

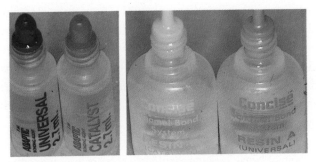

Figure 2-47 Typical unfilled self-cured bonding resins.

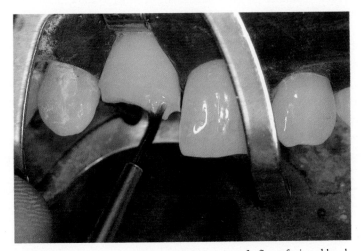

Figure 2-48 Bond resin carefully applied by means of a fine soft-tipped brush.

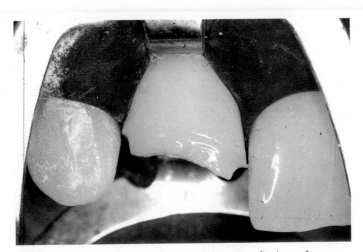

Figure 2-49 The air-inhibited layer presents a tacky reflective surface.

Insertion of the Composite Material

It is a well-known fact that composites cured against a matrix have a resin-rich surface that is the smoothest attainable (Chandler et al, 1971). A carefully controlled matrix technique, designed particularly to minimize the amount of labial finishing, is therefore conducive to an excellent result. A properly trimmed resin crown form greatly facilitates insertion of the composite, particularly in extensive incisal build-up techniques. Unfortunately, however, most crown forms (Odus-Pella[9] and IB[10] crown forms) are of minimal thickness and conducive to positive restoration of the contact area. The crown form should be carefully adapted to the prepared tooth with the following in mind (Fig. 2-50):

1. A minimum of labial finishing should be necessary after the composite material has polymerized.
2. A thin film of composite excess should extend no more than 1 mm beyond the marginal periphery of the chamfer-shoulder preparation.
3. Vent holes should be placed palatoincisally in order to allow for air escape during insertion (Fig. 2-51).

The crown form matrix is filled with composite material and seated into position over the prepared tooth (Fig. 2-52). An anatomically contoured wooden wedge (13X or 13XT Interdental[11]) is then placed into the gingival embrasure to compress the matrix form into tight adaptive contact with the proximogingival surface and to ensure a slight amount of separation to allow for the thickness of the matrix (Fig. 2-53). The crown form matrix should be lightly compressed labiolingually (Fig. 2-54). This expands the proximal portion of the matrix form into tight adaptive contact with the adjacent tooth, thereby ensuring tight proximal contact (Fig. 2-55).

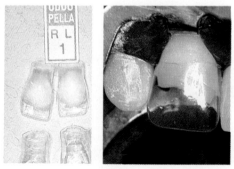

Figure 2-50 Thin crown form properly applied.

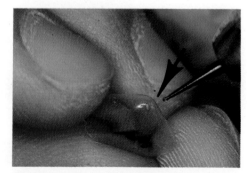

Figure 2-51 Four or five incisal vent holes are placed by means of a No. 1 round bur.

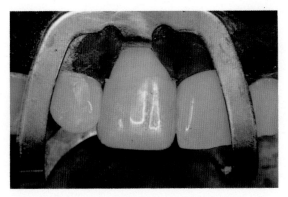

Figure 2-52 Composite filled crown form properly seated.

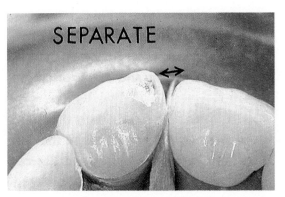

Figure 2-53 Anatomically contoured wooden wedge in position.

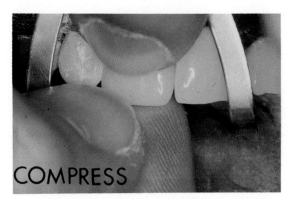

Figure 2-54 The crown form is compressed labiolingually between thumb and index finger.

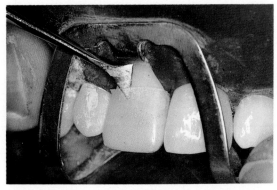

Figure 2-55 The thin crown form matrix is easily peeled away from the composite surface after polymerization without sticking.

A self-cured composite material must be allowed to undergo polymerization for a full 5-minute period, whereas polymerization of a light-cured material may be brought about in a fraction of that time (40 seconds).

In effecting proper cure of a light-cured composite material, six factors must be recognized and, if possible, controlled (Watts et al, 1984; Combe, 1983; Swartz et al, 1983). They are:

1. Time of application of light
2. The plane of direction of the light source
3. The distance from the end of the light source to the composite surface
4. The shade of the composite material
5. The nature of the filler particle within the composite material
6. The temperature of the composite material

All six factors are of extreme importance clinically in that they all singly and cumulatively affect the extent and depth of cure of the composite material.

Time. The more closely the time of application of the visible light source approximates *40 seconds*, the better will be the cure. In an incisal restoration, therefore, the application of light 20 seconds labially and 20 seconds lingually will result in optimal cure of the material. Although there are variations between the various types of composite materials, the average depth of cure resulting from a single-direction application of light is between *2.5 and 3 mm*.

In the event that the composite thickness exceeds 2.5 to 3 mm and visible light cannot be applied from two directions (i.e., in class II situations), the composite material must be placed by use of multiple increments, each of which must be sequentially light-cured before proceeding to the next addition.

Plane. The plane of application of the light source should not be directed obliquely against a composite surface, but should be at right angles to the surface being cured.

Distance. The optimal distance from the end of the light source to the composite surface being cured should be as close as possible to zero. In any event, the maximum distance from the end of the light source to the composite surface should not exceed 1 mm for most effective curing.

Shade. Dark composite materials are more difficult to cure than those of light shades since pigments present in the dark shades tend to absorb visible light. In the event that a dark shade is utilized, curing time should be extended 10 seconds.

Nature of the Filler. Microfilled composites are more difficult to fully cure than other composite types. It is essential, therefore, that the light application used with the microfilled systems be of adequate duration.

Temperature. A cool composite material subjected to visible light will cure to only a fraction of the depth of room temperature composite. Therefore a composite material must always be allowed to assume room temperature before it is light cured.

All six factors are important in that they cumulatively affect the cure depth of the composite material. Accordingly, control must be exercised relative to each. Overcure constitutes no problem with composite materials, but the clinician must exercise extreme caution to ensure that undercure does not result. Particular care should be taken to avoid the "skin effect". Suppose a dark microfilled material is taken directly from the refrigerator and subjected to a total of 20 seconds of light application. Multiple factors are accordingly compromised. The "skin effect" results. The composite surface is fully cured, but the subsurface material is only partially polymerized. The result may well be clinical failure of the restoration.

Finishing

Finishing of the microfilled composite material should be carried out by means of the following technique.

The finishing armamentarium includes tapering multifluted carbide burs (ET6 or ET9[12]; T–Burs, Spiral Fluted[13]), carbide hand finishing knives (150:17 to 150:20[14]), and aluminum oxide composite finishing discs (Sof-lex[15]) and strips (Sof-lex[16]).

The multifluted carbide bur is used at ultra high speed with a water coolant in order to remove gross excess and to effect *initial* marginal finish by means of a *premargination* technique (Fig. 2-56). Premargination refers to the use of the finishing bur to remove only enough marginal excess to allow a thin overlapping fin of excess marginal composite material, which can subsequently be removed readily by means of a combination of discs and a sharp knife (Fig. 2-57).

Final margination can be accomplished by the use of a sharp knife properly "guide-planed" in the marginal region. This is done by resting half of the instrument on the enamel adjacent to the marginal area, the other half on the composite material, and then using a shaving motion in a direction parallel to the marginal line in order to remove the final remnants of fin-type marginal excess (Fig. 2-58). The cutting instrument is thus "guide-planed" by the adjacent tooth structure, thereby preventing submargination of the composite material.

Carbide-tipped composite finishing knives are particularly useful for this purpose since they maintain their sharp cutting edges indefinitely (Fig. 2-59).

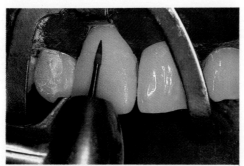

Figure 2–56 Proper alignment of tapering bur for the removal of gross excess.

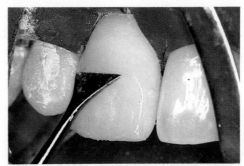

Figure 2–57 A sharp gold knife is used for final margin trimming.

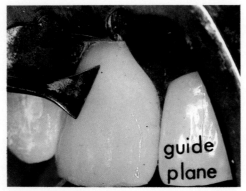

Figure 2–58 "Guide-planed" orientation of knife for margin finishing.

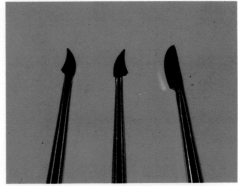

Figure 2–59 "Carbide-tipped" finishing knives[14]: (*left*) No. 150.18 and No. 150.19 interproximal knives; (*right*) No. 150.20 labial knife.

Proximogingival finishing is conveniently accomplished by the use of the thin tapering bur placed from both labio- and palatoproximal directions to premarginate (Fig. 2-60A), followed by the use of the interproximal knives, shaving from composite material gingivally to tooth structure in order to remove final marginal excess. A pair of carbide-tipped interproximal finishing instruments is shown in Figure 2-60B. The proximogingival region is then stripped carefully using aluminum oxide strips to complete the finish in this region (Fig. 2-61). In finishing the lingual concavity region, an appropriate donut-shaped stone (WPH No. 54[17]) may be used to incorporate proper anatomic detail (Fig. 2-62). Final finish of the labial contour is accomplished by the use of aluminum oxide discs—medium, fine, and superfine—in that order, at low speed with light intermittent contact, carefully avoiding heat generation (Fig. 2-63). Application of the superfine disc to the hybrid composite surface results in a smooth "high-sheen" reflective surface topography (Fig. 2-64). "Dry discing" the composite in such a manner enhances the polymerization of the material and results in a hard wear-resistant surface which has been described as the "smear layer" (Davidson et al, 1981).

A good deal of care must be taken to precisely adjust the occlusion in order to provide light group contact in centric, protrusive, and protrusive lateral positions. If the occlusion in inadvertently left slightly "high", particularly during eccentric movements, this will surely result in a cohesive fracture of the composite material (Fig. 2-65). This point is particularly critical with the microfilled composite materials since they are "lighter filled" than the conventional composites. Microfilled composites show a 15 percent to 20 percent reduction in tensile strength relative to other composite materials and accordingly demonstrate less resistance to impact forces when placed in stress-bearing situations.

A very thin articulating film (Truspot II[18]) is used to finally assess the occlusion in order to ensure light group contact on the palatoincisal aspect of the restoration (Fig. 2-66), particularly in protrusive and protrusive lateral movements.

The final composite restoration, comparable in both surface smoothness and reflectivity to the adjacent tooth structure (Fig. 2-67), does not require a glazing technique because the final disced surface presents a glassy smooth, highly reflective appearance.

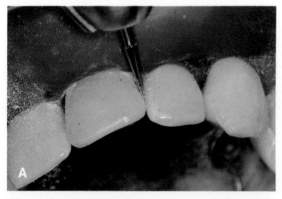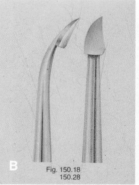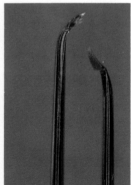

Figure 2-60   *A,* Use of tapering bur for removal of proximal gross excess. *B,* Interproximal knives No. 150.18 and No. 150.19 for final marginal finish.

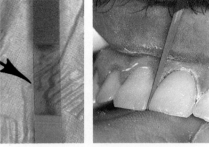

Figure 2–61 Use of interproximal strip (Sof-lex[1]) for final finish of gingival margin.

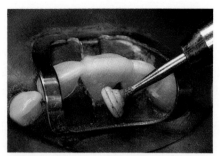

Figure 2–62 Use of donut-shaped stone (WPH No. 54[17]) for lingual concavity.

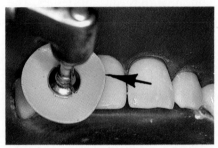

Figure 2–63 Aluminum oxide disc (Sof-lex[15]) for final contouring and surface finish.

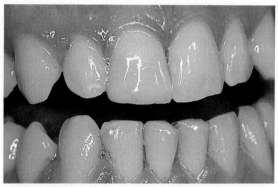

Figure 2–64 Composite restoration after final aluminum oxide disc finish.

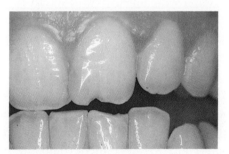

Figure 2–65 "Chip-type" fracture of a class IV microfilled composite restoration.

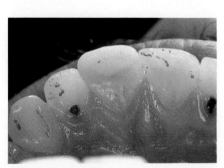

Figure 2–66 The palatoincisal surface of the composite restoration shows lighter contact than adjacent enamel surfaces.

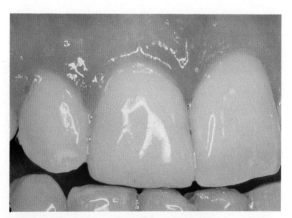

Figure 2–67 Close-up view of final composite restoration.

LABIAL VENEER RESTORATIONS

Composite resin materials may be successfully utilized as labial veneers for the interim treatment of hypoplastic, or worn, or discolored anterior teeth (Fig. 2-68). A technique similar to that already described for incisal fracture restorations is recommended for labial veneering.

Materials. The same considerations as have already been presented for cases of incisal fracture relate to the conservative use of labial veneer restorations in the *young patient* with discolored, worn, or hypoplastic teeth rather than full coverage in the form of porcelain jacket or porcelain fused to gold crowns. The three basic types of labial veneer restorations are (1) *direct* light-cured composites, (2) *indirect* (laboratory-processed) *composite*, and (3) *indirect porcelain* veneers. There are specific clinical indications for each type of veneering technique. Direct light-cured composite veneers are the simplest to place in terms of clinical technique and are the easiest for the general practitioner to fabricate with predictable results. The direct veneers are primarily indicated for the treatment of erosion-abrasion labial wear and extensive enamel hypoplasia.

Assuming that direct composite veneer restorations are indicated, the question quite naturally arises, "What is the best choice of composite material?"

If occlusion is normal and can be adjusted in protrusive or protrusive lateral movements to prevent inordinate stress on the restorations, the light-cured, *microfilled* composite materials are the best choice because of their superb polishing characteristics and overall esthetic acceptability. Should occlusal factors be more demanding, the *macrofilled* or *hybrid* materials would be the better choice.

The light-cured, microfilled composite materials are ideally suited for the labial resin veneering of the maxillary central incisors of the young patient shown in Figure 2-69. The central incisors demonstrate extreme abrasion-erosion wear together with incisal fracture. Occlusal factors are optimal. Labial resin veneer microfill (Durafill[19]) restorations were placed (Fig. 2-70), and the result at 3-year recall is shown in Figure 2-71. The color stability and wear resistance of the veneer restorations are self-evident. Another ideal clinical situation for direct microfilled composite labial veneer restorations is shown in Figure 2-72. The 36-year-old patient presented with severely hypoplastic anterior teeth. Hypoplasia is amenable to direct veneer treatment since the discolored tooth structure is confined almost entirely to the superficial enamel thickness. Accordingly, the defective tooth structure may be entirely removed by means of a simple chamfer preparation (Fig. 2-73) and esthetic composite veneer restorations placed without requiring opaquers, which significantly complicate the restorative procedure.

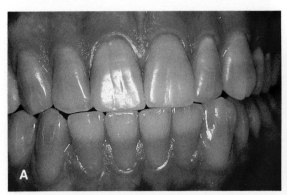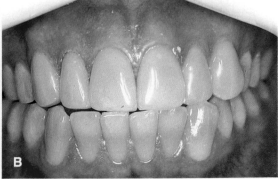

Figure 2–68   Discolored dentition before, *A*, and after, *B*, veneering treatment.

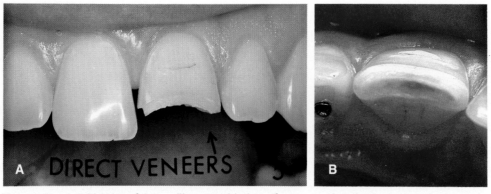

Figure 2-69   *A*, Labial view of the maxillary central incisors of a young patient showing erosion-abrasion wear in combination with incisal fracture. *B*, Incisal view of maxillary left central incisor.

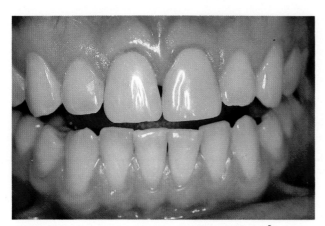

Figure 2-70   The same maxillary central incisors (as shown in Fig. 2-69) after labial veneer restoration using a light-cured microfilled composite (Durafil).

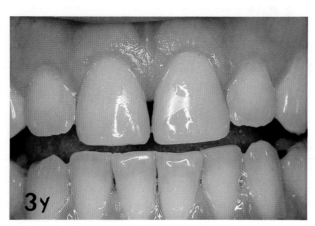

Figure 2-71   Three-year recall of the composite labial veneers.

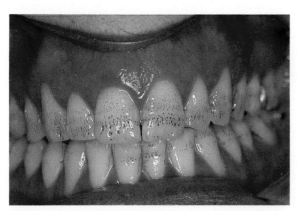

Figure 2-72   Severe hypoplasia involving the anterior dentition.

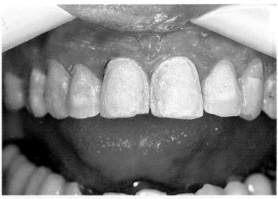

Figure 2-73   Labial chamfer preparations remove all of discolored tooth structure thereby obviating the use of opaquing materials.

DIRECT LIGHT-CURED COMPOSITE VENEER RESTORATIONS

Before isolation of the field, a tapering bullet-nosed diamond instrument is used to "rough out" labial chamfer-shoulder preparations (Figs. 2-74 to 2-76). The chamfer preparation should extend gingivally to just level with the crest of the gingival tissue, proximally to just labial to the mesial and distal contact areas, and incisally to the crest of the incisal ridge (Fig. 2-77).

Isolation of the Field. Proper *isolation of the field* is accomplished by placement of a rubber dam and a properly stabilized No. 212 gingival retraction clamp (Ivory 212 S.A.[20]) (Fig. 2-78). An alternate method of isolation involves the use of cheek retractors and of cotton rolls placed in the muco-labial fold. Careful placement of a double-strand thickness of retraction cord in the labial gingival crevice (Fig. 2-79) helps to control seepage in this area.

For multiple anterior veneer composite restorations, a useful cheek retraction apparatus (Self Span[21]) is shown in Figure 2-80. This, combined with properly modified gingival retraction clamps, allows excellent access to the operative field.

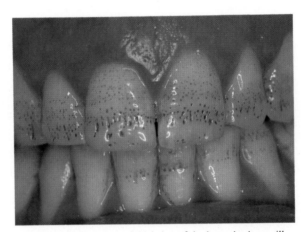

Figure 2-74   Preoperative labial view of the hypoplastic maxillary anterior dentition.

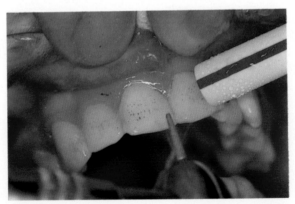

Figure 2-75   A bullet-nosed diamond at ultra high speed is used for labial chamfer preparation.

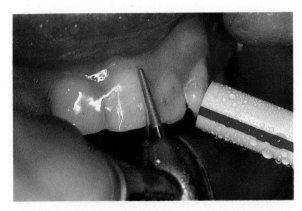

Figure 2-76 The chamfer preparation involves the removal of 0.5 to 1 full millimeter of labial enamel.

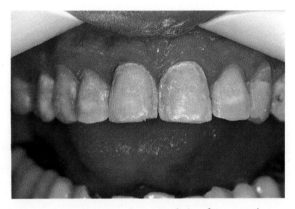

Figure 2-77 Labial view of completed chamfer preparations.

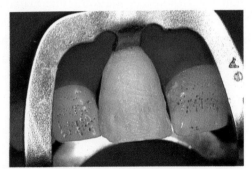

Figure 2-78 Close-up view of labial chamfer preparation with No. 212 clamp in position.

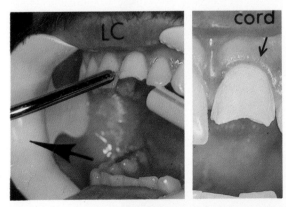

Figure 2-79 Cheek retractors (*left*) and gingival retraction cord (*right*).

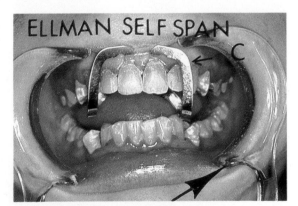

Figure 2-80 "Self-span" cheek retractor[21] in combination with modified clamps (Ivory 212 S.A.[20]).

Preparation. The *chamfer-shoulder* preparation is then completed on the labial enamel surface using a bullet-nosed diamond instrument (Fig. 2-81). Three important reference points serve as guidelines for the labial veneer chamfer-shoulder margins, namely, the free gingival crest, the proximal contact areas, and the incisal ridge (Fig. 2-82). The gingival margin of the preparation should extend cervically to just short of the free gingival margin. The mesio- and disto-proximal borders of the preparation end just slightly labial to the contact areas to allow convenient access for finishing purposes. Incisally, the preparation extends to the crest of the incisal edge usually without palatal overlap. Prior to making the preparation, scribing a proximocervical pencil line on the labial periphery of the tooth greatly facilitates the procedure.

The chamfer-shoulder labial veneer preparation serves all of the important functions of the incisal fracture preparation relative to enhanced retention and marginal integrity. In addition, it serves the important function in veneering of providing an acceptable labial thickness of composite restorative material without significantly *overcontouring* this surface. Long-term observations of labial resin veneer restorations indicate that overcontouring, with resultant gingival inflammation, is one of the major pitfalls associated with the technique (Fig. 2-83).

To provide adequate labial thickness of the composite material, optimal *depth* in the preparation is required. The preparation should extend as deep as possible into the labial enamel thickness without exposing dentin. Maximal thickness of composite material overlying the cut enamel surface is thus provided, thereby enhancing the esthetic acceptability of the restoration.

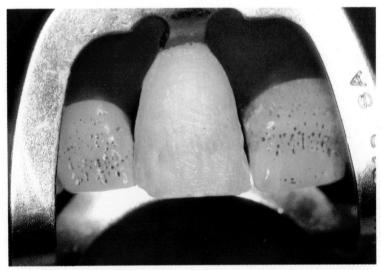

Figure 2–81 Completed chamfer preparation after refinement with retraction clamp in position.

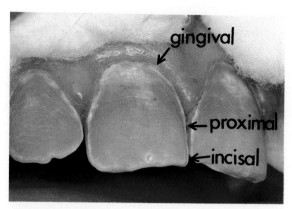

Figure 2-82 Reference points for location of chamfer preparation margins.

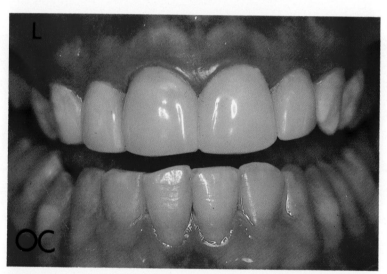

Figure 2-83 Overcontoured labial veneer restorations with resultant gingival inflammation.

Matrix. A careful matricing technique simplifies the finishing of the composite material and enhances the final result. The labial half of a thin crown form[9,10] is cut and subsequently trimmed to extend approximately 0.5 mm beyond the gingivoproximal margins of the preparation (Fig. 2-84). Accurate embrasure fitting of the crown form matrix to ensure restoration of the exact labial contour desired without requiring extensive labial finishing should be the primary goal of the matrix fabrication technique. A properly fitted crown form matrix is shown in Figure 2-85. When the entire anterior arch segment is restored with labial veneer restorations, appropriate crown form matrices (DenMat[22]) may be prefitted on a study model by the dental assistant (Fig. 2-86), and thereby a good deal of chair time is saved.

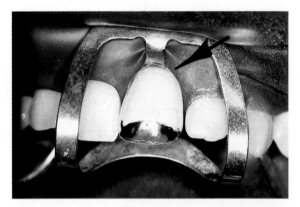

Figure 2-84 Labial crown form matrix trimmed to extend 0.5 mm beyond gingival margin of preparation.

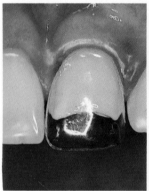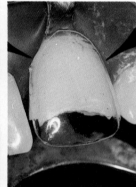

Figure 2-85 Proper embrasure fitting of the crown form matrix renders unnecessary the prolonged and extensive finishing of veneer restorations.

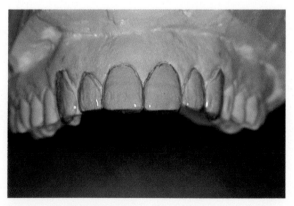

Figure 2-86 Multiple labial crown form matrices trimmed and fitted on study model.

Acid Etching. Many light-cured composite materials come with gel-type etchants. An etching gel is painted over the enamel surface area (Fig. 2-87) and left in place for a minimum of one minute; continuous stroking motion is not used. After 30 to 45 seconds of thorough water lavage, the labial enamel is thoroughly air dried (Fig. 2-88).

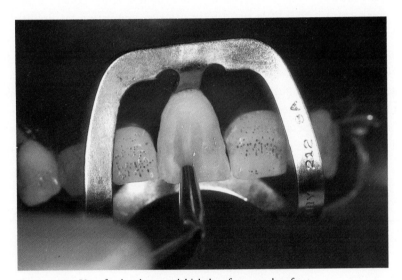

Figure 2-87   Use of gel etchant on labial chamfer enamel surface.

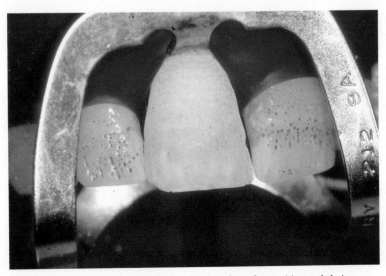

Figure 2-88   Etched labial enamel chamfered surface after washing and drying.

Bonding. A phosphonate enamel dentin bond resin (Scotchbond;[30] Prisma Universal Bond[47]) should be carefully applied to the enamel surface. A small ball of bond resin is applied to the midenamel region on the end of a soft fine-tipped brush (Fig. 2-89). Then it is thinly spread peripherally toward the enamel cavo-surface periphery and gently blown with air.

The composite material may be placed over the bond resin surface prior to light-curing or preferably after the bond resin has been cured by means of a 20-second exposure to visible light. The latter procedure is recommended since the composite material is much easier to control when placed on a prepolymerized surface. After the 20-second period of light cure, the air-inhibited layer is clearly evident (Fig. 2-90).

Insertion. A polyethylene strip is placed between the proximal chamfer margins and the adjacent teeth in order to control the placement of the composite material (Fig. 2-91). By means of a flat-bladed anodized aluminum-coated instrument (Felt No. 4[24]) (Fig. 2-92), the composite paste (Silux[23]) is then applied and contoured over the labial surface. Wetting the side of the instrument with a little bond resin prior to contouring facilitates the procedure and allows for proper shaping and forming of the composite material without "pull back" (Fig. 2-93). The prefitted crown form matrix is filled with additional composite material and subsequently placed in proper alignment over the labial surface (Fig. 2-94). Ideally, the composite material should be highly viscous, readily moldable, and free of "slumping" or uncontrolled flow. The flat-bladed composite instrument wetted with a slight amount of bond resin may be used to shape and form the marginal areas before curing, in which case it is unnecessary to remove gross excess during finishing or the excess composite may be allowed to squeeze between the matrix and the chamfer margins (Fig. 2-95).

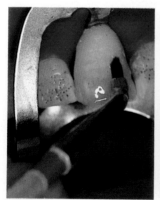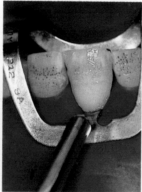

Figure 2–89 Application of bond resin; thin spread with fine-tipped brush (*left*), then air blown (*right*).

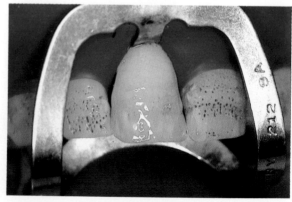

Figure 2-90 Bond resin surface after cure.

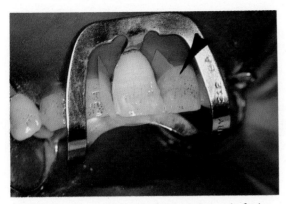

Figure 2-91 Proper placement of polyethylene strip for isolation.

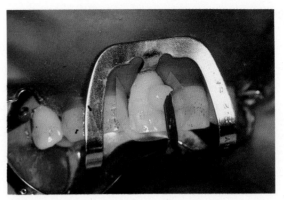

Figure 2-92 Bulk pack placement of composite material over labial surface.

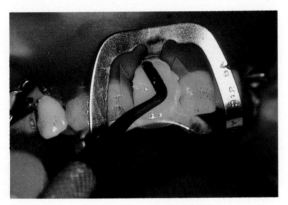

Figure 2-93 Shaping composite with Teflon instrument wetted with bond resin prevents "pull back".

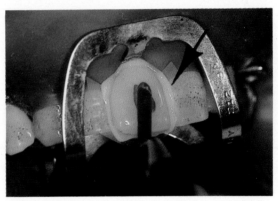

Figure 2-94 Composite filled crown form matrix initially adapts to labial surface.

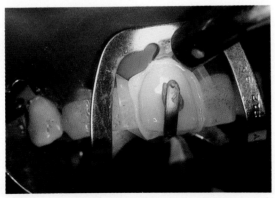

Figure 2-95 Precuring of the composite material by means of a 5-second application of visible light.

The composite material is then cured by means of a 40-second application of visible light from both labial and lingual directions, preferably using a light tip with an end diameter of 12 to 15 mm. After cure, the proximogingival excess composite material is "flaked" away using an explorer (Figs. 2-96 and 2-97). The crown form matrix is then "peeled off" the composite surface from which it separates cleanly (Fig. 2-98).

When the matrix crown form is removed, a smooth, highly reflective *matrix-cured surface* should be observed (Fig. 2-99), and if the matricing and insertion techniques have been carried out satisfactorily, only a small amount of composite marginal excess is observed.

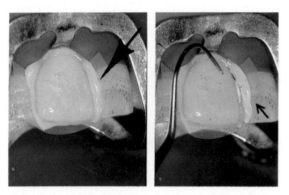

Figure 2-96 Proximogingival gross excess composite material flaked away with explorer, followed by 40-second final light cure.

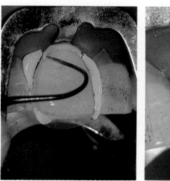
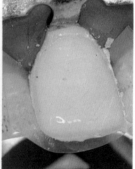

Figure 2-97 Labial composite veneer after final cure.

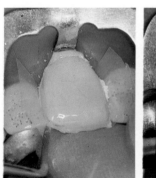
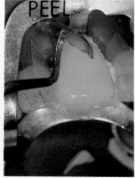

Figure 2-98 The matrix form is peeled away from the composite material.

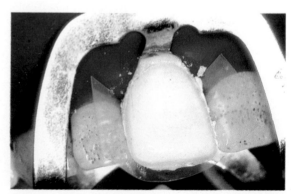

Figure 2-99 The "matrix-cured" labial surface prior to finishing.

Finish. In *finishing*, most of the smooth matrix-cured labial surface should be left intact if at all possible (Fig. 2-100). Marginal finishing should be carried out by means of a tapering, multifluted finishing bur (Fig. 2-101), and final finishing is carried out with aluminum oxide discs (Figs. 2-102 and 2-103). The use of ⅜-inch aluminum oxide discs on a small-headed snap-on mandrel[25] facilitates the finishing procedure in the gingival region. Careful adjustment of the occlusion in centric, protrusive, and protrusive lateral positions should follow. Group function is mandatory. The finished veneer restorations are shown immediately postoperatively in Figure 2-104 and at 18-month recall in Figures 2-105 to 2-108.

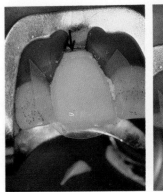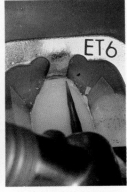

Figure 2–100 Marginal excess composite material is removed using a tapering carbide bur.

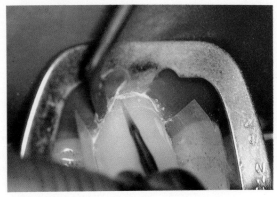

Figure 2–101 The fine tapering tip of the carbide bur allows easy access into "difficult to reach" areas.

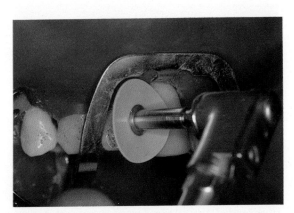

Figure 2–102 Three-eighths-inch aluminum oxide discs complete contouring and surfacing.

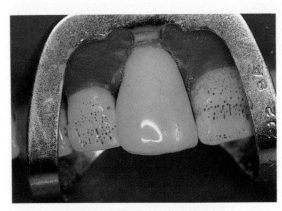

Figure 2–103 Finished labial veneer restoration.

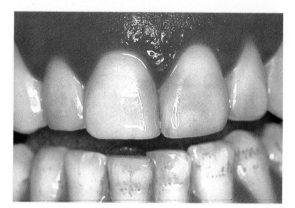

Figure 2-104 Completed labial veneer restorations, maxillary anterior arch at time of insertion.

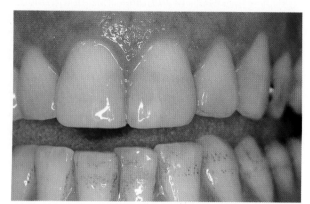

Figure 2-105 Veneer restorations at 18-month recall.

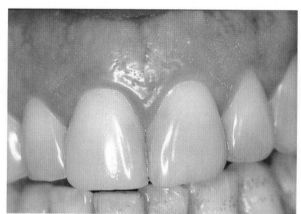

Figure 2-106 Close-up labial view of veneer restorations at 18-month recall.

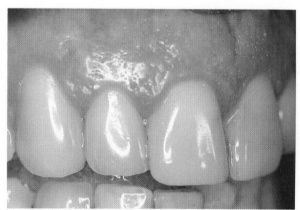

Figure 2-107 Right lateral view of veneer restorations at 18-month recall.

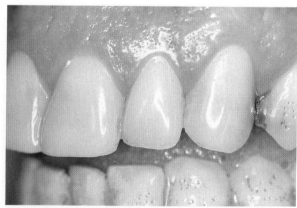

Figure 2-108 Left lateral view of veneer restorations at 18-month recall.

Microfilled composite materials demonstrate excellent durability relative to wear and fracture resistance, provided occlusal circumstances are normal and proper group function (i.e., light group contact) can be established. In the event that occlusal function is more demanding, macrofilled or hybrid-type composite materials should be utilized for direct composite veneer restorations (Figs. 2-109 to 2-111).

Direct light-cured composite veneer restorations are ideal for the conservative treatment of abrasion-erosion wear and/or enamel hypoplasia. Extremely dark tetracycline discoloration (Fig. 2-112) calls for advanced clinical techniques in the form of indirect veneer restorations or direct veneers in combination with opaquers and tints (see Chapters 3, 4, 5).

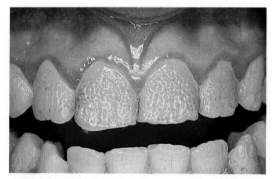

Figure 2–109 Maxillary hypoplastic dentition prior to veneer treatment.

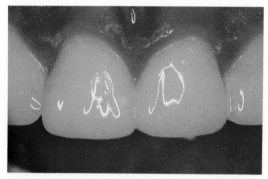

Figure 2–110 Maxillary hypoplastic dentition after labial veneer treatment using a macrofilled visible-light-cured composite material (Prismafil[26]).

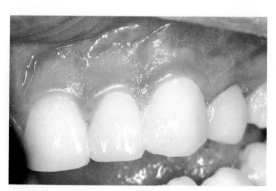

Figure 2–111 Lateral view of the dentition shown in Figure 2-110.

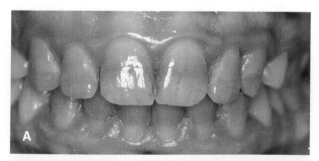

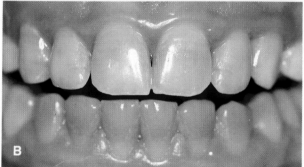

Figure 2–112 Dark tetracycline-discolored dentition before, *A*, and after, *B*, veneer treatment.

EXTENSIVE CROWN RESTORATIONS ON NONVITAL ANTERIOR TEETH

An extensive fracture of a maxillary central incisor in a 16-year-old patient is shown in Figure 2-113. The original trauma devitalized the pulp, and subsequent to root canal therapy, crown restoration is required.

Materials. Normally a cast post and core followed by a full-coverage restoration in the form of a porcelain jacket or porcelain fused to metal crown are the method of choice. However, full eruption of the anterior teeth is not yet complete in midadolescence, and the distinct possibility of a negative gingival response subsequent to crown placement must be anticipated (Fig. 2-114). An interim composite core metallic post restoration is probably the better choice at this stage since such an approach combines demonstrated durability with acceptable esthetics. Preoperative assessment of occlusal factors suggests an inordinately heavy occlusal load in protrusive and protrusive lateral movements. In addition, the patient is an active sports enthusiast. Both factors favor the choice of a small-particle macrofilled, light-cured composite (Prismafil[26]), rather than a microfilled material.

Preparation. Prior to extensive composite crown build-up of a nonvital anterior tooth, a prefitted metalic post (Fig. 2-115) should be luted into the root canal to provide a stable base for both the interim and final restorations. Under no circumstances should composite materials alone be used for the post portion of the restoration because the brittleness of these materials invites cohesive failure at the post-core interface.

A parallel-sided serated metallic post (Parapost[27]) should be prefitted into the root canal. Relative to *length*, the post should extend into the root canal a distance equal to at least half of the remaining alveolar bone support (Fig. 2-116). In fitting the post, care must be taken to avoid disturbing the apical 3 mm of root canal seal. The post should be loose-fitting without binding on the lateral walls of the prepared radicular pulp space.

Luting the Post. The clinician has two choices relative to the luting material for the prefitted post:

1. A fast-setting glass ionomer cement (Ketac–Cem[28]) (Fig. 2-117).
2. A heavy-filled, self-cured hybrid composite material (Conclude or P/10[29]) used in conjunction with a dentin bonding agent (Scotchbond[30]).

The glass ionomer cement provides a chemical bond to both post metal and root dentinal surfaces. The heavy-filled, self-cured composite material used with a dentin bonding agent provides a chemical bond to dentin (but not metal) and demonstrates a comparatively high shear strength.

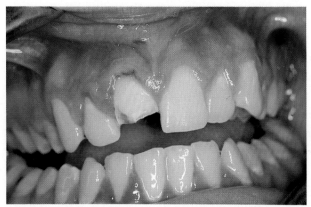

Figure 2-113 Fractured nonvital maxillary right central incisor.

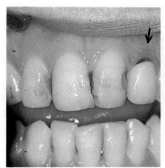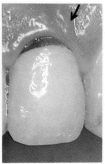

Figure 2–114 Full crown restoration, maxillary left lateral incisor at 3-year recall.

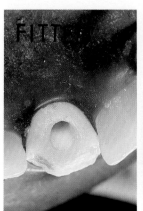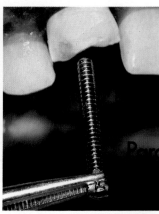

Figure 2–115 A serrated parallel-sided metallic post (Parapost[27]) fitted loosely into the root canal.

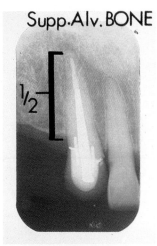

Figure 2–116 Optimal post distance should be at least one-half the cervicoapical length of the supporting alveolar bone.

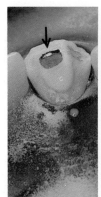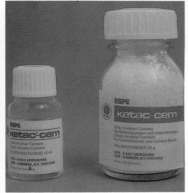

Figure 2–117 A fast-setting glass ionomer cement (Ketac-Cem[28]) suitable for luting.

In the restoration under consideration, the glass ionomer cement was used to lute the metallic post (Fig. 2-118). After properly opaquing (Helicolor Opaque[31]) the metallic surface of the post projecting from the pulp space, a chamfer preparation is made (Fig. 2-119), and after etching and bonding, the coronal restoration is built up using macrofilled composite in a thin crown form. The interim composite crown restoration is shown in Figure 2-120. Such a restoration may indeed be "long-term" in nature since little can go wrong that cannot be easily reversed by conservative means. For example, if fracture should occur subsequent to new trauma (Fig. 2-121), the composite crown may be easily reveneered with the composite material of choice (Fig. 2-122) (see Chapter 9).

Nonvital teeth that have undergone discoloration subsequent to root canal therapy may be esthetically restored using composite materials in conjunction with "walking" bleach techniques. For example, Figure 2-123 shows a discolored nonvital maxillary right central incisor with a large discolored composite restoration. The use of "opaquers" on such teeth prior to composite restoration frequently results in a "shine-through" problem which may seriously compromise the esthetic acceptability of the restoration (Fig. 2-124). A "walking" bleach technique carried out prior to composite crown restoration provides a more reliably predictable esthetic result.

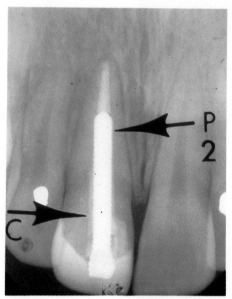

Figure 2-118 Metal post luted with glass ionomer cement.

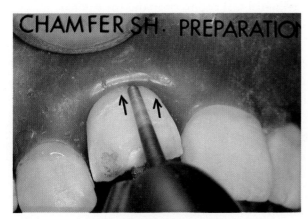

Figure 2–119   Chamfer preparation prior to crown build-up.

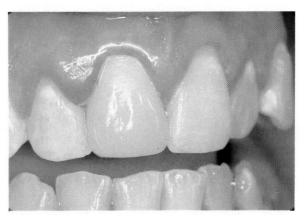

Figure 2-120   Full crown build-up in macrofilled light-cured composite. (Prismafil[36]).

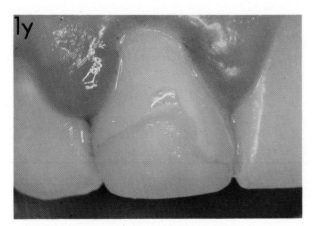

Figure 2-121   Composite fracture at 1-year recall.

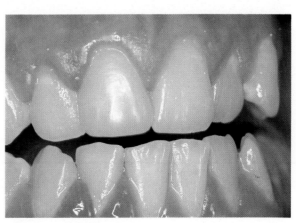

Figure 2-122   Reveneered composite restoration.

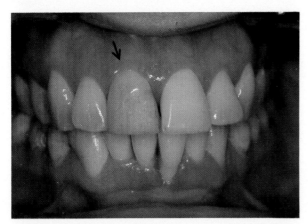

Figure 2–123   Discolored nonvital maxillary central incisor with discolored composite restoration.

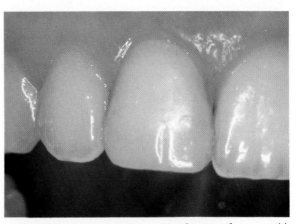

Figure 2–124   "Shine-through" resulting from use of opaquer with composite veneer restoration.

A diamond instrument is used to remove the lingual seal and to clean out the coronal contents of the pulp chamber (Fig. 2-125). Approximately 1.5 mm of the root canal filling is removed in the cervical region, and a "plug" of polycarboxylate (Poly–F–Plus[32]) or fast-setting glass ionomer cement is inserted into the cervical space thus created; this seals the radicular root canal filling from the coronal pulp space. A small cotton pledget is soaked in phosphoric acid, placed into the coronal pulp space for one minute, and removed; the area is then thoroughly washed and dried. The dentin tubules on the walls of the coronal pulp space are thereby widened (Fig. 2-126), allowing greater diffusion of the bleaching material through the dentinal tissue. A "walking" bleach is mixed, consisting of oral perborate powder[33] added to 2 drops of 30 percent hydrogen peroxide (Superoxol[34]) to form a stiff white paste (Fig. 2-127). The walking bleach paste is inserted into the coronal pulp space to completely cover the labial dentinal wall, and this is subsequently covered with a dry cotton pledget. The lingual opening is sealed with polycarboxylate or glass ionomer cement (Figs. 2-128 and 2-129). The patient is recalled within 5 to 7 days and reassessed, and if necessary another walking bleach is placed. After two or three appointments, the natural crown color is attained (Fig. 2-130), and the tooth is subsequently restored with composite (Visiodispers[35]) (Fig. 2-131).

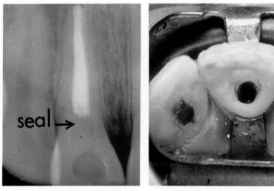

Figure 2-125 The coronal pulp space is prepared (*right*), and the cervicogingival region (*left*) is sealed with cement.

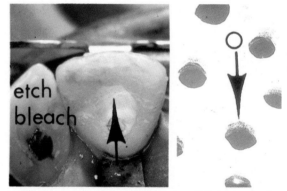

Figure 2-126 The coronal pulp chamber (*left*) is phosphoric acid-etched, and thereby the dentinal tubules are widened (*right*).

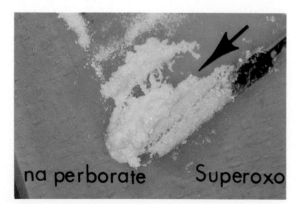

Figure 2-127 Sodium perborate powder is mixed with Superoxol into a stiff paste.

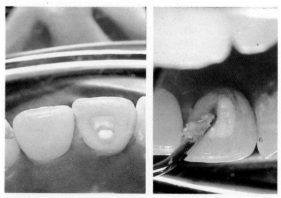

Figure 2-128 The "walking bleach" is then condensed into the pulp chamber.

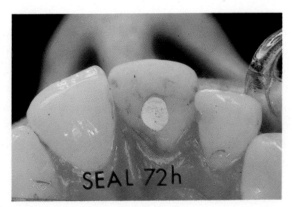

Figure 2-129 A lingual seal is placed.

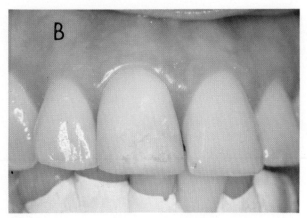

Figure 2-130 Maxillary right central incisor after bleaching.

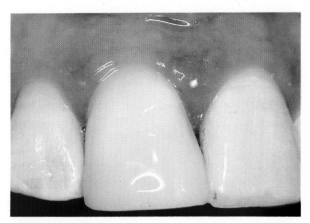

Figure 2–131 The maxillary incisor shown in Figure 2-130 after composite restoration.

MANDIBULAR INCISAL RESTORATION

A mandibular incisal edge presents a special problem in composite restoration since extremely heavy function combined with a restricted labiolingual thickness of restorative material both predominate. Although occasionally microfilled materials may be successfully utilized for incisal restoration (Figs. 2-132 to 2-135), the composite materials of choice should be heavy-filled, macrofilled (Prismafil[36]), or hybrid systems (Figs. 2–136 and 2–137). One of the most demanding retention situations relates to mandibular incisal erosion lesions in patients of advanced age who have lost vertical dimension (Figs. 2-138 and 2-139). For best results relative to retention, two self-threading 0.0017-inch incisal pins[37] (Fig. 2-140) in combination with circumferential chamfer-shoulder preparations are recommended. Particularly when oral hygiene is less than adequate, heavy-filled, light-cured, hybrid composite materials (Command Ultrafine[38]) are best indicated because of their combined smooth polishability and fracture resistance (Figs. 2-141 to 2-145).

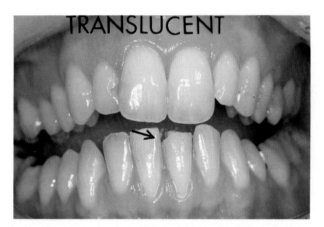

Figure 2-132 Fractured mandibular left central incisor.

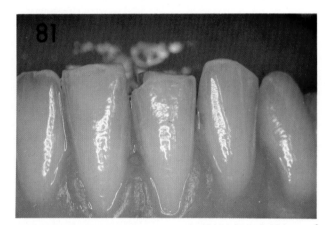

Figure 2-133 Close-up view shows restricted labiolingual thickness of incisal area to be restored.

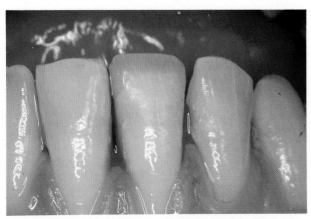

Figure 2–134 Incisal restoration with microfilled light-cured composite (Visiodispers). (note translucency at baseline.)

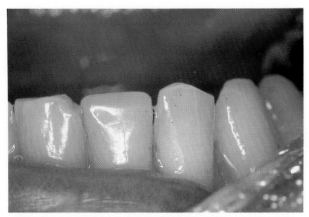

Figure 2-135 Three-year recall of incisal restoration.

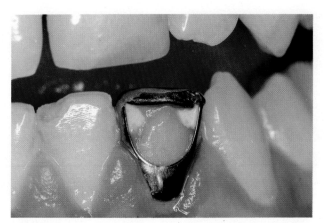

Figure 2–136 An "open-faced" metallic crown placed on a mandibular lateral incisor preoperatively.

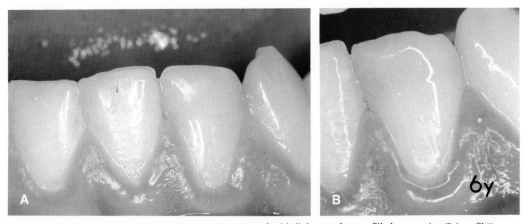

Figure 2–137 *A,* The tooth shown in Figure 2-136 restored with light-cured macrofilled composite (Prismafil[26]) at 2-year recall. *B,* The same tooth shown in Figures 2-136 and 2-137A at six year recall.

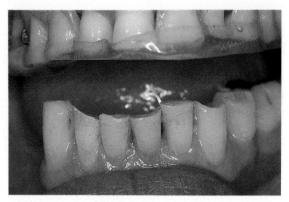

Figure 2-138 Mandibular incisal erosion-abrasion lesions in geriatric patient.

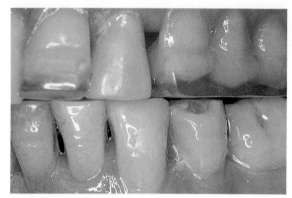

Figure 2-139 "Bite plane" in position for vertical opening.

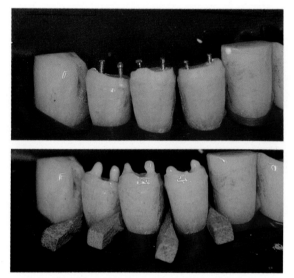

Figure 2-140 Pins (.0017 inch) and chamfer preparations (*top*). Pins masked by opaquer (Helicolor Opaque[31]) (*bottom*).

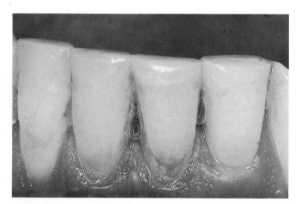

Figure 2-141 Finished incisal restorations using a heavy-filled, light-cured hybrid composite material (Command Ultrafine[38]).

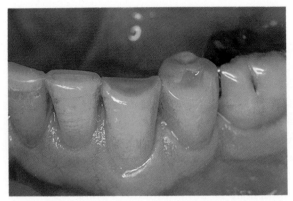

Figure 2-142   Incisal erosion lesion of mandibular left cuspid.

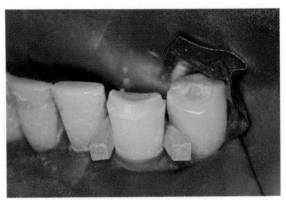

Figure 2-143   Chamfer preparation.

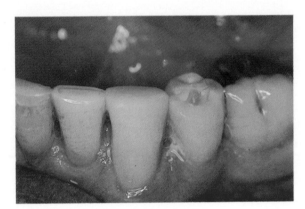

Figure 2-144   Hybrid composite restoration.

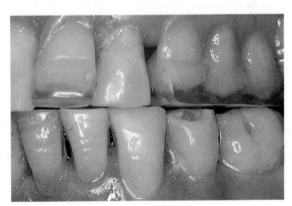

Figure 2-145   Bite-plane in position.

DIASTEMA CLOSURE

Materials. Given the advent of resin-enamel bonding techniques together with vastly improved composite materials, rarely are full-coverage or full labial veneer restorations indicated for diastema closure. Composite materials, because of their direct add-on bondability to enamel surfaces, are by far the most appropriate materials for the purpose.

If the diastema spaces are small and occlusal factors normal (Fig. 2-146), light-cured, microfilled materials are best indicated (Fig. 2-147). However, when the diastema spaces are large (Fig. 2-148), heavy-filled, light-cured hybrid (Command Ultrafine[38]), or macrofilled (Prismafil[36]) materials are indicated, particularly when demanding occlusal factors predominate (Fig. 2-149).

Technique. Irrespective of the type of composite material utilized for the purpose, the technique of diastema closure (Fig. 2-150) is as follows:

1. The proximal enamel surfaces adjacent to the diastema space are lightly disced up to and including the proximolabial line angles (Fig. 2-151).
2. After phosphoric acid etching, washing, and drying of the proximal enamel surfaces, a thin layer of bonding resin is applied and cured.
3. A thin crown form matrix is trimmed and fitted to the proximal area and pre-stabilized using an anatomically contoured wooden wedge to fill the gingival embrasure.
4. The crown form matrix is removed, filled with composite, placed, stabilized, light-cured and finished using the instrumentation technique previously described.

Occasionally, an extremely wide midline diastema is seen. Direct add-on build-out of composite to the two mesial proximal surfaces adjacent to the space would unnaturally widen the central incisors, thus causing a bovine appearance. The technique of choice in such cases is to partially close the diastema by means of minor tooth movement, followed by the direct add-on build-out of multiple proximal surfaces using a hybrid-type composite material (Command Ultrafine[38]), thus widening slightly all four (or six if necessary) anterior teeth. Figures 2-152 to 2-156 illustrate the procedure.

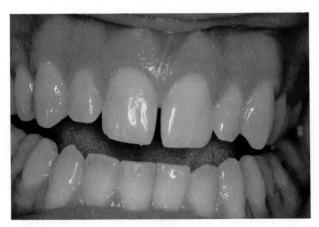

Figure 2-146 Midline diastema shown preoperatively.

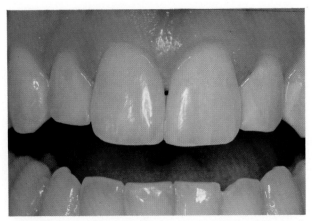

Figure 2-147 Diastema closed using direct add on light-cured microfilled composite (Silux[23]).

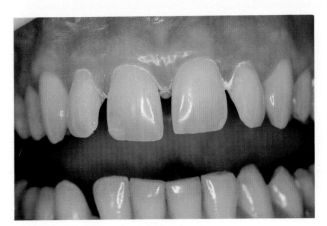

Figure 2-148 Large anterior diastemas.

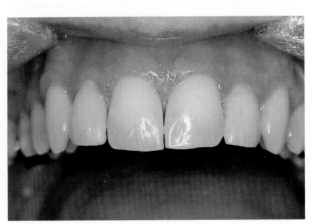

Figure 2-149 Spaces closed with macrofilled composite material (Prismafil[36]).

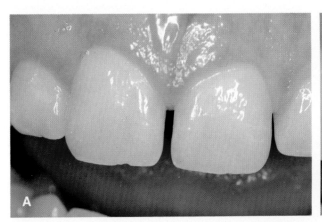

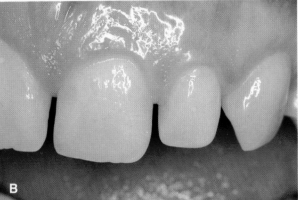

Figure 2-150 *A*, Midline diastema, front labial view. *B*, Midline diastema, left lateral view.

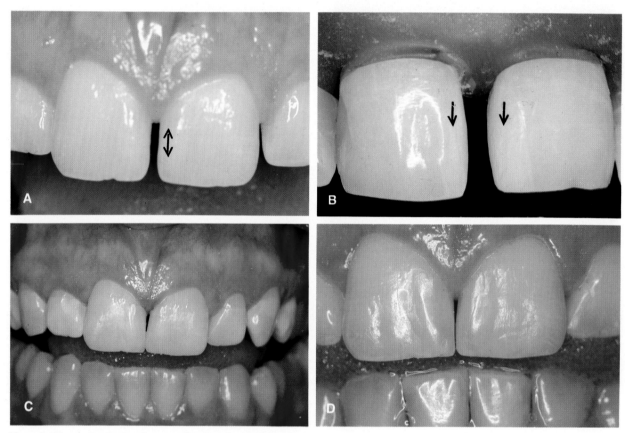

Figure 2-151 *A*, Proximal surfaces are disced to the labial line angle (*arrow*). *B*, Arrows indicate finish lines at the mesiolabial line angles. *C*, Diastema closure completed using light-cured microfilled composite[2w]. *D*, Restorations at 2-year recall.

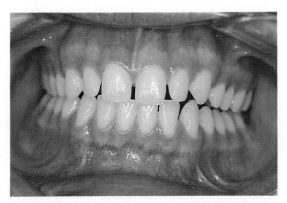

Figure 2-152   Wide midline diastema between maxillary central and lateral incisors, after minor tooth movement.

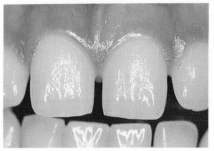

Figure 2-153   Preoperative close-up view of diastema.

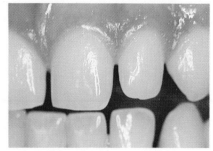

Figure 2-154   After minor tooth movement, composite (Command Ultrafine[38]) was directly bonded to the mesial surfaces of both central and lateral incisors.

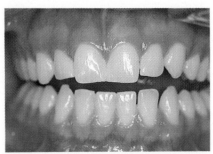

Figure 2-155   Composite (Command Ultrafine[38]) directly bonded to mesial surfaces of central and lateral incisors.

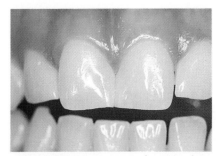

Figure 2-156   Close-up view of completed composite restorations.

PEG LATERAL BUILD-UP

Peg lateral build-up (Fig. 2-157) is similar in all respects to diastema closure, particularly relative to materials and technique utilized:

1. The enamel surfaces are lightly disced (Fig. 2-158), phosphoric acid etched, washed, and dried (Fig. 2-159).
2. After bond resin placement, a thin crown form matrix is fitted (Fig. 2-160), filled with composite, placed, and stabilized.
3. After visible-light-curing from both labial and lingual directions, thin tapering carbide finishing burs are used to remove excess and contour, and then aluminum oxide discs are used to finally finish (Fig. 2-161). Depending on occlusal factors, either microfilled or macrofilled composite materials may be utilized for the direct crown build-up technique. Long-term recall results are shown in Figures 2-162 to 2-165.

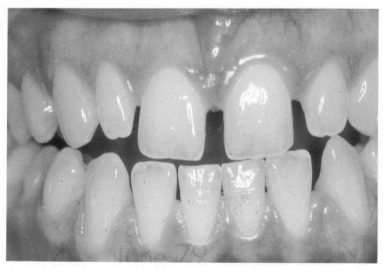

Figure 2-157 Maxillary left and right peg lateral incisors.

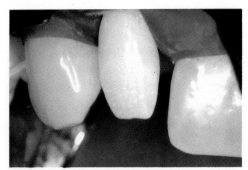

Figure 2-158 The enamel surface is lightly disced.

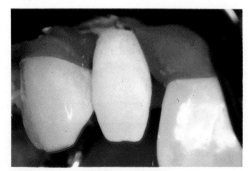

Figure 2-159 Phosphoric acid etching.

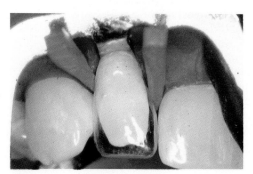

Figure 2-160 Thin crown form matrix.

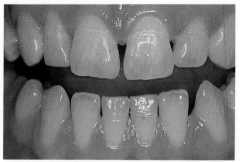

Figure 2-161 Postoperative view of left and right peg lateral build-up.

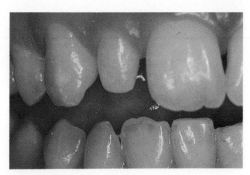

Figure 2-162 Right maxillary peg lateral as seen preoperatively.

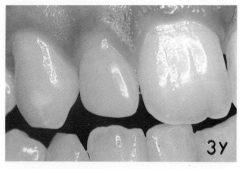

Figure 2-163 Restoration with microfilled composite (Phaseafil[1]) at 3-year recall.

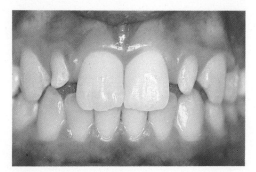

Figure 2-164 Peg lateral incisors as seen preoperatively.

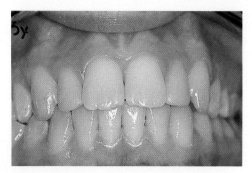

Figure 2-165 Restoration with macrofilled composite (Nuvafil[41]) at 5-year recall.

WHITE SPOT LESIONS AND HYPOPLASTIC DEFECTS

Both white spot lesions and hypoplastic defects are treated in a similar fashion.

Materials. Since such lesions usually are encountered on the labial enamel surfaces in predominantly nonfunctional situations, light-cured, microfilled materials are normally indicated (Fig. 2-166). Hypoplastic defects involving the functional incisal surfaces of anterior teeth should be restored with heavy-filled, macrofilled, or hybrid-type materials, particularly when heavy occlusal function predominates (Fig. 2-167).

Technique. Whatever material is utilized, the technique is as follows:

1. Opaquers should be avoided if possible because of the associated "shine-through" effect (Figs. 2-168 and 2-169). A bullet-nosed diamond is used to remove all of the discolored enamel (Figs. 2-170 and 2-171) even if this necessitates exposure of the superficial labial dentin (Fig. 2-172). If this occurs, the dentin should be protected by application of a thin layer of synthetic varnish or, alternatively, a light-cured dentin bonding resin (see Chapter 6).
2. Using a viscous gel-type etchant (Scotchbond Etching Gel or Control Etch[39]), the enamel should be etched for a one minute period, washed, and dried.
3. After bonding, composite is placed, cured, and finished. Figures 2-173 and 2-174 show the restored tooth at 5- and 10-year recall.

   Treatment of a typical white spot lesion by means of enamel plasty and composite restoration is illustrated in Figures 2-175 to 2-180.

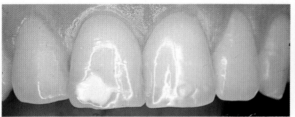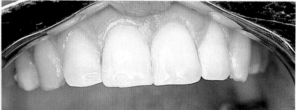

Figure 2-166   White spot lesion on maxillary right central incisor (*left*) restored with microfilled composite (Silux[23]) (*right*).

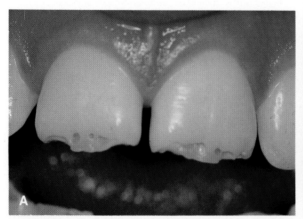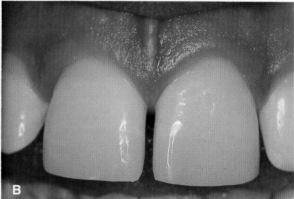

Figure 2-167   *A*, Hypoplastic central incisors. *B*, After restoration with macrofilled composite (Prismafil[26]).

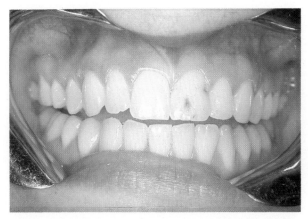

Figure 2-168 Hypoplastic defects on maxillary left central incisor.

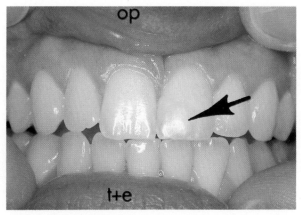

Figure 2-169 Use of opaquer results in a "shine through" effect.

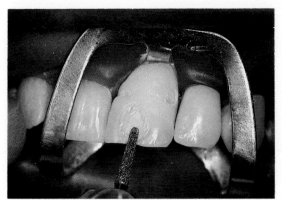

Figure 2-170 Use of bullet-nosed diamond to remove discolored enamel.

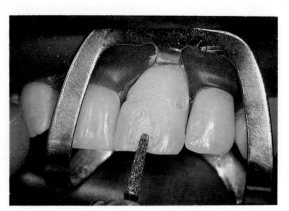

Figure 2-171 Sufficient tooth structure is removed so that opaquer is unnecessary.

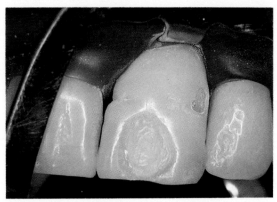

Figure 2-172 Close-up view of preparation.

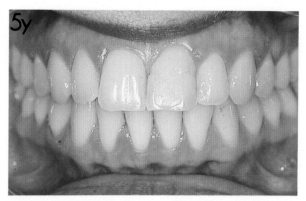

Figure 2-173 Labial composite restoration at 5-year recall; before reveneering.

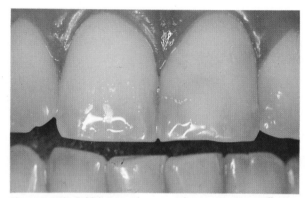

Figure 2-174 Labial composite restorations at 10-year recall.

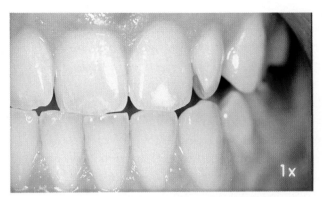

Figure 2-175 White spot lesion, maxillary left central incisor.

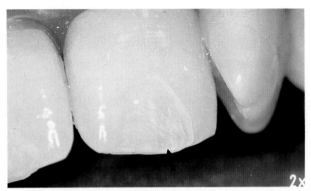

Figure 2-176 Preparation approximately halfway through enamel thickness.

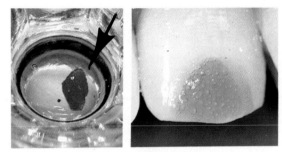

Figure 2-177 Controlled gel etching.

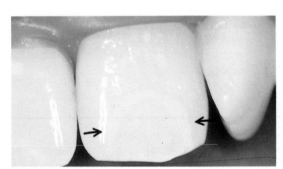

Figure 2-178 Results of gel etching.

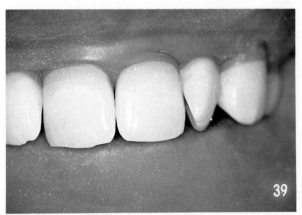

Figure 2-179 Completed restoration, light-cured microfilled composite (Visiodispers[35]).

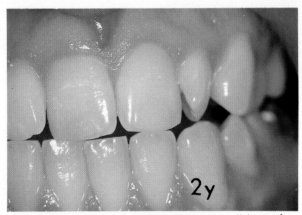

Figure 2-180 Close-up of completed restoration, light-cured microfilled composite (Visiodispers[35]).

CERVICAL DEMINERALIZED LESIONS

A cervical demineralized lesion *totally surrounded by enamel* may be conservatively treated by the use of composite materials in combination with an ultraconservative cavity preparation that is almost exclusively confined to the enamel (Roberts, 1982). For example, a typical early demineralizing lesion is shown in Figure 2-181. It involves a small central area of cavitation (where the carious process extends to include the dentin enamel junction) surrounded mesially and distally by linear areas of demineralization extending toward the proximal line angles.

The cavity design includes a small conventional preparation in the central area of cavitation, necessitated by the removal of carious material involving the dentin enamel junction. The peripheral demineralized enamel, however, is only superficially removed with a blunt-nosed diamond instrument. The traditional box-shaped undercut cavity design is not attempted; a simple "saucer preparation" involving the removal of superficially demineralized enamel is used (Fig. 2-182). After the exposed dentin is protected with a glass ionomer cement liner,[44] the preparation is acid-etched and the area restored using a light-cured composite resin (Nuvafil[41]) (Fig. 2-183). Clinical observations carried out over recall periods of up to 10 years indicate that this is a highly reliable clinical technique (Fig. 2-184).

Because the major prerequisite to successful retention is that the area to be restored must be *totally surrounded by enamel*, cervical erosion lesions treated in this manner do not have a high degree of reliability since the cervical margin of most erosion lesions is located in cementum. In such cases, dentin bonding agents may be utilized in combination with composite materials or alternately the composite-ionomer sandwich restoration may be used (see Chapter 6).

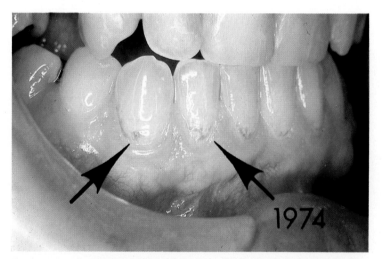

Figure 2-181   Cervical demineralizing lesions, mandibular right lateral and cuspid.

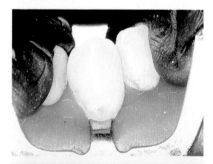

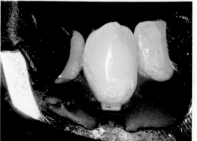

Figure 2-182 Cuspid lesion isolated with retraction clamp (Ivory 212 S.A.[20]) (*top*). "Saucer" preparation (*bottom*).

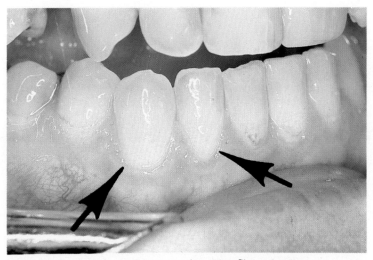

Figure 2-183 Bonded composite restorations (Nuvafil[41]) at baseline.

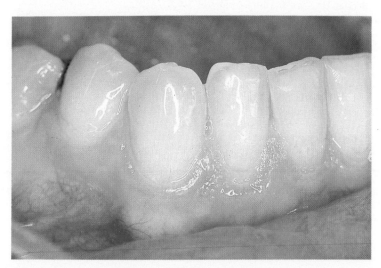

Figure 2-184 Cervical composite restorations (Nuvafil[41]) at 4-year recall.

References

Baum L. Personal communication, 1982.

Buonocore MG. A simple method of increasing the adhesion of acrylic filling materials to enamel surfaces. J Dent Res 1955; 34:849.

Chan RC, Boyer DB. Repair of conventional and microfilled composite resins. J Prosthet Dent 1983; 50:345.

Chandler HH, Bowen RL, Paffenbarger GC. Method for finishing composite restorative materials. J Am Dent Assoc 1971; 83:344.

Combe EC. Personal communication, 1983.

Davidson CL, Duysters PPE, Delange C, Bausch JR. Structural changes in composite surface material after dry polishing. J Oral Rehabil 1981; 8:431.

Dello Russo NM. Replacement of crown margins in patients with altered passive eruption. Int J Periodont Restor Dent 1984; 4(1):59.

Goto G, Jordan RE. Pulpal response to composite resin materials. J Prosthet Dent 1972; 28(6):601.

Gwinnett AJ. Personal communication, 1982.

Gwinnett AJ. Bonding factors in technique which influence clinical success. NY State Dent J 1982; 48:223.

Hembree JH, Andrew JT. In vivo microleakage of several acid etch composite resins. J Dent Res 1976; 55:139.

Hormati AA, Fuller JL, Denehy GE. Effects of contamination and mechanical disturbance on the quality of acid-etched enamel. J Am Dent Assoc 1980; 100:34.

Hwas M, Sandrik JL. Acid and water solubility and strength of calcium hydroxide bases. J Am Dent Assoc 1984; 108:46.

Jendresen MD, Stanley HR. IADR Abstracts, March, 1981.

Jordan RE, Suzuki M, Gwinnett AJ. Conservative applications of acid etch resin techniques. Dent Clin North Am 1981; 25(2):307.

Jordan RE, Suzuki M, Gwinnett AJ, Hunter JK. Restoration of fractured and hypoplastic incisors by the acid etch technique. J Am Dent Assoc 1977; 95:795.

Mitchem JC, Turner LR. The retentive strength of acid etched retained resins. J Am Dent Assoc 1974; 1107.

Newman JG, Nevaste M. The intermediate effect of low viscous fissure sealants on the retention of resin restoratives in vitro. Proc Finn Dent Soc 1975; 71:96.

Roberts GJ. The saucer preparation. Part I. Clinical evaluation over three years. Br Dent J 1982; 153:96.

Rock W. The effect of etching enamel upon bone strengths with fissure sealant resins. A Oral Biol 1974; 19:875.

Silverstone LM. The acid etch technique. Proc Int Symp Acid Etch Tech, St. Paul: North Central Publishing Co, 1975.

Soetopo, Beech DR, Hardwick J. Mechanism of adhesion of polymers to acid etched enamel. J Oral Rehabil 1978; 5:69.

Suzuki M, Goto G, Jordan RE. Pulpal response to pin placement. J Am Dent Assoc 1973; 87:636.

Swartz ML, Phillips RW, Rhodes B. Visible-light-activated resins. Depth of cure. J Am Dent Assoc 1983; 106:634.

Watts DC, Amer O, Combe EC. Characteristics of visible-light-activated composite systems. Br Dent J 1984; 156(6):209.

Product Information

Product	Manufacturer/Distributor	Purpose
1. Herculite XR	Kerr-Sybron Co. P.O. Box 455 Romulus MI 48174	Heavy filled polishable hybrid composite material for stress bearing situations
2. RCBIIK 4–5 Duet Diamond and carbide pair	Brasseler USA Inc. 800 King George Blvd. Savannah, GA 31419	Prepare chamfer-shoulder
3. 201.3F Tapering Diamond	ESPE-Premier Sales Corp. Romano Dr., P.O. Box 111 Norristown, PA 19401	Prepare chamfer interproximally
4. Hydroxyline	G. Taub Products 277 New York Ave. Jersey City, NJ 07307	Thin suspension of calcium hydroxide for coating pins
5. Caviline	L.D. Caulk Co. P.O. Box 359 Milford, DE 19963	Synthetic varnish for sealing dentin
6. Universal (nitrocellulose) Cavity Varnish	S.S. White Co. Three Parkway Philadelphia, PA 19102	Synthetic varnish for sealing dentin
7. Fine-tipped brush	Dental Products/3M Company 3M Center 270–5N–02 St. Paul, MN 55144	For controlled application of calcium hydroxide and/or bond resin
8. Handi-Dry warm air dryer	Lancer Pacific Box 819 Carlsbad, CA 92008	For warm air drying of enamel after etching
9. Odus Pella Thin Crown Forms	Svedia Inc. 9 Bowl St., Box 609 Newport, RI 02849	For large crown composite build-up; diastema closure
or		
10. IB Thin Crown Forms	Clinical Research Publications 34 Ullswater Cresc. London, Ont., N6G 3Y8	For large crown composite build-up; diastema closure
11. 13X; 13XT Interdental "anatomically contoured" wooden wedges	ESPE-Premier Sales Corp. Romano Dr., P.O. Box 111 Norristown, PA 19401	For wedging and separation for large crown composite build-up
12. ET 6; ET 9 Carbide Burs	Brasseler USA Inc. 800 King George Blvd. Savannah, GA 31419	Gross finishing of composite materials
13. T Burs, Spiral Fluted	Ritter/Midwest Co. 901 W. Oakton Des Plaines, IL 60018	Gross finishing of composite materials
14. 150:17 to 150:20 Carbide Finishing Knives	Brasseler USA Inc. 800 King George Blvd. Savannah, GA 31419	Precise marginal finish
15. Sof-lex Aluminum Oxide Composite Finishing Discs Coarse; Medium; Fine; Superfine	Dental Products/3M Company 3M Center 270–5N–02 St. Paul, MN 55144	Final finish and contouring of composite materials

Product Information

Product	Manufacturer/Distributor	Purpose
16. Sof-lex Aluminum Oxide Finishing Strips	Dental Products/3M Company 3M Center 270–5N–02 St. Paul, MN 55144	Final interproximal finish of composite materials
17. WPH No. 54 White Stone	J. M. Ney Co. International Maplewood Ave. Bloomsfield, CT 06002	Finish of lingual concavity on incisor restorations
18. Truspot II Thin Articulating Film	MDS Products 1440 South State College Blvd. Anaheim, CA 92806	Precise marking of contact relationships in centric and protrusive
19. Durafil VS	Kulzer Inc. 10005 Muirlands Blvd., Unit G Irvine, CA 92714	Light-cured, microfilled composite material
20. Ivory 212 S.A. Retraction Clamp	Columbus Dental Mfg. Co. 1000 Chouteau Ave. St. Louis, MO 63188	Gingival retraction in labial veneer and class V restorations
21. Self-Span Cheek Retractor	Ellman Mfg. Co. 1135 Railroad Ave. Hewlett, NY 11557	Cheek and lip retraction during bonding procedure
22. DenMat Labial Crown Forms	DenMat Inc. 3130 Skyway Dr., Unit 501 Santa Maria, CA 93456	Matrix for labial veneer restorations
23. Silux	Dental Products/3M Company 3M Center 270–5N–02 St. Paul, MN 55144	Light-cured, microfilled composite material
24. Flat-Bladed Anodized Aluminum Composite Instrument Felt No. 4	American Dental Instrument Mfg. Co. P.O. Box 4546 Missoula, MT 59801	Insertion and precure contouring of composite materials
25. 3/8″ Discs; Pop-On Mandrel	Dental Products/3M Company 3M Center 270–5N–02 St. Paul, MN 55144	Composite finishing in the cervical region
26. Prismafil	L.D. Caulk Co. Box 359 Milford, DE 19963	Heavy-filled (76% small macro-filled) composite material for stress-bearing situations
27. Parapost Plus	Whaledent International 236 5th Ave. New York, NY 10001	Parallel-sided, serrated metallic post for post-core restorations
28. Ketac-Cem	ESPE-Premier Sales Corp. Romano Dr., P.O. Box 111 Norristown, PA 19401	Multipurpose fast-setting, glass ionomer cement
29. Conclude or P/10	Dental Products/3M Company 3M Center 270–5N–02 St. Paul, MN 55144	Heavy-filled, self-cured, hybrid composite materials
30. Scotchbond	Dental Products/3M Company 3M Center 270–5N–02 St. Paul, MN 55144	Dentin-enamel bonding agent
31. Helicolor Opaque	Vivadent USA Inc. P.O. Box 304 Tonawanda, NY 14150	Multipurpose opaquer
32. Poly-F-Plus	DeTreys/A.D. Intl. Ltd. Weybridge, Surrey, England	Multipurpose fast-setting polycarboxylate cement
33. Oral Perborate	Squibb 2365 Côte de Liesse St. Laurent, Quebec H4N 2M7	Walking bleach

Product Information

Product	Manufacturer/Distributor	Purpose
34. Superoxol	Union Broach Co., Inc. 36–40–37th Street Long Island City, NY 11101	30% hydrogen peroxide for bleaching techniques
35. Visiodispers	ESPE-Premier Sales Corp. Romano Dr., P.O. Box 111 Norristown, PA 19401	Light-cured, microfilled composite material
36. Prismafil	L.D. Caulk Co. Box 359 Milford, DE 19963	Heavy-filled, macrofilled composite material for stress-bearing situations
37. 0.0017-in. Pins Bondent	Whaledent International 236 5th Ave. New York, NY 10001	Pin-retained restorations
38. Command Ultrafine	Kerr-Sybron Co. P.O. Box 455 Romulus, MI 48174	Heavy-filled (76%), hybrid light-cured composite
39. Scotchbond Etching Gel	Dental Products/3M Company 3M Center 270-5N–02 St. Paul, MN 55144	Viscous gel etchant
or Control Etch	DenMat Inc. 3130 Skyway Dr., Unit 501 Santa Maria, CA 93456	Viscous gel etchant
40. Dycal Advanced Formula	L.D. Caulk Co. Box 359 Milford, DE 19963	Calcium hydroxide pulp-protective material
41. Nuvafil	L.D. Caulk Co. Box 359 Milford, DE 19963	Ultraviolet-light-cured composite material
42. Life	Kerr-Sybron Co. P.O. Box 455 Romulus, MI 48174	Acid-resistant, pulp-protective material
43. Reolit	Vivident USA Inc. P.O. Box 304 Tonawanda, NY 14150	Acid-resistant, pulp-protective material
44. G–C Lining Cement	G.C. International Corp. 7830 East Redfield Rd. Scottsdale, AZ 85260	Fast-setting, glass ionomer cement for pulp protection
45 Valux	Dental Products/3M Company 3M Center 270-5N-02 St. Paul, MN 55144	Heavy-filled, macrofilled composite material for stress-bearing situations
46 VLC Dycal	L.D. Caulk Co. Box 359 Milford DE 19963	A visible light cured calcium hydroxide material
47 Prisma Universal Bond	L.D. Caulk Co. Box 359 Milford DE 19963	Dentin-enamel bonding agent
48 Bondlite	Kerr-Sybron Co. P.O. Box 455 Romulus, MI 48174	Dentin-enamel bonding agent

3

RONALD E. JORDAN
MAKOTO SUZUKI

CONSERVATIVE TREATMENT
OF THE DISCOLORED DENTITION

Discolored young dentitions present the dental practitioner and the patient with frustration and outright discouragement. On the one hand, young patients are understandably anxious for immediate remedial treatment. On the other hand, practitioners must weigh carefully the clinical variables of large pulp chambers in young teeth and the unpredictable gingival response as they relate to full-coverage restorations for adolescent patients (Fig. 3-1).

There are four conservative treatment alternatives to full-coverage restorations:

1. Vital and nonvital bleaching techniques
2. Direct composite labial veneer restorations
3. Direct composite veneer restorations combined with vital bleaching
4. Indirect labial veneer restorations (laboratory-fabricated) using either fused porcelain or laboratory processed composite

Before selecting one of the treatment alternatives, the clinician must diagnose the exact nature of the discoloration. In general, the most common causes of discoloration are as follows:

1. Hypoplasia, either generalized or localized
2. Tetracycline
3. Fluorosis
4. Acquired superficial stain of unknown etiology
5. Hemorrhagic discoloration

Whatever the nature of the discoloration, the practitioner must determine whether it is confined to the *superficial enamel thickness* or concentrated within the *deep dentin layers*. The differentiation between the two is important for it will determine not only the complexity and extent of conservative treatment, but in addition the choice of treatment. A description of treatment alternatives and indications for their use follows.

VITAL BLEACHING

Vital bleaching is by far the most conservative treatment alternative. The results of this particular procedure are effective, reliable, and long-term in nature (Fig. 3-2). Indications for vital bleaching include:

1. Light yellow to gray uniform tetracycline staining
2. Fluorosis discoloration
3. Acquired superficial staining
4. Hemorrhagic discoloration

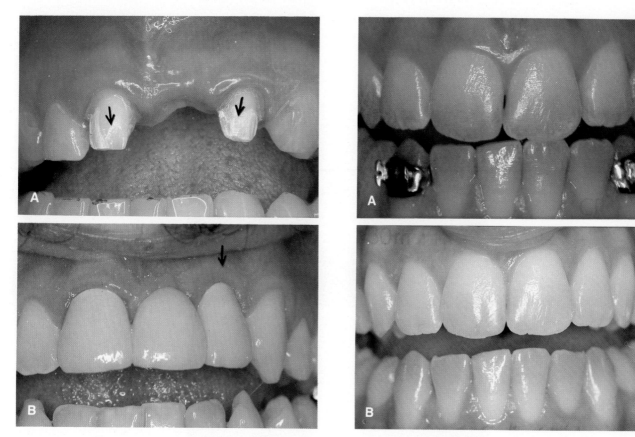

Figure 3-1 *A*, Near pulp exposures incurred during preparation of anterior teeth for full-coverage restorations. *B*, Gingival inflammation in association with the placement of full-coverage restorations in a young patient.

Figure 3-2 *A*, Tetracycline-stained dentition in a young patient before treatment. *B*, Two and one-half years after vital bleaching on the maxillary anterior teeth.

Tetracycline Stain

The extent of tetracycline staining may be classified as slight, moderate, or severe.

Slight tetracycline staining is observed as a light yellow or light grey uniform discoloration of the entire dentition (Fig. 3-3). This type, slight in extent and uniformly distributed throughout the crown without "banding" or concentration of stain in localized areas such as the cervical or middle third regions, is highly amenable to vital bleaching and usually requires no more than three appointments.

Moderate tetracycline staining demonstrates a darker or deeper hue of uniform yellow or grey staining without banding (Fig. 3-4). This type is responsive to vital bleaching, but usually requires three to six appointments.

Severe tetracycline staining, the most extensive expression of the affliction, is characterized by dark grey or blue to purple discoloration, usually in combination with "banding", in which the stain is heavily concentrated in the cervical regions (Fig. 3-5). Bleaching does lighten these teeth to a certain extent (Fig. 3-6), but in order to arrive at a satisfactory clinical result, veneering techniques with concomitant use of opaquers are usually necessary. When doubt exists as to which treatment procedure to use, vital bleaching should be attempted initially. Regardless of what treatment follows, direct or indirect veneers, the result invariably is enhanced by the initial vital bleach treatment.

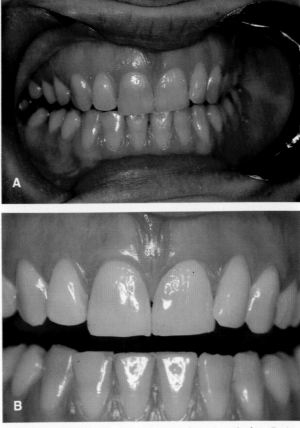

Figure 3-3   *Slight* tetracycline staining before, *A*, and after, *B*, three appointments for vital bleaching of the maxillary anterior teeth.

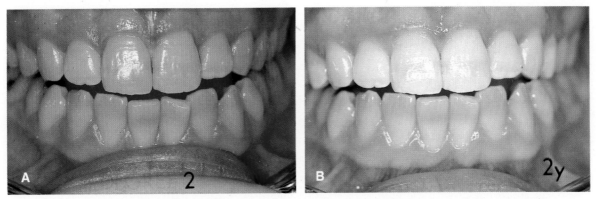

Figure 3-4 *Moderate* tetracycline staining before, *A*, and two years after, *B*, vital bleaching of the maxillary anterior teeth.

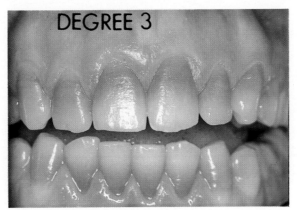

Figure 3-5 *Severe* tetracycline staining.

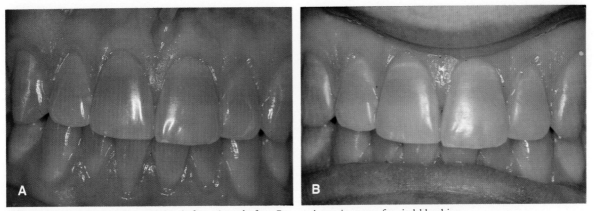

Figure 3-6 *Severe* tetracycline staining before, *A*, and after, *B*, several appointments for vital bleaching.

Vital Bleaching Technique

This technique must be carefully time- and temperature-controlled to prevent possible pulp complications and patient discomfort. Bleaching is carried out over several short appointments, as follows. The teeth are given a thorough prophylaxis with a paste that does not contain oil bases or fluoride (Fig. 3-7). A pumice slurry is suggested. To protect soft tissues from the caustic effects of the bleaching solution, Vaseline[1] or Kenalog[2] is liberally applied to the mucosa and gingival tissue immediately adjacent to the teeth that are to be bleached.

The rubber dam holes should be punched approximately 5 mm apart so that the gingival papillary tissues are adequately covered. The rubber dam is carefully inverted by means of an air syringe or with the help of dental floss ligatures. Rubber dam clamps should not be used since the dam may not cover the tissues adequately around the beaks of the clamp. Dental floss may be left between the contact areas of the posterior teeth in order to stabilize the rubber dam. The use of profound local anesthesia is contraindicated during vital bleaching since the response of the vital tooth to applied heat dictates the temperature level used during bleaching procedures. Great variation exists in this regard because of the size of the pulp chamber, age of the patient, porosity of the enamel, patency of dentin tubules, and pain threshold of the individual. Minimal soft tissue anesthesia is warranted to facilitate rubber dam placement, but pulp anesthesia should be carefully avoided.

After proper rubber dam isolation, the teeth should be etched with 30 to 40 percent phosphoric acid. The phosphoric acid etchant should be applied for *one minute*, and this is followed by a thorough water lavage and air drying. After etching, the enamel presents a surface porosity that enhances the penetrability of the bleaching solution (Fig. 3-8). The bleaching procedure is then initiated; warm Superoxol[3] (30% hydrogen peroxide) is used as the bleaching agent. Superoxol should be used fresh, stored in the refrigerator when not used, and marked with the purchase date. It should not be stored for more than 3 months after the date of first use. Since Superoxol is potentially caustic, the patient *must* wear safety glasses throughout the procedure.

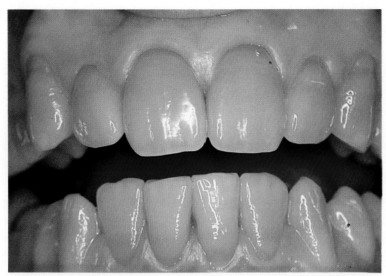

Figure 3-7 *Moderate* tetracycline discoloration prior to vital bleaching treatment.

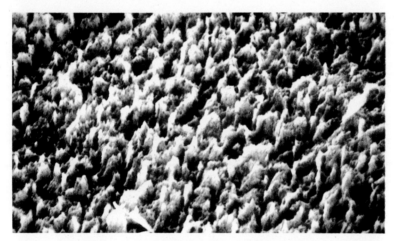

Figure 3-8 Scanning electron micrograph (1000 ×) of a phosphoric acid-etched enamel surface.

A Superoxol-ether bleaching mixture is used for the bleaching technique. One drop of ethyl ether is mixed with five drops of Superoxol in a dappen dish. Ethyl ether lowers the surface tension and enhances the penetration of the bleaching solution through inter-prismatic enamel spaces and dentin tubules. It is claimed that Superoxol-ether is an explosive combination, but only if the chemicals are exposed to high temperatures well above those required for this procedure. A Superoxol-sodium perborate bleaching mixture is equally as effective as the Superoxol-ether combination (Arzt, 1981). A large No. 3 cotton pledget or a small square cut from a 4 × 4-cm gauze sponge is soaked in the bleaching mixture, wrung out, and then applied to the labial surface of one of the discolored teeth. The flat plate tip of the warming instrument[4] is then applied to the cotton pledget (Fig. 3-9). The temperature of the tip is gradually increased by slowly turning the control dial clockwise until the "sensitivity point" is reached. This is the heat level at which the patient just begins to experience sensitivity. Once the patient indicates sensitivity, the heat is decreased below the sensitivity point to a level at which no sensitivity is experienced, the "toleration point". Heat should be applied to each tooth at the toleration point for a maximum of 3 minutes. Each tooth in the anterior arch should be treated sequentially in the same fashion. Under no circumstance should heat be applied for prolonged periods. The patient should experience no discomfort whatsoever during or after bleaching, otherwise the treatment must be discontinued to prevent possible pulp sequelae. The procedure is repeated on a *once-weekly* basis until the treatment is complete (Figs. 3-10 to 3-12). A successful result requires three to six appointments, depending on the degree of involvement. Once treatment is begun it is important to have the patient return once weekly so that regression does not occur.

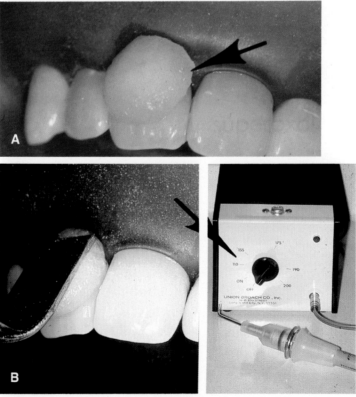

Figure 3-9 *A*, Superoxol-soaked pledget applied to the labial surface of the maxillary right central incisor. *B*, Application of the warming instrument.

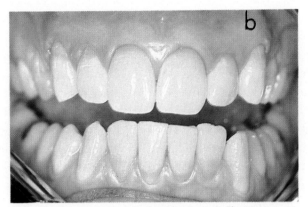

Figure 3-10 Appearance of the dentition shown in Figure 3-7 immediately after rubber dam removal at the final bleaching appointment. Note opacity of dehydrated enamel.

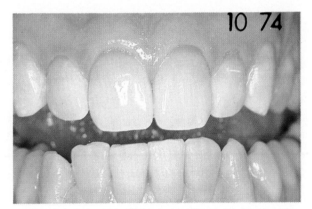

Figure 3-11 Appearance of bleached teeth 2 weeks after bleaching treatment.

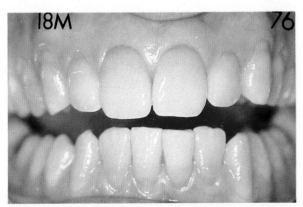

Figure 3-12 Sixteen-month recall appearance of the dentition shown in Figures 3-7 and 3-11.

Thermal sensitivity postoperatively in a patient undergoing bleaching treatment is a danger signal which indicates that the heat level used during the procedure has been excessive or the treatment has been carried out for too long on each tooth. Usually thermal sensitivity disappears within 24 hours. Careful monitoring of each step in the process with a stopwatch significantly decreases the number of postoperative complications and deleterious effects on the pulp. Treatment *must* be monitored carefully since the young pulp is most sensitive to thermal and/or chemical irritation associated with this procedure. Vital bleaching should not be carried out prior to age 14 years. In more than 300 cases of tetracycline discoloration treated at The University of Western Ontario by means of the vital bleach technique over a 5-year period, there have been no instances of irreversible pulpitis or loss of vitality. Further, histologic studies indicate that the vital bleaching technique is innocuous, provided a properly controlled technique is used (Cohen, 1979).

Vital bleaching should also be considered as an adjunctive treatment for teeth requiring veneer restorations since preveneer brightening of the discolored teeth invariably enhances the clinical result (Figs. 3-13 to 3-15). The combined bleaching-veneer technique will be discussed in more detail subsequently.

Fluorosis Staining

Enamel hypoplasia due to fluoride (fluorosis), or mottled enamel (Fig. 3-16), is caused by an interference with the calcification process of the enamel matrix. The result is incomplete maturation accompanied with opacity and/or porosity (Kerr and Ash, 1973). Whereas there is little or no mottling of any clinical significance at a level below 0.9 to 1.0 part per million of fluoride in the water, it becomes progressively evident above this level (Minister for National Health and Welfare, 1979). There is a wide range of severity in the appearance of mottled teeth, from minor involvement characterized by intermittent white flecking or spotting of the enamel to severe manifestations which involve pitting and brownish staining of the surface (Fig. 3-17). Since the staining involved in fluorosis affects only the superficial enamel thickness, significant improvement may be achieved with vital bleaching (Fig. 3-18) or, alternatively, by use of a combination of vital bleaching and direct composite veneers (Figs. 3-19 and 3-20).

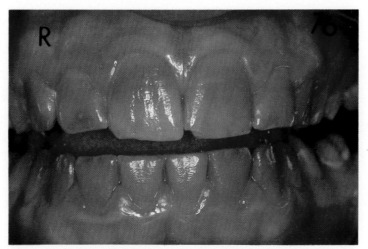

Figure 3-13 Severe tetracycline staining before bleaching treatment.

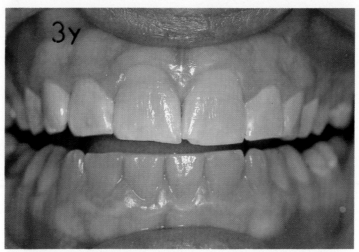

Figure 3-14 The dentition shown in Figure 3-13, 3 years after bleaching of the maxillary anterior teeth.

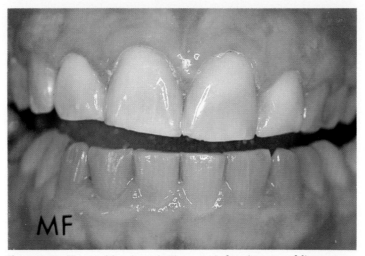

Figure 3-15 The dentition shown in Figure 3-14 after placement of direct composite veneers.

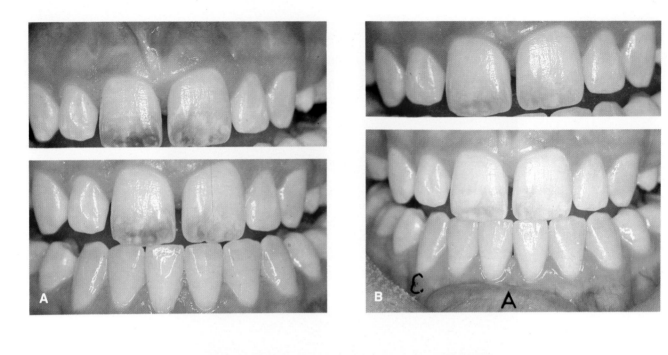

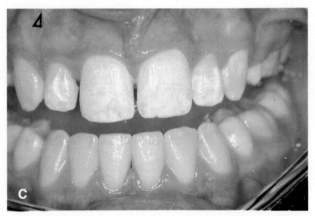

Figure 3-16 *A*, Fluorosis staining before treatment (*top*) and after one bleaching appointment (*bottom*). *B*, After two bleaching appointments (*top*) and after three bleaching appointments (*bottom*). *C*, After four bleaching appointments.

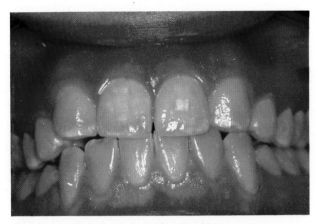

Figure 3-17   Fluorosis staining before bleaching treatment.

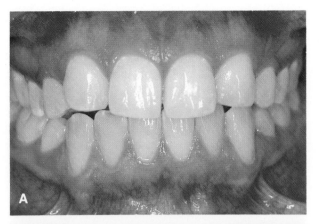

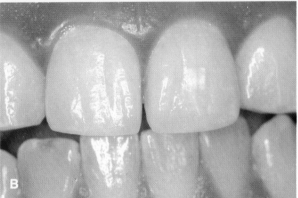

Figure 3-18   *A*, The dentition shown in Figure 3-17, 3 years after vital bleaching. *B*, Close-up view of the bleached teeth at 3-year recall.

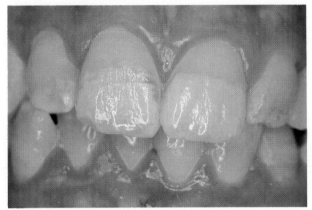

Figure 3-19   Severe fluorosis staining.

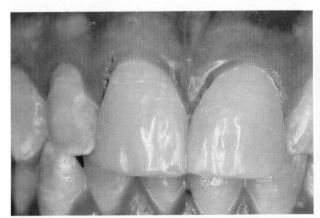

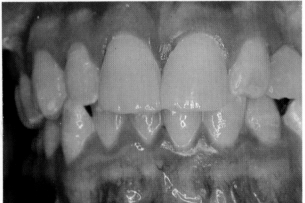

Figure 3-20   The dentition shown in Figure 3-19 after bleaching followed by the placement of direct composite veneers.

Acquired Superficial Stain of Unknown Etiology

Not uncommonly, staining is seen for which the exact etiology is unknown. For example, the discolored maxillary central incisors of the 36-year-old patient shown in Figure 3-21 were vital with no radiographic evidence of periapical pathology. Although it was unknown whether a history of osteogenesis imperfecta in this patient was in any way contributory, the discoloration was entirely removed after three appointments of vital bleaching (Fig. 3-22).

Hemorrhagic Discoloration

Discoloration of single or multiple anterior teeth may result from a severe blow at an early age associated with rupture of pulp blood vessels and extravasation of erythrocytes into the dentin tubules. The tooth quickly takes on a pink hue and, in many cases, remains vital but discolored throughout life (Fig. 3-23). Such teeth do not respond well to ordinary vital bleaching procedures since the entire pulp chamber and dentin tubules are usually fully calcified (Fig. 3-24). A normal color may be restored by preparing a lingual access opening and cutting an artificial coronal pulp chamber prior to internal and external bleaching (Fig. 3-25), as described in the next section.

NONVITAL BLEACHING TECHNIQUES

Discoloration of pulpless teeth may occur as the result of a number of combined circumstances. However, darkening or discoloration of endodontically treated teeth is not inevitable, but should it occur, it can be successfully treated by means of conservative bleaching techniques.

Hemorrhage in the pulp chamber may result from a blow, from death of the pulp, or from failure to control bleeding during endodontic therapy; this allows blood to penetrate the dentin tubules. The hemolysis of the red cells with the release of hemoglobin produces a yellowish brown discoloration when the iron pigment degrades to iron sulfide. This discoloration may appear some months after endodontic treatment is completed and is similar to hemorrhagic discoloration previously described.

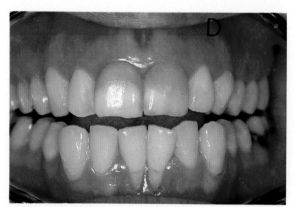

Figure 3-21 Acquired superficial stain of unknown etiology involving the maxillary central incisors.

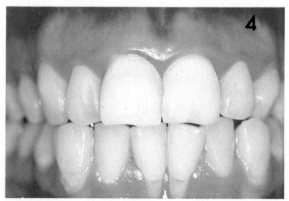

Figure 3-22 The incisors shown in Figure 3-21 after vital bleaching treatment.

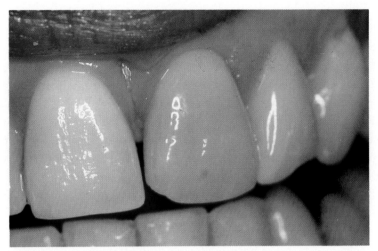

Figure 3-23   Hemorrhagic discoloration of the left central incisor.

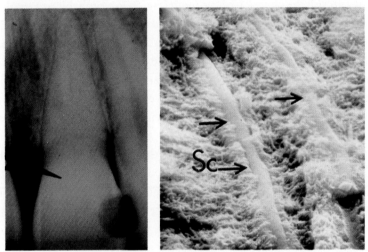

Figure 3-24   Radiograph (*left*) of the left central incisor showing total calcification of pulp space and (*right*) scanning electron micrograph showing calcification of dentinal tubules.

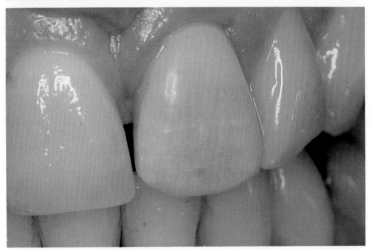

Figure 3-25   The left central incisor shown in Figure 3-23 after bleaching. A direct labial veneer using light cured microfilled composite material may now be placed resulting in a highly esthetic restoration (see Figure 3-15).

The majority of postendodontic discoloration is caused by the failure of the operator to completely remove blood or other organic material from the pulp chamber during treatment (Ingle and Beveridge, 1976). Should the access opening to the pulp chamber be inadequate, shelves of dentin are left which make it difficult, if not impossible, to remove the debris from the pulp horns and the lingual area of the pulp chamber. Adequate access for complete debridement of the pulp chamber is therefore essential.

Medicaments and sealing pastes must be removed from the coronal pulp space subsequent to completion of root canal therapy. Many of these agents contain silver which, if left in the crown, will cause discoloration (Cohen and Burns, 1980). Even zinc oxide and eugenol, which is considered by many to be an innocuous material, stains tooth structure if left in contact with dentin for a protracted period. Medicaments cause stains that are usually more pronounced in the cervical region of the tooth and are identified by a bluish grey discoloration (Cohen and Burns, 1980).

Silver amalgam, which has been used extensively in the past for restoration of lingual access openings subsequent to root canal therapy, is contraindicated for that purpose. The material causes a greyish discoloration of the tooth (Fig. 3-26), probably as a result of penetration into the dentinal tubules of sulfidized by-products of the corrosion process. The use of resin materials without an acid-etch technique usually results in marginal percolation with eventual internal staining of the crown. The lingual access opening subsequent to root canal therapy should be sealed by means of a carefully controlled phosphoric acid-etch technique with a microfilled composite material (Fig. 3-27). A heavy-filled composite material should not be used for the lingual seal because it is extremely difficult to remove should postoperative circumstances (e.g., bleaching) dictate.

Although extensively discolored nonvital teeth are highly receptive to bleaching techniques, the clinical situation must be carefully assessed before bleaching treatment is considered. Of prime importance is the quality and type of root canal filling that has been employed. The canal must be apically sealed adequately to prevent percolation of the bleaching agents into the periapical tissues. Accordingly, if a poorly condensed gutta-percha or an otherwise inadequate root canal filling exists, retreatment is indicated before bleaching is attempted. Further, the crown should be relatively intact since a crown with large carious lesions or restorations may be better treated by means of a cast post and core together with full coverage.

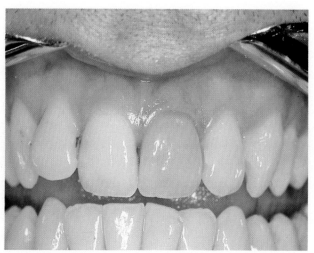

Figure 3-26   A discolored, nonvital maxillary left central incisor.

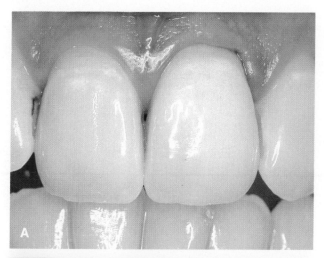

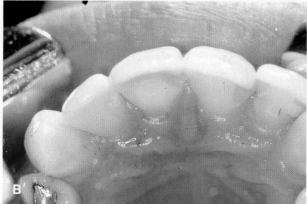

Figure 3-27   *A*, The incisor shown in Figure 3-26 after bleaching treatment. *B*, Lingual view of the same tooth after placement of a lingual seal using microfilled composite material.

Technique. Figure 3-28 shows a discolored maxillary left central incisor 5 years after root canal therapy. Prior to rubber dam application, the soft tissues surrounding the tooth should be liberally coated with petroleum jelly to avoid the caustic effects of the bleaching agent. The rubber dam is placed and carefully inverted to ensure an adequate seal. The coronal contents of the pulp chamber are removed by means of an appropriate instrument, and particular care is taken to remove pulp horn remnants and all stained dentin (Fig. 3-29). Approximately 1.5 mm of radicular filling is removed beyond the cervical region (Figs. 3-30 and 3-31), and a "plug" of polycarboxylate or glass ionomer cement is placed in order to isolate the radicular root canal filling from the coronal pulp space (Fig. 3-32). This will ensure that the bleaching agent will not be forced along the lateral borders of the root canal filling during treatment. In addition, the placement of a cement plug in the cervical region helps to prevent external resorption (Lado et al, 1983).

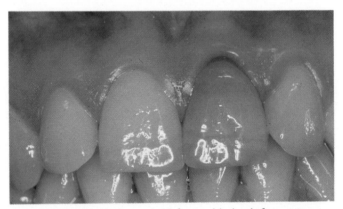

Figure 3-28   A discolored, nonvital left central incisor before treatment.

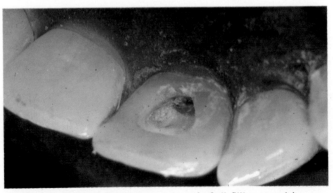

Figure 3-29   The coronal pulp space cleaned of all filling material.

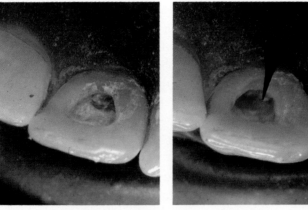

Figure 3-30 One and one-half millimeters of radicular filling is removed.

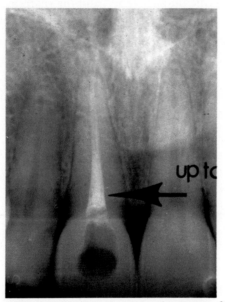

Figure 3-31 Radiograph showing the amount of radicular filling material removed.

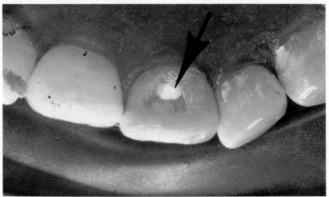

Figure 3-32 A ''plug'' of polycarboxylate or glass ionomer cement separates the coronal pulp space from the radicular root canal filling.

The pulp chamber should now be cleaned with an organic solvent such as ether, alcohol, acetone, xylene, or chloroform, applied on a cotton pledget. A small cotton pledget soaked in 30 to 40 percent phosphoric acid is then placed in the pulp chamber for one minute (Fig. 3-33). A large cotton pledget soaked in phosphoric acid is simultaneously placed on the external enamel surface for one minute (Fig. 3-34); this is followed by a 30-second water lavage and careful air drying. As a result of the "internal and external" phosphoric acid-etching procedures, the dentin tubules (internally) are widely opened (Fig. 3-35) and the enamel shows a microporous surface externally (Fig. 3-36); the permeability of the bleaching agent through both tissues is thereby enhanced.

As in the vital bleaching technique, Superoxol is used as the bleaching material. Since a high-heat technique is used in this procedure, the use of ethyl ether is not recommended. A suitable bleaching instrument (University of Indiana Bleaching Instrument or Holt-Monarch Instrument[4]) should be used to apply heat to the Superoxol. A pledget of cotton soaked in Superoxol is placed into the pulp chamber, and the sharp narrow point of the bleaching instrument is used to apply high heat, approximately 140°C to 160°C, for one minute (Fig. 3-37). This should be repeated three times using a fresh Superoxol-soaked cotton pellet. The external surface of the tooth is now bleached labially by applying a large Superoxol-soaked pledget to the enamel surface and applying high heat for one minute using the wide spoon-shaped blade of the instrument (Fig. 3-38). This "external bleaching" is repeated three times using a fresh Superoxol-soaked pledget.

After the bleaching treatment is completed, a thick mixture of sodium perborate and Superoxol is now placed into the pulp chamber (Fig. 3-39). A layer of this material is condensed over the labial dentin and subsequently covered with a dry cotton pledget (Fig. 3-40). This has been referred to as a "walking bleach" (Hyasaki et al, 1980). The access opening

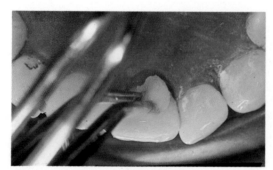

Figure 3-33 "Internal" etching using phosphoric acid.

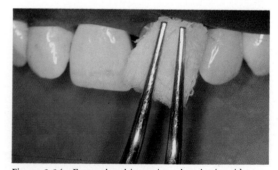

Figure 3-34 External etching using phosphoric acid.

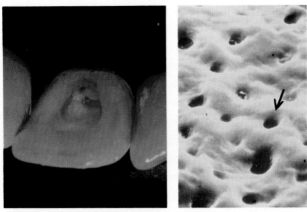
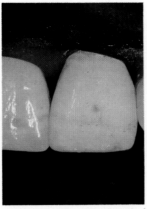
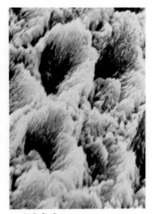

Figure 3–35 The internally etched dentin (*left*) is characterized by wide open tubules (*right*).

Figure 3–36 The externally etched enamel (*left*) demonstrates a porous surface (*right*).

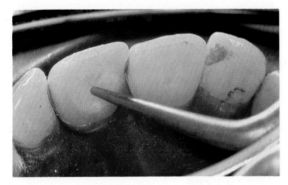

Figure 3-37 Internal bleaching.

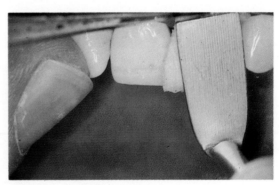

Figure 3-38 External bleaching.

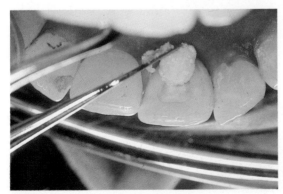

Figure 3-39 Insertion of ''walking'' bleach.

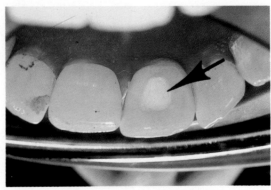

Figure 3–40 ''Walking'' bleach applied to labial dentin wall of coronal pulp space.

is now sealed with either glass ionomer (Ketac Bond[5]) or Term Composite[6] (Fig. 3-41). The foregoing procedure is repeated at weekly intervals until the desired shade (or a shade slightly lighter than the adjacent teeth) is achieved. Normally, two or three appointments are more than ample for the purpose. The walking bleach technique after intentional endodontics has been advocated for the esthetic treatment of severe tetracycline discoloration (Abou-Rass, 1982).

After the desired shade has been attained (Fig. 3-42), the rubber dam is placed and all contents of the pulp chamber are removed. The external and internal phosphoric acid etching techniques are repeated, followed by thorough washing and drying. A bonding agent (Durafill Bond[7]) is placed on the internal dentin walls of the coronal pulp space as well as the enamel walls of the lingual access opening, and restoration of the lingual access opening is completed using a microfilled resin material (Durafill[8]). The use of the acid-etch technique with a bonding resin virtually eliminates marginal leakage of the lingual seal restoration. The labial enamel surface is now finally sealed by means of the application of a thin film of a filled glaze resin (Complus[9]) in order to prevent extrinsic staining of the porous enamel surface (Fig. 3-43). Such sealing markedly enhances the long-term results of the procedure (Figs. 3-44 and 3-45). Slight recurrence of the discoloration may be treated successfully using a walking bleach technique (Figs. 3-46 and 3-47).

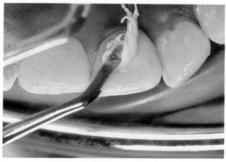

Figure 3-41 Lingual seal using Term Composite.[6]

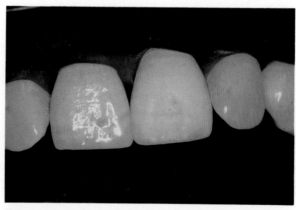

Figure 3-42 Maxillary left central incisor after final bleaching treatment.

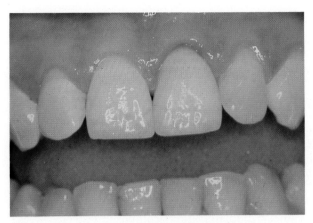

Figure 3-43 ''Glaze'' resin applied to labial surface.

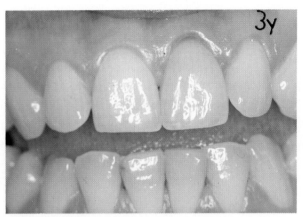

Figure 3-44 Appearance of bleached left central incisor at 3-year recall.

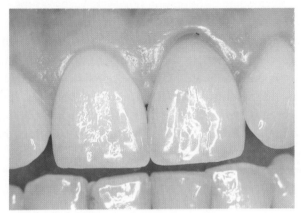

Figure 3-45 Close-up view of bleached central incisor at 3-year recall.

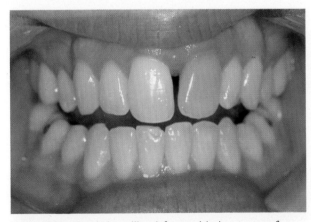

Figure 3-46 Nonvital maxillary left central incisor 3 years after bleaching showing extensive regression.

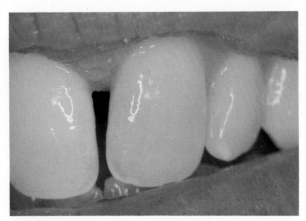

Figure 3-47 The tooth shown in Figure 3-45 after two walking bleach appointments.

DIRECT COMPOSITE LABIAL VENEER RESTORATIONS

Direct composite labial veneer restorations are indicated for patients who have either extreme labial wear or severe localized or generalized enamel hypoplasia (Fig. 3-48). Both can be treated satisfactorily by direct light-cured composite veneer techniques since the worn or discolored tooth structure is mainly external, that is, it is confined to the superficial enamel thickness and rarely involves deep dentin (Fig. 3-49). In the event that superficial dentin is involved in the wear or hypoplastic process, dentin bonding agents (Scotchbond,[10] Durafill Dentin Bond,[11] J & J Dentin Bond[12]) may be effectively used in combination with light-cured microfilled composite materials (Durafill,[8]Silux,[13]Certain[14]) to attain a highly satisfactory esthetic result (Figs. 3-50 to 3-52). Since the discoloration or wear involves only the superficial enamel thickness in cases of labial erosion or enamel hypoplasia, direct composite veneer restorations constitute the treatment of choice. A clinical approach involving labial chamfer preparations (Chapter 2) followed by the placement of light-cured composite materials gives a normally contoured esthetic result without the need for opaquers. The direct composite veneer technique for such cases has been described in Chapter 2.

Extremely dark tetracycline discoloration (Fig. 3-53) is by far the most difficult to treat because it is highly resistant to vital bleaching and the discolored tooth structure is primarily confined to the deep dentin (Fig. 3-54). Accordingly, the discoloration cannot be removed by means of labial chamfer preparations, and opaquers must be used to mask the discoloration prior to placement of veneer restorations. With this approach, however, it is difficult to attain a predictable esthetic result because of a persistent "shine-through" problem (Fig. 3-55).

Direct composite veneer restorations for severe tetracycline discoloration call for a meticulously controlled technique involving the use of opaquers and tints. In Chapters 4 and 5, such techniques are discussed in detail.

In many cases, vital and nonvital bleaching techniques may be used in combination with direct composite veneer restorations to provide an excellent clinical result.

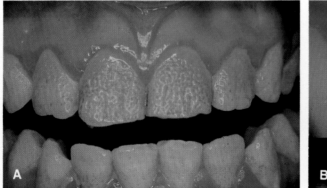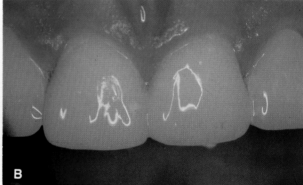

Figure 3-48 Generalized hypoplasia, *A*, treated by means of direct composite veneers, *B*.

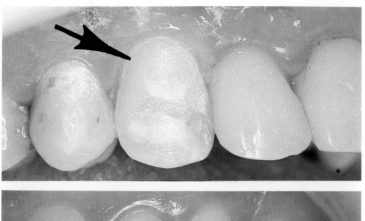

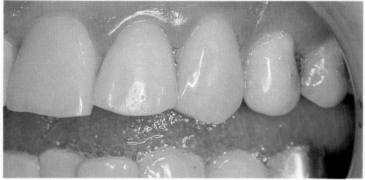

Figure 3–49 Labial chamfer preparation halfway through the enamel thickness on a hypoplastic canine *(top)* almost totally removes discolored tooth structure prior to direct veneer placement *(bottom)*.

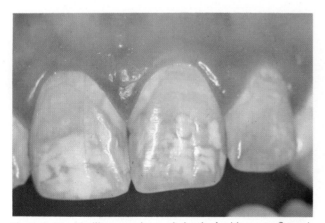

Figure 3–50 Maxillary anterior teeth involved with severe fluorosis staining.

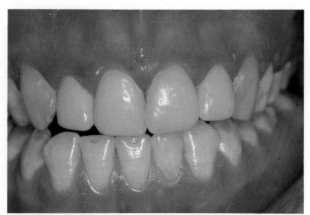

Figure 3–51 Labial resin veneer restorations on the maxillary anterior teeth shown in Figure 3-50 (Silux and Scotchbond).

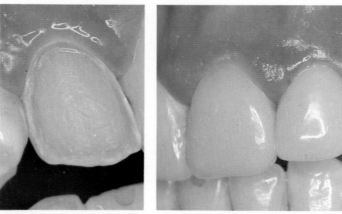

Figure 3-52   The dentin bonding agent may be safely applied to superficial exposed dentin *(left)* before placement of the microfilled veneer *(right)*.

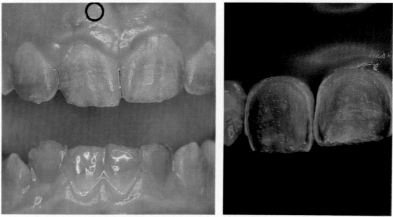

Figure 3-53   Severe tetracycline discoloration *(left)*. After a labial chamfer preparation *(right)* is made, the discoloration persists.

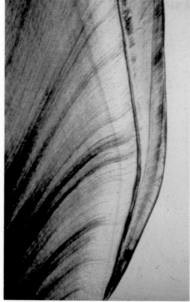

Figure 3-54   Tetracycline discoloration is concentrated in the deep dentin layers *(D)* rather than in the enamel *(E)*.

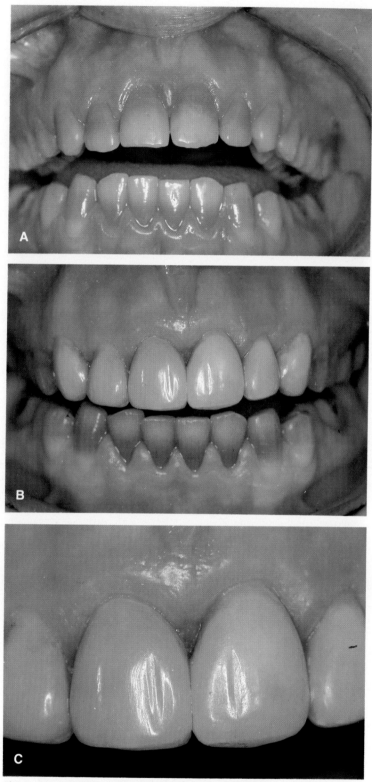

Figure 3-55 *A,* Severe tetracycline staining. *B* and *C,* Treated by means of direct composite veneers. Note the ''shine-through'' appearance.

DIRECT COMPOSITE VENEER RESTORATIONS COMBINED WITH VITAL BLEACHING

Some cases of tetracycline discoloration are most amenable to a conservative treatment approach of vital bleaching followed by direct composite veneers (Fig. 3-56). After three vital bleaching appointments, the appearance is considerably improved, but the teeth retain a greyish cast (Fig. 3-57). After acid etching and placement of direct microfilled composite veneers (Extra Smooth[15]), the appearance is markedly improved (Fig. 3-58).

Discolored nonvital teeth may also be treated satisfactorily by means of this combined procedure (Figs. 3-59 to 3-64).

The combined bleaching-veneer technique gives satisfactory esthetic results only if the discoloration can be properly ''masked'' by the composite materials.

Tetracycline discoloration which is dark grey or blue and shows ''banding'' or heavy concentration of stain in the cervical region (i.e., severe staining) is probably most predictably treated by means of indirect (laboratory-processed) labial veneer restorations.

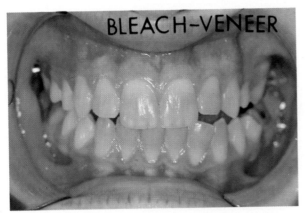

Figure 3-56 Tetracycline-stained anterior teeth before treatment.

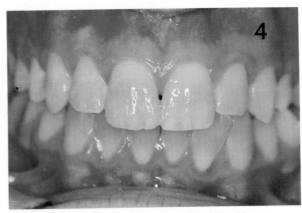

Figure 3-57 After four appointments of vital bleaching.

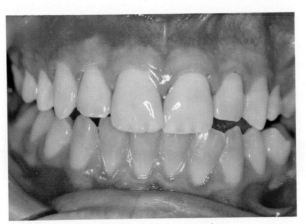

Figure 3-58 After direct labial veneer restorations.

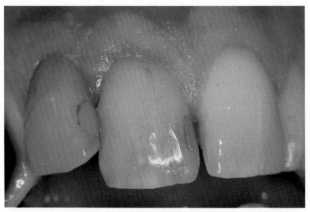

Figure 3-59 Discolored, nonvital maxillary right central incisor.

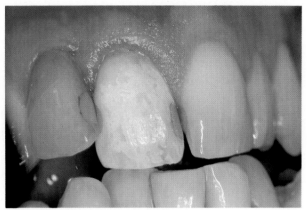

Figure 3-60 The same incisor after bleaching.

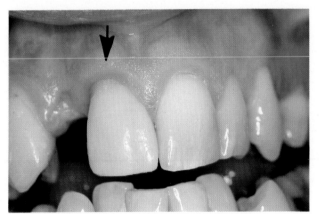

Figure 3-61 After placement of direct microfill veneer.

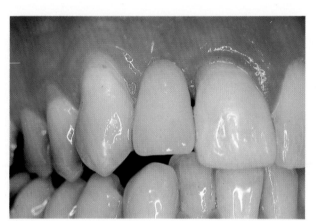

Figure 3-62 Resin-bonded retainer replacing maxillary right lateral incisor.

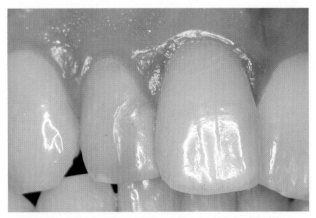

Figure 3-63 Discolored, nonvital maxillary right lateral incisor.

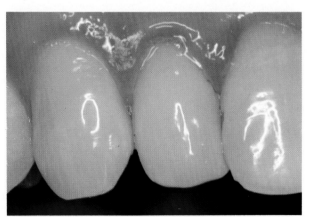

Figure 3-64 The lateral incisor shown in Figure 3-63 after bleaching and labial veneering with microfill composite (Paste Laminate[20]).

INDIRECT LABIAL VENEER RESTORATIONS

Indirect labial veneer restorations (laboratory-processed) are particularly indicated for the conservative treatment of extremely dark tetracycline discoloration or other cases of staining which involve the deep dentin (see Figs. 3-53 and 3-54). In such instances, laboratory-processed veneer restorations are usually associated with a more predictable esthetic result than direct veneer techniques since they are more effective in masking the underlying discoloration. Accordingly, the dependency on opaquers is not nearly so critical as in direct veneer procedures.

Materials. Either fused porcelain (Cerinate Veneers[16]) or laboratory-processed, light-cured, composite materials (Dentacolor,[17] Visio-Gem[18]) may be used for the indirect veneer restorations. Porcelain veneers are highly satisfactory from an esthetic standpoint, but not easily repaired should fracture occur. Indirect composite veneers, although not as esthetic as porcelain veneers, are more amenable to a direct repair technique should fracture or wear occur postoperatively. This is an important consideration, since indirect composite veneers are more prone to cohesive ("Chip-Type") fracture than porcelain veneers. Whatever material is chosen, the technique is essentially the same.

INDIRECT PORCELAIN VENEERS

A typical indication for porcelain veneer treatment is shown in Figure 3-65. The 18-year-old patient presented with severe tetracycline discoloration with pronounced "banding" or localized concentration of stain in the middle third areas. After three appointments of vital bleaching of the maxillary anterior teeth, although they were considerably lightened, the esthetic result was far from satisfactory. Light-cured composite was placed in the form of partial veneers over the midlabial areas, but unfortunately such a "patchwork" approach is of little value in improving the appearance. Porcelain veneers (Cerinate™ 16) are the next option.

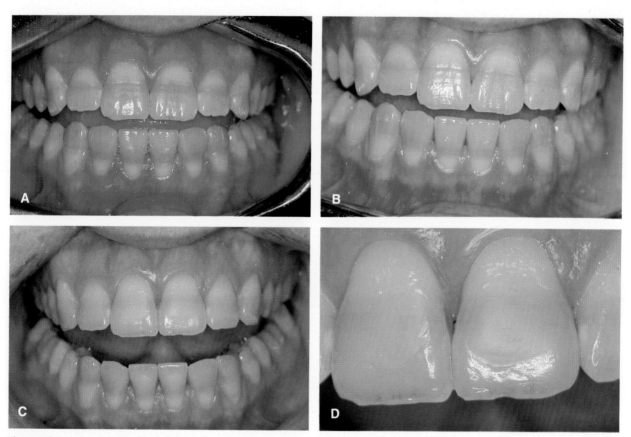

Figure 3-65   *A,* Severe tetracycline staining before treatment. *B,* After vital bleaching. *C and D,* After placement of light-cured composite partial veneers.

Technique

Preparation. A tapering bullet-nosed diamond carbide instrument pair (RCBIIK 8–9 Diamond Carbide Duet[19]) is used to chamfer-shoulder the labial enamel, as previously described (Fig. 3-66). The diamond instrument is used to "rough out" the preparation, and the carbide is used to refine it. Sufficient enamel thickness must be removed (i.e., at least 0.5 mm) to avoid overcontoured restorations. Controversy exists regarding the necessity for preparation of any kind. If no preparation is used, the inevitable result is overcontoured restorations to which gingival tissues do not usually respond positively. Accordingly, preparation should be omitted only when the anterior teeth present relatively flat labial contours or are in linguoversion. The chamfer-type labial preparation is strongly recommended for full-contoured anterior teeth since little if any overcontouring results. The esthetic result is inevitably superior when chamfer preparations are made and so is the gingival response to the normally contoured restorations. After preparation, retraction cord is gently positioned into the crevicular regions (Fig. 3-67) in order to displace the gingival tissues away from the marginal areas. The preparation may now be refined by use of the bullet-nosed carbide bur. Figure 3-68 shows the close-up details of the labial chamfer preparation. It will be remembered that the gingival cavosurface margin is placed level with the free gingival crest; the mesial and distal proximal margins are placed just labial to the proximal contact areas; and the incisal margin is located at the crest of the incisal ridge. A full arch impression is taken, and the master model is poured in diestone (Fig. 3-69). The marginal periphery of the chamfer preparation should be carefully assessed for proper detail. A proper shade should be selected, and the laboratory prescription should clearly indicate that a precise marginal adaptation is required.

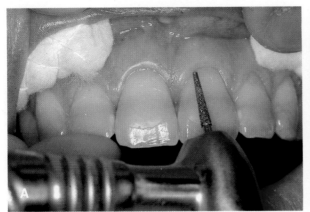 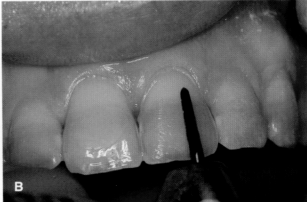

Figure 3-66 *A,* Use of a bullet-nosed diamond to prepare a labial chamfer. *B,* The chamfer preparation is refined using a carbide bur.

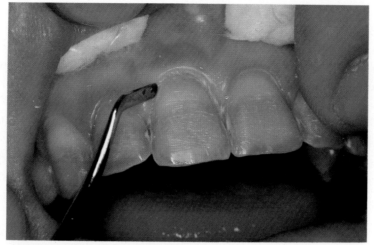

Figure 3-67 Placement of gingival retraction cord.

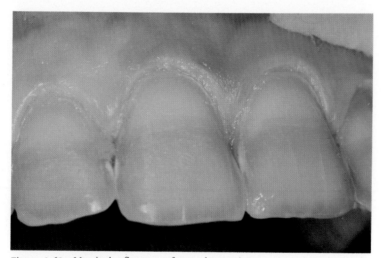

Figure 3-68 Marginal refinement after cord retraction.

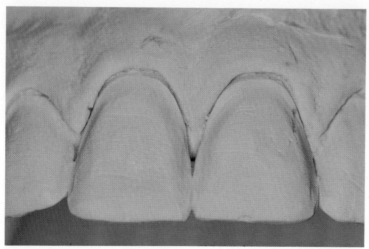

Figure 3-69 Diestone model showing clean-cut marginal detail of chamfer preparations.

Temporization. Temporary veneer restorations are not only time consuming but they add considerably to the cost of the restorative procedure. Accordingly, temporary veneer restorations should be avoided if at all possible. However, if temporary veneers are an absolute requirement, visible-light-cured, microfill materials may be used for the purpose. A small amount of gel etchant is placed on two or three internal enamel areas (Fig. 3-70). After washing and drying light-cured microfill, temporary veneer restorations (Paste Laminate[™][20]) are placed (Fig. 3-71). The small internal areas of acid-etched enamel "tack" the veneers onto the enamel surfaces so that they can be easily removed prior to final veneer insertion.

Insertion. The laboratory time with indirect veneer restorations usually requires 7 to 10 days, and the cost is approximately sixty dollars per unit. The highly glazed labial porcelain

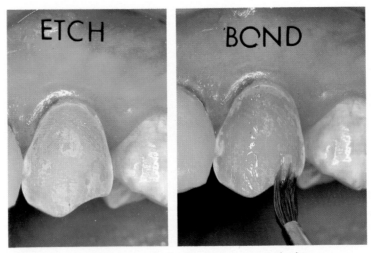

Figure 3-70 Proper placement of gel etchant prior to temporization.

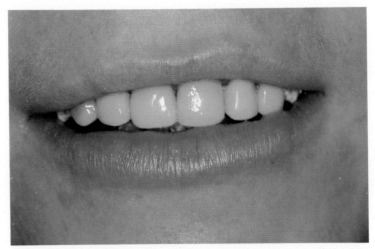

Figure 3-71 Temporary microfill veneers.

surfaces are highly esthetic (Fig. 3-72). The internal surfaces present a dull frosty opaque appearance (Fig. 3-73) since they have been etched in the laboratory using hydrofluoric acid. A scanning electron micrograph of the etched porcelain surface is shown in Figure 3-74. The etched internal porcelain surfaces are highly microporous and thereby provide the basis for micro-mechanical retention. The veneer restorations precisely fit the cavo-surface periphery of the stone dies (Fig. 3-75). For cases of dark tetracycline discoloration, porcelain veneers should not be opaqued in the laboratory because a false appearance usually results. Rather, opaquer should be applied to the discolored enamel surfaces prior to insertion of the veneer restorations. The use of opaquers in veneer techniques is discussed fully in Chapters 4 and 5.

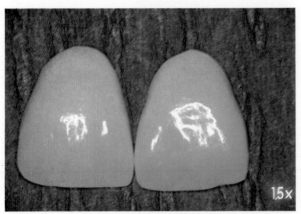

Figure 3-72   Indirect porcelain veneers.

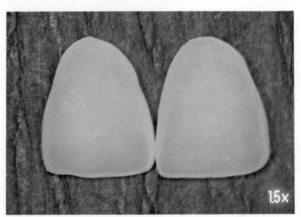

Figure 3-73   Internal hydrofluoric acid-etched surfaces of porcelain veneers.

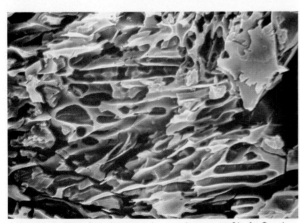

Figure 3-74   Scanning electron micrograph (100 x) of hydrofluoric acid-etched internal porcelain surface.

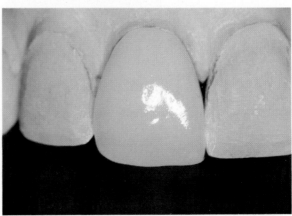

Figure 3-75   Porcelain veneer precisely fits cavo surface chamfer margin on die.

The method of insertion is as follows:

1. The porcelain veneers are dipped in water (in order to provide capillary attraction) and seated into position over the chamfer preparations (Fig. 3-76).

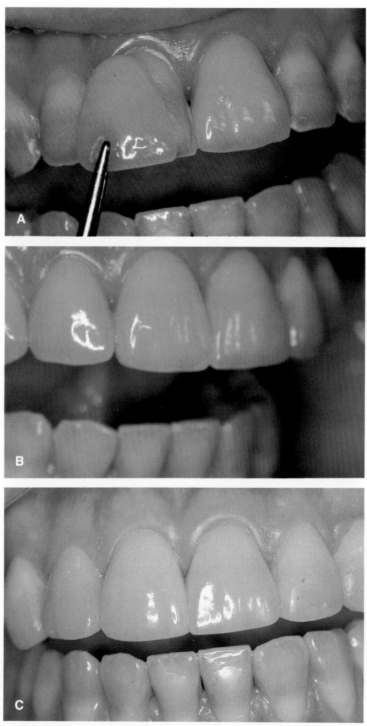

Figure 3–76 "Try-in" of porcelain veneers. *A,* Water-wetted veneer placed. *B,* Lateral view of veneers at try-in. *C,* Frontal view of veneers at try-in.

2. The margins are carefully examined for precise fit.

3. A *prebonding* procedure is now carried out by the dental assistant. Note: porcelain veneers must be handled carefully because they are extremely fragile prior to bonding.

    a. The porcelain veneers are phosphoric acid etched for 30 seconds (Fig. 3-77), washed with water, and dried. The phosphoric acid removes from the veneers contaminant salivary protein adherent pellicle that may have accumulated at the try-in stage.

    b. A *silane*-type porcelain bonding agent (Porcelain Bonding Agent[21]) is carefully applied to the internal porcelain surfaces by means of a fine-tipped brush (Fig. 3-78) and, after 30 seconds, gently air-blown.

    c. A thin layer of light-cured bond resin (Light-Cured Bonding Resin[22]) is then spread over the internal porcelain surfaces, air blown and left uncured (Fig. 3-79).

4. The veneers are now bonded to the prepared teeth by use of the following technique:

    a. The interproximal contact areas are cleared by use of thin finishing strips (Fig. 3-80).

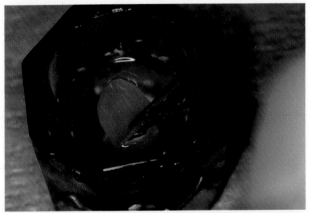

Figure 3-77 Prior to insertion, the porcelain veneers are cleaned in phosphoric acid.

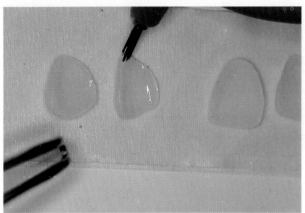

Figure 3-78 Application of silane porcelain bonding agent (Porcelain Bonding Agent[21]).

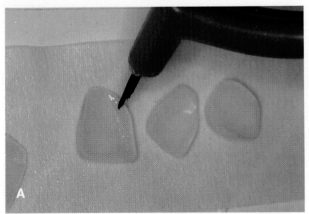
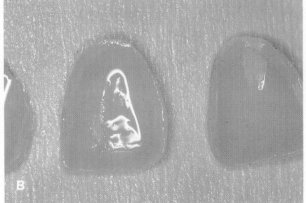

Figure 3-79 *A,* Thin application of light-cured bond resin to internal porcelain surface. *B,* The bond resin is left uncured.

b. The chamfered enamel surfaces are thoroughly cleaned using a flour of pumice slurry (Fig. 3-81), washed with water, and dried.

c. A thin, dead soft metal matrix strip (Dead Soft™ Metal Matrix Strip[23]) is then placed interproximally (Fig. 3-82).

d. The chamfered enamel surface of the right central incisor is acid-etched with a gel etchant (Convenience,™[24] Scotch Bond Etching Gel[25]) (Fig. 3-83) for a 60-second period.

e. After washing with water for 45 seconds and thorough air drying, the enamel should appear frosty and opaque (Fig. 3-84).

f. A bonding resin (Light-Cured Bonding Resin[22]) is thin-spread over the enamel surface and air-blown (Fig. 3-85).

g. In cases of dark tetracycline staining, a thin layer of opaquer (see Chapters 4 and 5) should be applied to the dark area in order to mask the stain. This should be followed by the application of another thin-spread layer of bond resin.

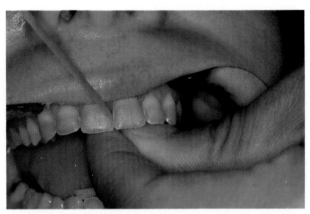

Figure 3-80 Interproximal areas stripped.

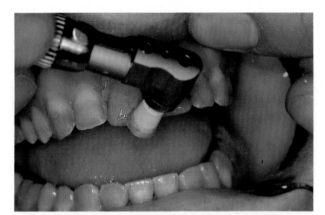

Figure 3-81 Prophylaxis using flour of pumice slurry.

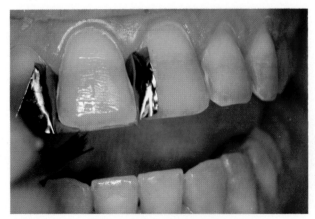

Figure 3-82 Application of dead soft matrix metal.

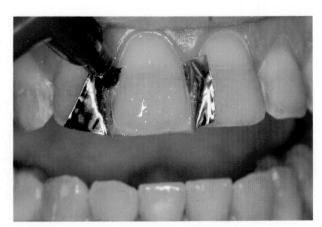

Figure 3-83 Gel etch applied for one minute.

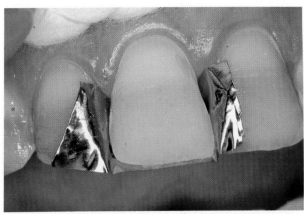

Figure 3-84 Frosty opaque appearance of labial enamel after etching.

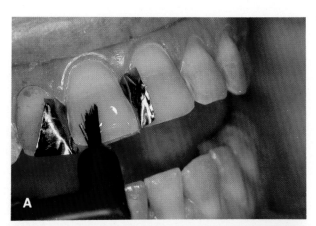

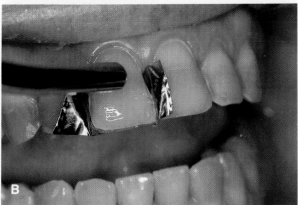

Figure 3-85 The bond resin is carefully thin-spread, *A*, and blown with air, *B*.

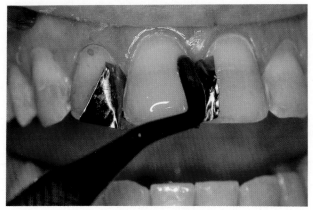

Figure 3-86 Direct application of composite to labial surface.

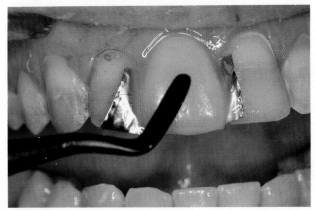

Figure 3-87 Veneer seated into position.

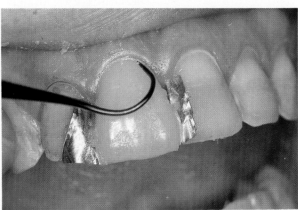

Figure 3-88 Removal of gross excess composite material.

h. A heavy-filled light-cured hybrid composite material (Ultrabond[®26]) is used to finally bond the porcelain veneers.

i. The composite material is applied to both the internal surface of the porcelain veneer and the chamfered enamel surface (Fig. 3-86) and the veneer carefully seated into position (Fig. 3-87).

j. After the removal of gross excess composite material interproximally and gingivally (Fig. 3-88), the bonding composite material should be precured by means of a 5-second application of light to the incisal region (Fig. 3-89).

k. The excess partially polymerized composite material may now be removed from the gingival and interproximal regions by means of an explorer or scaler (Fig. 3-90), after which the composite material is finally cured by means of a 30- to 40-second application of visible light both labially and palato-incisally.

l. Any remaining composite excess is removed by means of a sharp scaler and, finally, a thin-tapered carbide finishing bur (E T –6; E T –9;[27] T Burs[28]) (Fig. 3-91).

m. The interproximal regions are finally stripped (Soflex Strips[29]) (Fig. 3-92) and the entire marginal region carefully examined by means of an explorer (Fig. 3-93) to ascertain that all excess composite material has been removed.

n. The left central incisor porcelain veneer is then bonded using exactly the same protocol.

o. Both lateral incisor veneers are bonded, and then both canines, using the same procedure.

p. The protrusive and protrusive lateral occlusion is carefully equilibrated (Fig. 3-94) and incisal finish is accomplished by use of aluminum oxide discs (Soflex Discs[30]) and a donut-shaped white polystone (No. 54 White Stone[31]) (Fig. 3-95).

q. To finish the veneer margins, porcelain veneer polishing paste (Porcelain Veneer Polishing Paste,[32] command Luster Paste[33]) is applied on a rubber prophylaxis cup (Fig. 3-96). The finished Cerinate[16] porcelain veneers are shown in Figures 3-97 and 3-98. The patient should be cautioned to avoid extreme masticatory stress for a period of 6 to 8 hours.

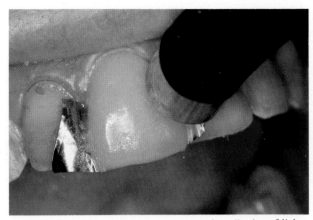

Figure 3-89 "Precuring" by means of 5-second application of light.

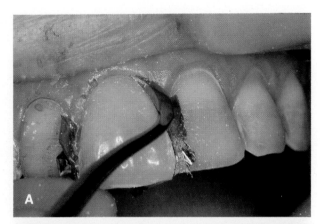

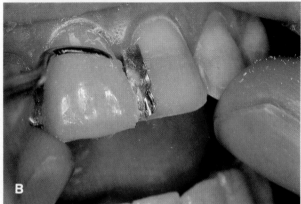

Figure 3-90 An appropriate sharp scaler is used to remove gross excess from gingival area, *A*, and interproximal areas, *B*.

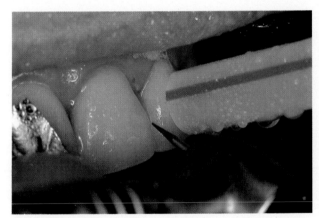

Figure 3-91 Use of a tapering carbide bur for removal of last composite excess.

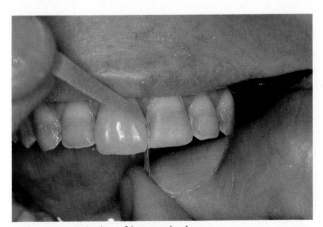

Figure 3-92 Stripping of interproximal areas.

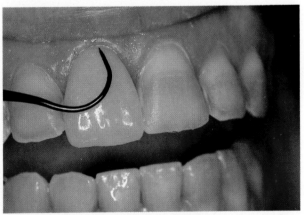

Figure 3-93 The marginal region is carefully explored to ensure that no excess composite material exists.

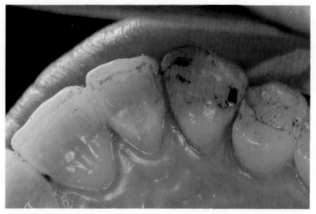

Figure 3–94   Protrusive and protrusive lateral contacts are carefully checked.

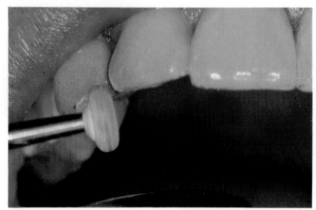

Figure 3-95   Use of white stone to finish incisal margins.

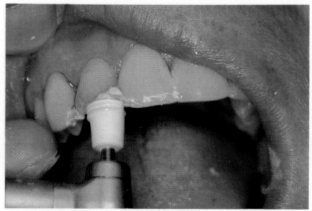

Figure 3-96   Application of polishing paste.

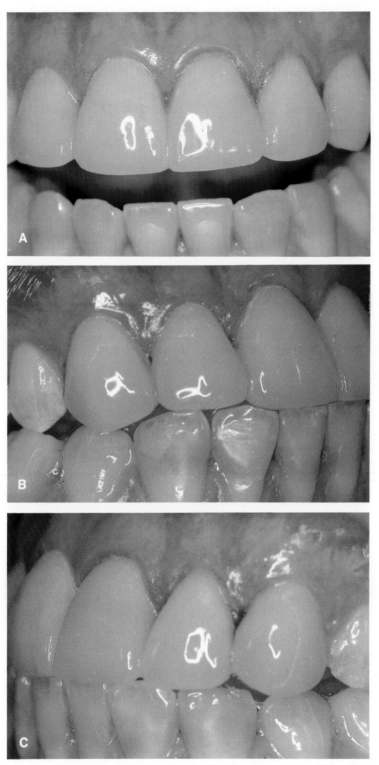

Figure 3-97   Porcelain veneers immediately after placement. *A*, Frontal view. *B*, Right lateral view. *C*, Left lateral view.

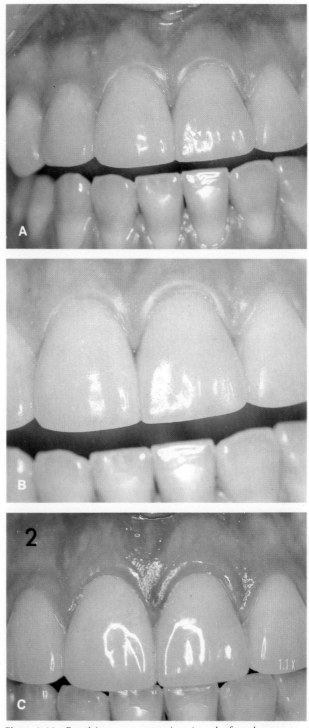

Figure 3-98   Porcelain veneer restorations 1 week after placement. *A*, Full labial arch view. *B*, Close-up view. *C*, At 2 year recall.

INDIRECT COMPOSITE VENEERS

Indirect laboratory-processed composite veneers (Dentacolor,[17] Visio-Gem[18]) have the same indications as porcelain veneers. These materials are essentially laboratory light-cured, microfilled systems which are often vacuum-cured under strictly controlled laboratory conditions. Accordingly, they may demonstrate superior physical properties when compared to their *direct* light-cured counterparts (Durafill,[8] Visiodispers[34]). The work of Lutz et al (1984) suggests an improvement in durability from the self- to light- to heat-cured composite systems. The clinical technique for indirect composite veneers is similar to that already described for porcelain veneers. A typical case of dark tetracycline discoloration is shown in Figure 3-99. The laboratory-cured composite veneers (Dentacolor[17]) are shown in Figure 3-100. The insertion technique is identical to that already described for composite veneers except that a porcelain bonding agent is not required. A thin layer of light-cured bond resin (Durafill Bond[7]) is applied to the internal surfaces of the composite veneers (Fig. 3-101) as well as to the acid-etched chamfered enamel surfaces. Unlike the porcelain veneers, the bonding resin provides a chemical bond to the composite veneers. The veneers are then bonded into position using a light-cured, microfill composite material (Durafill Flow[35] for Dentacolor[17] or Visiodispers[34] for Visio-Gem[18]) and light-cured. Figure 3-102 shows the finished composite veneer restorations.

Although both porcelain and composite laboratory-processed veneers are indicated for the severe tetracycline-discolored dentition, the clinician, when making a choice, must consider *esthetics, technique-sensitivity*, and *cost*.

Porcelain veneers provide the ultimate in esthetic acceptability. However, they are more *technique-sensitive* and more costly than indirect composite veneers. Porcelain veneers are more technique-sensitive in two respects: (1) a primarily micro-mechanical bond exists at the composite-porcelain interface, and (2) should fracture of the porcelain occur, it is difficult to repair simply by the addition of composite material. As for cost, the laboratory fee for a porcelain veneer is usually somewhat higher than that for an indirect composite veneer.

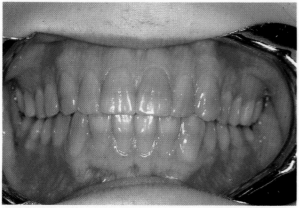

Figure 3-99 Severe tetracycline staining prior to indirect composite veneering.

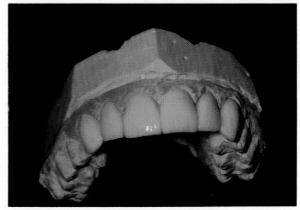

Figure 3-100 Indirect composite veneers on master model.

Despite the excellent esthetic results, indirect composite veneers lack the super enamel-like reflectivity of fused porcelain surfaces. However, composite veneers are less technique-sensitive than porcelain veneers for a chemical bond is attainable at the composite-veneer interface. In addition, should fracture occur, the indirect composite veneers are easily repaired by means of a direct add-on composite technique (Figs. 3-103 and 3-104). The laboratory cost for indirect composite veneers is usually somewhat lower than that for porcelain veneers, that is, between forty and sixty dollars per unit.

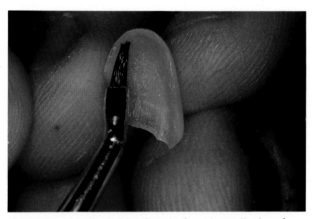

Figure 3-101 A chemical bond results from the application of bond resin to internal surface of the composite veneer.

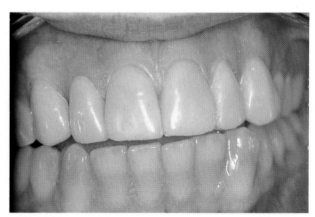

Figure 3-102 Postoperative appearance of indirect composite veneers.

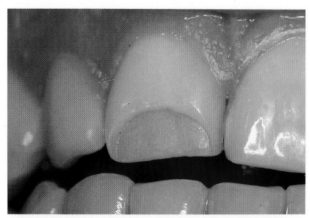

Figure 3-103 Fractured indirect composite veneer, maxillary right central incisor.

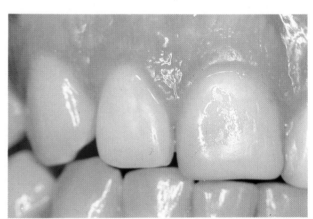

Figure 3-104 Indirect composite veneer repaired.

This chapter has described five conservative treatment alternatives available to the practitioner in treating the discolored dentition. See Chapters 4 and 5 for a description of an additional conservative treatment approach, *Direct Composite Labial Veneers Using Opaquers and Tints*.

Table 3–1 provides an over-all summary of the indications, advantages, and limitations of each treatment approach.

TABLE 3–1   Over-All Summary of Conservative Treatment of the Discolored Dentition

Treatment	Indications	Advantages	Limitations
Vital bleaching	Light yellow; light grey tetracycline stain Fluorosis Acquired superficial stain Hemorrhagic discoloration	Ultraconservative Predictable Least costly Little or no regression	Cannot be used alone for extremely dark tetracycline stain
Nonvital bleaching	For all discolored nonvital teeth	Ultraconservative Predictable Least costly	Slight regression may occur
Direct composite labial veneers	Labial wear Hypoplasia Fluorosis	Conservative Excellent esthetics Normal labial contours Excellent gingival response Easily repairable Affordable cost Not highly technique-sensitive	Difficult to attain predictable esthetic result with extremely dark tetracycline stain
Direct composite labial veneers using opaquers and tints	Hypoplasia Fluorosis Dark tetracycline discoloration	Conservative Excellent esthetics Normal labial contours Excellent gingival response Easily repairable Moderate cost	Technique-sensitive Requires extensive clinical experience regarding proper use of opaquers and tints
Direct composite labial veneers combined with bleaching	Moderate tetracycline stain Fluorosis	Ultraconservative Predictable Affordable cost Little or no regression Easily repairable Not highly technique-sensitive	Not usually applicable to extremely dark tetracycline stain
Indirect porcelain veneers	Dark tetracycline discoloration and otherwise extensive involvement	Conservative Excellent esthetics Excellent gingival response	Technique-sensitive Most costly of conservative alternatives Repair difficult
Indirect composite veneers	Dark tetracycline discoloration and otherwise extensive involvement	Conservative Very good esthetics Not highly technique-sensitive Easily repairable Moderate cost	Esthetic result not quite so good as porcelain veneers

References

Abou-Rass M. The elimination of tetracycline discoloration by intentional endodontics and internal bleaching. J Endo 1982; 8:101.

Arzt AH. Updating tetracycline stained teeth bleaching technique. Quintessence Int. 1981; 12:15.

Cohen SC. Human pulpal response to bleaching procedures on vital teeth. J Endo 1979; 5:134.

Cohen SC, Burns RC. Pathways of the Pulp. St. Louis: CV Mosby Co, 1980.

Hyasaki F, Takamizu M, Mumoi Y, Kusunoki G, Kono A. Bleaching teeth discolored by tetracycline therapy. Dent Surg 1980; 56:17.

Ingle J, Beveridge E. Endodontics. 2nd ed, Philadelphia: Lea & Febiger, 1976.

Kerr DA, Ash MM. Oral Pathology. 3rd ed, Philadelphia: Lea & Febiger, 1977.

Lado EA, Stanley HR, Weisman MI. Cervical resorption in bleaching teeth. Oral Surg 1983; 55:78.

Lutz F, Phillips RW, Roulet JF, Setcos J. In vivo and in vitro wear of potential posterior composites. J Dent Res 1984; 63:914.Minister for National Health and Welfare. Preventive Dental Services, September, 1979. Minister for Supply and Services Canada, 1980. Catalogue No. H39-4, 1980 E.

Product Information

Product	Manufacturer/Distributor	Purpose
1. Vaseline	Chesebrough-Ponds Canada Ltd. 150 Bullock Drive Markham, Ontario L3P 1W3	Petroleum jelly for lubrication of soft tissues prior to bleaching
2. Kenalog	Squibb 2365 Côte de Liesse St. Laurent, Quebec H4N 2M7	Topical corticosteroid for lubricating soft tissues prior to bleaching
3. Superoxol	Union Broach Co. Inc. 36–40–37th Street Long Island City, NY 11101	30% hydrogen peroxide for use in vital bleaching techniques
4. University of Indiana Bleaching Instrument	Union Broach Co. Inc. 36–40–37th Street Long Island City, NY 11101	Bleaching instrument
or Holt-Monarch Instrument	Almore International P.O. Box 25214 Portland, OR 97225	Bleaching instrument
5. Ketac Bond	ESPE-Premier Sales Corp. Romano Dr., P.O. Box 111 Norristown, PA 19401	Glass ionomer interim seal for lingual opening
6. Term-Temporary Endodontic Restorative Material	L.D. Caulk Co. Box 359 Milford, DE 19963	A light-cured composite interim seal for lingual opening
7. Durafill Bond	Kulzer Inc. 10015 Muirlands Blvd., Unit G Irvine, CA 92714	Bond for internal dentin, lingual and enamel
8. Durafill	Kulzer Inc. 10015 Muirlands Blvd., Unit G Irvine, CA 92714	Light-cured, microfilled composite for lingual seal
9. Complus	Parkell Co. 155 Schmitt Blvd. Farmingdale, NY 11735	Filled glaze for labial seal
10. Scotchbond	Dental Products/3M Company 3M Center 270-5N-02 St. Paul, MN 55144	Self-cured, dentin bonding agent
11. Durafill Dentin Bond	Kulzer Inc. 10015 Muirlands Blvd., Unit G Irvine, CA 92714	Light-cured, dentin bonding agent

Product Information

Product	Manufacturer/Distributor	Purpose
12. J&J Dentin Bond	Johnson and Johnson 20 Lake Drive, CN7060 East Windsor, NJ 08520	Self-cured, dentin bonding agent
13. Silux	Dental Products/3M Company 3M Center 270–5N–02 St. Paul, MN 55144	Light-cured microfill
14. Certain	Johnson and Johnson 20 Lake Drive, CN7060 East Windsor, NJ 08520	Light-cured microfill
15. Extra Smooth	DenMat Inc. 3130 Skyway Dr., Unit 501 Santa Maria, CA 93456	Microfill labial veneering after vital bleaching
16. Cerinate Veneers	DenMat Inc. 3130 Skyway Dr., Unit 501 Santa Maria, CA 93456	Indirect porcelain veneer
17. Dentacolor	Kulzer Inc. 10015 Muirlands Blvd., Unit G Irvine, CA 92714	Indirect composite veneer
18. Visio-Gem	ESPE-Premier Sales Corp. Romano Dr., P.O. Box 111 Norristown, PA 19401	Indirect composite veneer
19. RCBIIK 8–9	ESPE-Premier Sales Corp. Romano Dr., P.O. Box 111 Norristown, PA 19401	Diamond-carbide duets for labial chamfer preparation
20. Paste Laminate	DenMat Inc. 3130 Skyway Dr., Unit 501 Santa Maria, CA 93456	Light-cured microfill for direct veneer restoration
21. Porcelain Bonding Agent	DenMat Inc. 3130 Skyway Dr., Unit 501 Santa Maria, CA 93456	Silane porcelain bonding agent
22. Light-Cured Bonding Resin	DenMat Inc. 3130 Skyway Dr., Unit 501 Santa Maria, CA 93456	Light-cured bonding resin
23. Dead Soft Metal Matrix Strip	DenMat Inc. 3130 Skyway Dr., Unit 501 Santa Maria, CA 93456	Isolating single teeth during veneer insertion
24. Convenience	DenMat Inc. 3130 Skyway Dr., Unit 501 Santa Maria, CA 93456	Gel etchant
25. Scotchbond Etching Gel	Dental Products/3M Company 3M Center 270–5N–02 St. Paul, MN 55144	Gel etchant
26. Ultrabond	DenMat Inc. 3130 Skyway Dr., Unit 501 Santa Maria, CA 93456	Heavy-filled, powder-liquid, hybrid composite for bonding porcelain veneers
27. ET 6; ET 9	Brasseler USA Inc. 800 King George Blvd. Savannah, GA 31419	Thin tapering carbide burs for removal of excess composite
28. T Burs	Ritter/Midwest Co. 901 W. Oakton Des Plaines, IL 60018	Thin tapering carbide finishing burs for removal of excess composite

Product Information

Product	Manufacturer/Distributor	Purpose
29. Soflex Strips	Dental Products/3M Company 3M Center 270–5N–02 St. Paul, MN 55144	Interproximal finish of porcelain veneer margins
30. Soflex Discs	Dental Products/3M Company 3M Center 270–5N–02 St. Paul, MN 55144	Finish of porcelain veneer margins
31. No. 54 White Stone	J. M. Ney Co. International Maplewood Ave. Bloomfield, CT 06002	Final polish of porcelain veneer margins
32. Porcelain Veneer Polishing Paste	DenMat Inc. 3130 Skyway Dr., Unit 501 Santa Maria, CA 93456	Final polish of porcelain veneer margins
33. Command Luster Paste	Kerr-Sybron Co. P.O. Box 455 Romulus, MI 48174	Final polish of porcelain veneer margins
34. Visiodispers	ESPE-Premier Sales Corp. Romano Dr., P.O. Box 111 Norristown, PA 19401	Light-cured microfill for direct veneers
35. Durafill Flow	Kulzer Inc. 10015 Muirlands Blvd., Unit G Irvine, CA 92714	Free-flowing, light-cured microfill for bonding indirect veneers

4

N O R M A N L. F E I G E N B A U M
K. W I L L I A M M O P P E R

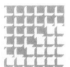

COLORING WITH RESINS

Along with the introduction of the visible-light-cured resins came new demands on the dentist. In the past, laboratory technicians have been primarily responsible for tooth color and anatomy. Today, by means of direct application techniques, the dentist has assumed full responsibility of tooth duplication. The dentist must therefore develop new skills in color manipulation as well as a revitalized sense of anatomy. In this chapter a step-by-step technique for direct composite restoration of tetracycline-stained teeth as well as tips and guidelines for the use of colored resin products will be presented.

PRINCIPLES OF COLOR

The principles of color must be restricted to resins only. Understanding color is a vast art and science of its own, and the reader is assumed to have some basic knowledge of color science. Much has been written about the use of color with dental porcelains (Preston and Bergen, 1980). There are some differences in color diffusion, refraction, and reflection when compared to resins which should be clarified and understood so that these materials can be used to best advantage.

Coloring From Within

It is a well-known fact that most of the coloring of teeth is a result of the color(s) of the dentin. The dentin color shines through the overlying enamel which is translucent. Enamel is generally *colorless*, but because it is physically laid down in rods, it transmits the color of the underlying dentin and tones it down somewhat. With composite restorations, therefore, coloring must be placed underneath the final layer of the restorative material used. Surface staining of teeth rarely accomplishes its goals and never stays in place very long.

Resin coloring uses combinations of colors and restoratives. It is essential that the clinician comprehend exactly how certain combinations are useful as well as the differences in the opacity and translucency of various composite materials.

Opacity and Translucency

Opacity: the quality of not allowing light to pass through.

Translucency: the quality of permitting light to pass through, but diffusing the light.

All restorative resins available are somewhat translucent. They must be, because natural teeth are translucent. Normal tooth structure is not at all opaque. In fact, opaquers help the clinician to change a tooth color, not to mimic one. Using an opaquer to cover a given color causes another problem called opacity or "shine-through". Incisal thirds are generally more translucent than middle and cervical thirds because there is a preponderance of translucent enamel at the incisal area. It is necessary to think of teeth in degrees of translucence rather than opacity.

There are four main areas that must be understood in order to become adept at using resin color:

1. Blocking out the undercolor (stains, metals, developmental defects, and old dentistry)
2. Multichromatic color transitions (cervical, body, and incisals)
3. Maverick coloring (areas of color differences)
4. Characterizing with tints (incisal translucence, crazing, checklines, and other unusual anomalies)

General Guidelines of Resin Color Mixing and Application

Light-cured opaquers and tints are available in a variety of colors and viscosities. They are either Bis-GMA or urethane-based Dimethacrylates containing various dyes or pigments. They are interchangeable with each other for the most part, although logic dictates that staying within the same system is more reliable.

Opaquers[1-4] are designed to block out the light with titanium dioxide and other opaque pigments. The intensity of an opaquer is dependent on the ratio of pigment to resin. The more intense the opaquer, the thinner the layer necessary to cover an unwanted color. *Tints,*[5-8] on the other hand, are designed to alter the existing shade or characterize a specific area. They are generally translucent. Some are colored with pigment and the particles are sometimes large enough to see. Others are colored with dyes and appear to be homogeneous in nature.

It is important to understand the differences and to use the appropriate materials for the job at hand. Tints and opaquers can be combined in the following instances: (1) when it is necessary to slightly modify an opaque to decrease the intensity in a brown, yellow, orange, or grey direction, and (2) when it is desirable to increase the opacity of a given tint.

Classification of Viscosities

Self-Drying Paint-On. This type of opaquer (Heliocolor[9]) must be mixed and brushed on the surface to be color-corrected. This covers best with the least amount of thickness. However, it creates the most intensity and requires a greater thickness of restorative material to recreate translucence. This material must be placed with a disposable brush.

Syrup-Like Liquid. There are both tints (Rembrandt Natural[6]) and opaquers (Estilux;[2] J & J;[3] Visiopaquers[4]) of this type. These may be placed with a brush or a ball-type instrument. They tend to accumulate in concavities and thin out over convexities. It is best to place these materials in thin multiple layers, polymerizing each layer separately.

Gelatinous Liquids. Both tints (Creative Color Tints[5]) and opaquers (Creative Color Opaquer[1]) are available in this type. These materials can be spread evenly with either a nylon or acrylic bristled brush. They can be placed with metal instruments or even the edge of a plastic strip. This type should also be placed in thin layers.

COLOR SELECTION

Factors Affecting Shade Matching

Any discussion of color selection must include the ambient lighting as well as the office decor. Apparent colors are affected by the color of the office walls and equipment and the type of lighting in the room. Natural light is the most reliable and, if possible, should be used as the standard. There are fluorescent lights available that are closely matched in wave lengths to natural daylight, and these are helpful.

A second variable is the operator's visual perceptions. The eyes are not always accurate in reporting information to the brain and can easily become fatigued. Some dentists are more or less color-blind. For these reasons it is helpful to make color choice a consensus of several opinions.

Matching existing shades is the most difficult of tasks with the greatest number of variables. The following suggestions are therefore presented:

1. Use shade guides made out of the materials to be used.
2. Move shade guides in and out quickly.
3. Use daylight when possible.
4. Let the patient participate in the shade-matching process.
5. Stare at a light blue object to rest the eyes.
6. Observe the multichromatic changes.
7. Warn the patient of the difficulty of shade selection.
8. Record your findings.

OFFICE PROCEDURE IN COLOR SELECTION

Shade Guides

Most of the shade guides included in resin kits are actually made of unfilled acrylic. They are inaccurate because they are not made of the composite material and therefore are not from the same batch of resin. A practical solution to this problem is to make shade guides from the material itself. Take an amount equal to the width of the syringe and form it on the end of a cottonwood stick. Shape it into an elliptical form and polymerize it. Polish it, and your first guide is finished.

Another technique is to fill a small celluloid crown form with the material and place a cottonwood stick into the material. Polymerize and strip off the celluloid crown. No polishing is necessary. By means of proper basic-shade blending, an infinite number of new shades can be created in this way.

Color Mock-Ups

Resins make possible a degree of color matching that exists with no other material. Since the material does not harden until it is "command-cured", the composite material can be placed directly on *unetched* enamel, light-cured, and then easily displaced. This unique quality allows color selections to be made directly on the teeth involved.

Filled resins are influenced color-wise by the surrounding tooth structure. The final shade is really a combination of the tooth structure and the resin. Results can be predicted more reliably if the color mock-up is used:

1. Choose the appropriate resin shades and mold them on the unetched tooth structure. Use the thickness you intend to use in the final product. If you are using several shades, you can make your mock-up with the colors blended. Polish the surface and assess the result.
2. If it is necessary to block out the undercolor, place the chosen opaquer(s) and polymerize it. Then cover it with the composite restorative material and polymerize. Remember to use the correct thickness, and finally polish. This may be done with several different combinations used at the same time on different teeth. The patient should be asked to express a preference.

Checklist

1. Remember that most patients want whiter and brighter and do not understand the meaning of "natural".
2. Understand the patient's needs.
3. Make sure the communication with the patient is clear.
4. When several teeth are involved, color one tooth first and have the patient approve the color before continuing.
5. Each experience with color changing increases the operator's ability to achieve better results.

VENEERING TETRACYCLINE-STAINED TEETH

Tetracycline stain is common; a new case is encountered almost every week. The severity of the discoloration determines the intensity of the treatment. The range of discoloration can be divided roughly into three categories: mildly stained, moderately stained, and severely stained (see Chapter 3). The moderately and severely stained tetracycline cases are the most difficult to treat and call for careful advance planning relative to the amount of tooth preparation.

PREPARATION: WHAT TO EVALUATE (Fig. 4-1)

Darkness of Color

The darker the discoloration, the more opaquer necessary to block out the undercolor. The more opaquer used, the thicker the resultant veneers. To avoid a protruded result, more tooth removal is necessary. *Rule:* The darker the teeth, the greater the tooth preparation (0.25 mm more for dark teeth).

Arch Form and Tooth Direction

Protruded Teeth Need More Preparation. If the teeth are flared labially, they must be more deeply prepared in order to avoid undue protrusion. If the teeth are lingually inclined, it may be possible to veneer them without any preparation. A diamond bur is used to create a *depth groove* 0.5 mm to 1.0 mm deep (Fig. 4-2). *Rule:* Determine thickness of the veneers (minimum 1.25 mm) and make a judgment of correct tooth thickness removal before starting the case.

Extent of the Proximal Boundaries

Note how far interproximally the preparation must be made in order to completely mask the discoloration, leaving room for opaquer as well as restorative. *Rule:* When it is possible, do not break the contact (Fig. 4-3).

Extent of Gingival Margin

There are two schools of thought here. The gingival margin should be prepared with a chamfered finish line. If a subgingival finish line is preferred, this is facilitated by reflecting the tissue (free margin) with an appropriate plastic instrument (8A[10]) (Fig. 4-4). In color change cases, it is important to eliminate the dark line at the gingival. In many cases, a successful result may be attained by preparing the chamfered margin just level with the free gingival crest rather than below it. Both ways should be tried.

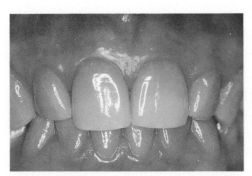

Figure 4-1 Preoperative view of severe tetracycline discoloration.

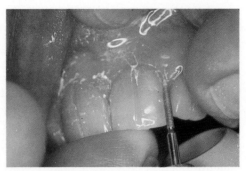

Figure 4-2 Depth grooves 0.5 to 1 mm, are prepared with a diamond instrument.

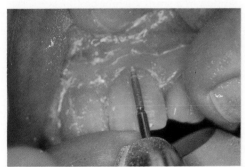

Figure 4-3 Removal of enamel with diamond instrument.

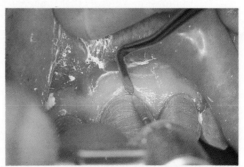

Figure 4-4 Gingival tissue is reflected during preparation of gingival margin.

Incisal Area Preparation

If lengthening of the tooth is not intended, the preparation is brought to the incisal edge at a depth of 0.5 mm. If lengthening is intended, the margin is extended to cover the incisal edge and chamfer-finished on the lingual.

Opaquing and Tinting (Blocking out the Undercolor)

Starting with a properly prepared tooth that has been etched on the enamel and coated with a dentin (Scotchbond;[11]Durafill Dentin Adhesive[12]) and/or an enamel bonding agent (Durafill Bond Resin;[13]Enamel Bond[14]), we are at last ready to begin the opaquing process.

1. The choice of opaque shade has been made in the mock-up stage. There are two methods for achieving a "natural" tooth color on the lighter end of the shade guide. First, an *ivory colored opaquer* (Creative Color 62 or 67[1]) covered by a medium light shade may be used or, alternatively a *darker opaquer* (Visiopaquer Brown or Yellow[4]) that is altered by the addition of a small amount of *honey yellow* (Creative Color[5]) tint may be used and overlaid with a light shade of *microfill resin*(Silux L or XL[15] or Visiodispers Standard[16] or Durafill G[17]). Both methods produce an excellent coloring result. Application of the opaquer is begun near the cervical margin (Fig. 4-5). A small instrument is used for this purpose. The material is spread incisally as well as toward the interproximals. It is not necessary to totally cover the tooth with one layer (Fig. 4-6).
2. Since the pigments in the opaquer will make it more difficult for the light to penetrate the heavier layers, each layer should be separately polymerized for 40 seconds. Two or three thin coats should be adequate. *Rule:* If there appears to be any patchy coloring at this stage, another coat of opaquer is needed. This layer should be no more than 0.5 mm. All visible surfaces should be coated (Fig. 4-7). If the opaquing layer extends beyond the margins of the preparation, the excess is removed with a fine diamond (Fig. 4-8). If too much debris is thus created, a thin coat of bonding agent is painted over the opaque layer before continuing.

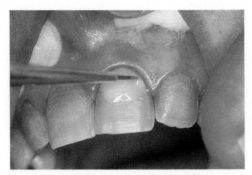

Figure 4-5 Initial application of opaque layer.

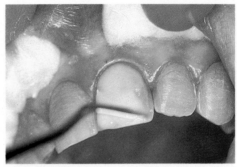

Figure 4-6 The opaquer is spread interproximally and toward the incisal.

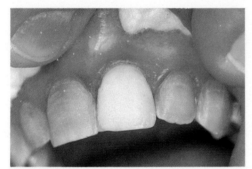

Figure 4-7 Final opaque layer in place.

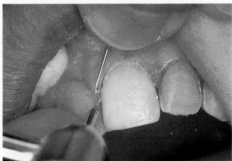

Figure 4-8 Excess opaque is removed from margins.

3. *Optional.* Polychromacity of the final result may now be achieved. In order to slightly darken the cervical third, a thin coat of a light-to-honey-yellow tint (Creative Color Tints[5]) may be placed or, alternatively, *light brown* (Creative Color Tints;[5] Rembrandt Natural[6]) and orange, depending on the result required (Fig. 4-9). Polymerize this with 20 seconds of visible light. If an opaquer is used for this purpose, the final result will be too opaque.

4. *Optional.* If the illusion of translucence is required, a slight hint of incisal translucence may be provided by using a thin coating of *grey opaquer* (J & J Grey Opaquer[18]) at the incisal third (Figs. 4-10 and 4-11).

5. *Optional.* If there is a need to further characterize the tooth with maverick colors, it should be done at this stage before the restorative resin is placed.

6. All of these artistic endeavors can be practiced on old crown and bridge shade guides.

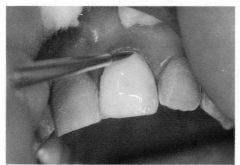

Figure 4-9 Application of gingival tint.

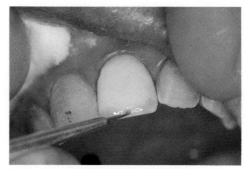

Figure 4-10 Application of grey incisal tint.

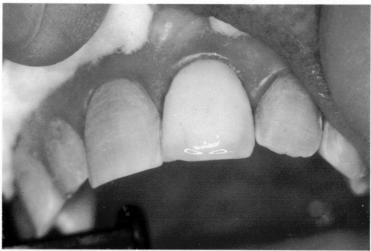

Figure 4-11 Completed incisal tint.

SCULPTING THE VENEER

The use of a microfill that has the consistency of putty is preferred (Durafill G[17]). There are many microfilled materials that are equally acceptable (Silux L or XL;[15] Visiodispers ST;[16] Certain[19]). An amount sufficient to completely veneer the tooth is rolled into a ball with clean fingers. This is our convenience form (Fig. 4-12). The composite ball is placed on the tooth with an instrument (8A Plastic Instrument[10]) (Fig. 4-13). The material is sculpted from the cervical (Fig. 4-14) to the interproximal (Fig. 4-15) and finally to the incisal contours (Fig. 4-16). Make certain that the tooth is slightly overcontoured.

Finishing of the veneer demands the same techniques used to finish all microfill resins (see Chapter 2). Figure 4-17 shows the treated dentition 2 weeks postoperatively.

Composite Restorative Overcoatings

Having done the color mock-up beforehand, one can clearly ascertain the exact type of composite restorative to be used as the final layer of the direct bonded veneer. Microfills are polishable to a surface that is as smooth as enamel, and as homogeneous in nature. Their increased translucence allows the undercolor to appear as it did when placed. This remarkable characteristic of microfills renders them the choice material for veneers of this type.

If macrofill or hybrid-type composite materials are used as the surface, it will be found that the diffusion of the light causes most of the color placement to be obliterated.

Final Words About Final Finishing

There is no substitute for proper anatomy, a textured surface, and final high gloss surfacing. All are necessary to a truly fine-quality result. Our well-finished microfill veneers have endured more than 5 years to date without discoloration of the resin, provided the surface is pure microfill and is polished and brushed by the patient.

Dealing with Other Color Problems

1. Blocking out metals is handled like the preceding case with one change. Mechanical retention must be achieved.
2. White and yellow spots can be eliminated by removal of the surface spotting. A bevelled preparation does the job.
3. Characterization is accomplished with creativity and techniques similar to those employed by ceramists.

AN APPRAISAL

Direct resin veneering is a fairly recent development in our profession. The technology is moving with such speed that it is difficult to keep abreast of current thought. We have made an attempt to describe a "state of the art" procedure that will have value in the future, if not as the final word at least as a building block for future techniques.

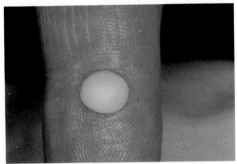

Figure 4-12 Ball of composite material (convenience form).

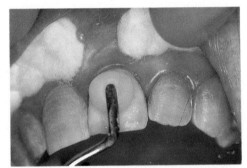

Figure 4-13 Initial application of composite ball.

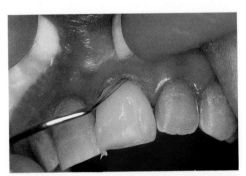

Figure 4-14 Cervical sculpture of composite material.

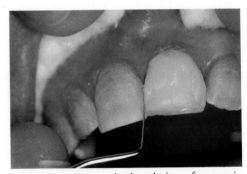

Figure 4-15 Interproximal sculpting of composite material.

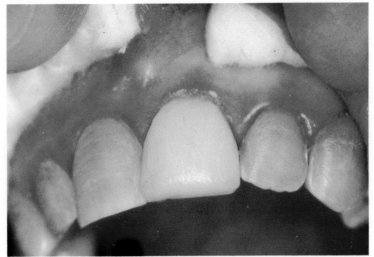

Figure 4-16 Final contour.

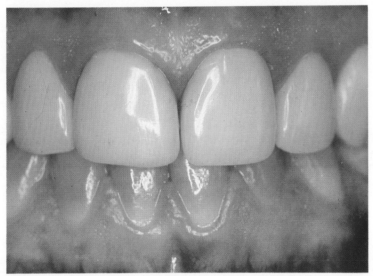

Figure 4-17 Completed veneer restorations 2 weeks postoperatively.

Reference

Preston JD, Bergen SF. Color Science and Dental Art. St. Louis: CV Mosby Co, 1980.

Product Information

Product	Manufacturer/Distributor	Purpose
1. Creative Color Opaquer	Cosmedent Inc. 5419 N. Sheridan Rd. Chicago, IL 60640	Masking undercolor (stains, metals, developmental defects)
2. Estilux Color Modifiers	Kulzer Inc. 10015 Muirlands Blvd., Unit G Irvine, CA 92714	Masking undercolor (stains, metals, developmental defects)
3. J&J Color Modifiers	Johnson and Johnson 20 Lake Drive, CN7060 East Windsor, NJ 08520	Masking undercolor (stains, metals, developmental defects)
4. Visiopaquers	ESPE-Premier Sales Corp. Romano Dr., P.O. Box 111 Norristown, PA 19401	Masking undercolor (stains, metals, developmental defects)
5. Creative Color Tints	Cosmedent Inc. 5419 N. Sheridan Rd. Chicago, IL 60640	Alter existing shade and characterization
6. Rembrandt Natural	DenMat Inc. 3130 Skyway Dr., Unit 501 Santa Maria, CA 93456	Alter existing shade and characterization
7. Durafill Intensive Color	Kulzer Inc. 10015 Muirlands Blvd., Unit G Irvine, CA 92714	Alter existing shade and characterization
8. Command Color	Kerr-Sybron Co. P.O. Box 455 Romulus, MI 48174	Alter existing shade and characterization
9. Heliocolor	Vivadent USA Inc. P.O. Box 304 Tonawanda, NY 14150	Self-drying paint-on opaquer
10. 8A Plastic Instrument	American Dental Instrument Manufacturing Co. 2800 Reserve St., P.O. Box 4546 Missoula, MT 59801	For reflecting gingival tissue
11. Scotchbond	Dental Products/3M Company 3M Center270-5N-02 St. Paul, MN 55144	Dentin adhesive
12. Durafill Dentin Adhesive	Kulzer Inc. 10015 Muirlands Blvd., Unit G Irvine, CA 92714	Dentin adhesive
13. Durafill Bond Resin	Kulzer Inc. 10015 Muirlands Blvd., Unit G Irvine, CA 92714	Enamel bond resin
14. Enamel Bond	Dental Products/3M Company 3M Center 270-5N-02 St. Paul, MN 55144	Enamel bond resin
15. Silux L or XL	Dental Products/3M Company 3M Center 270-5N-02 St. Paul, MN 55144	Light-cured, microfilled composite
16. Visiodispers ST	ESPE-Premier Sales Corp. Romano Dr., P.O. Box 111 Norristown, PA 19401	Light-cured, microfilled composite
17. Durafill G	Kulzer Inc. 10015 Muirlands Blvd., Unit G Irvine, CA 92714	Light-cured, microfilled composite
18. J&J Grey Opaquer	Johnson and Johnson 20 Lake Drive, CN7060 East Windsor, NJ 08520	For incisal translucence
19. Certain	Johnson and Johnson 20 Lake Drive, CN7060 East Windsor, NJ 08520	Light-cured, microfilled composite

5

PART ONE
MARK J. FRIEDMAN
PART TWO
ISAAC COMFORTES

PART ONE
OPAQUERS AND TINTS
WITH DIRECT VENEERS

$\mathbf{M}$any patients are seeking improvement of their smiles through conservative means. The esthetic correction of discolored teeth presents one of the most difficult challenges for the dental practitioner.

Stains and discoloration can be categorized into two groups: (1) intrinsic, and (2) extrinsic. The extrinsic stains are easier to manage and frequently can be removed with minor enamelplasty followed by resin veneering (either partial or full coverage).

The intrinsic stains, or developmentally dark teeth, present a more complex set of problems. If possible, as is the case with endodontically treated teeth, bleaching should be considered to reduce the undesirable color of the affected teeth (see Chapter 3). Usually, however, bleaching has some degree of "relapse", and a period of several weeks should be allowed to determine the final "stable" tooth color. If bleaching is not possible or does not give the desired results, some form of opaquing becomes necessary.

By definition, opaques block the transmission of light through the tooth structure, thus changing the optical characteristics of the tooth and giving it a "flat" and lifeless appearance. The opaque, by its nature, reflects light rays and reduces the depth to which rays of light may penetrate. At the same time, however, the undesirable color is also hidden from the observer, and this is why the addition of opaque is advocated.

To ensure a tooth-like appearance that closely resembles enamel and dentin, the opaque layer must *not be placed too close to the external surface*, but rather should be as "deep" as possible.

When opaque is used in resin veneering, the restoration must be properly planned. A trial wax-up is helpful in the planning of enamelplasty and final veneer thickness.

CONCEPTS OF OPAQUING

Color changes should always be evaluated on the basis of both the absolute color of the tooth in question (value is the most important parameter) and the color of the surrounding teeth. In other words, teeth vary in *value, chroma,* and *hue* (Preston and Bergen, 1980) within the same arch; thus an exact match is often difficult to achieve. It is easier to decide on a value range and try to create that range for the teeth in question. It is also important to "mimic" proper outline form and surface texture characteristics to develop undetectable veneers. Basically, the darker the tooth, the more room needed to "cover" that discoloration. This is achieved by *controlled enamelplasty*, which can be defined as the removal of surface enamel in a prescribed manner according to specific guidelines:

1. Enamelplasty should conform to the three planes found on all teeth, i.e., gingival, body, and incisal. Particular attention is paid to the gingival plane since overcontouring in this area can lead to deleterious gingival sequelae (Kuwata, 1980).
2. Perforation into dentin should be allowed to occur when necessary to provide adequate opaque layering together with a suitable thickness of surface composite. These dentin perforations, however, need to be "mapped" in the practitioner's mind so as to protect them from possible etching.
3. A periphery of enamel should be maintained to maximize the resin tag retention or seal circumferentially.
4. A gentle chamfer should be established at the height of the free gingival margin and should extend beyond the proximal transitional line angles. The proximal contacts should be maintained in enamel whenever possible. A supragingival margin will ensure:

    a. Maximum retention if ending on etched enamel rather than dentin or cementum
    b. Nonviolation of the tooth-tissue relationship, i.e., healthier periodontal tissue
    c. Easier finishing with diamonds, rubber cups, and the like
    d. Reduced hard and soft tissue trauma such as "ditching" of cementum or abrasion of gingiva

This supragingival margin may compromise the esthetic result when marked discoloration occurs in the gingival third of a tooth as in severe tetracycline discoloration. This may necessitate extensive enamel removal which may eliminate all traces of gingival enamel for etching. To ensure adequate gingival retention, a mechanical retention form should be placed. This can be placed with a ¼ round bur or 33½ inverted cone. The retention form should be approximately 0.5 mm axially to the external tooth surface and should extend the entire mesiodistal width of the enamelplasty preparation. The use of a dentin bonding agent (Scotchbond[1]) helps to ensure marginal integrity and reduces microleakage. Ideally the composite increment, which includes the dentin area of the retention form, should be *polymerized first* to prevent "pulling" toward the enamel during polymerization shrinkage (see Chapter 6).

THE OPTIPHYSICS OF MASKING DISCOLORATIONS

Ideally, undesirable shades should be masked gradually (within the given space) with an opaque composite rather than an opaquer. If the composite alone can be used to lighten the tooth adequately, the gradual opaquing effect will give the resulting restoration lifelike depth. This concept has been discussed in relation to porcelain crown fabrication by McLean (1979) and by others. McLean states, "Natural teeth always exhibit and permit diffuse and regular transmission of light." The use of a strong opaque layer will eliminate most light transmission and thus reduce the lifelike character of the composite veneer. This is due in part to the highly reflective nature of the opaquer. If this layer is too close to the tooth surface, almost total light reflection occurs, reducing the possibility of diffraction or transmission of light rays. The net result is a flat and nontranslucent (artificial) appearance uncharacteristic of natural teeth.

I have developed a concept of *opaque zoning*, which will be described in the following text.

There are two components to opaque zoning. The first is to try to use opaquers (when they are absolutely necessary) very sparingly, using only enough opaquer to block 50 to 75 percent of the undesirable discoloration and remembering to keep the opaquer from pooling in the gingival sulcus and proximal regions. In addition, opaquer should be kept to a bare minimum on the incisal edge in order to maintain some translucency in this area.

The remainder of the opaquing of the undesirable discoloration is accomplished by choosing an *overlying composite* which has an adequate opaque "ranking" (i.e., has opaque particles incorporated in the shade). Frequently these composites are designated by the manufacturers with an "O" after the shade name (Silux UO;[2]Durafill GO[3]).

Thus the opaque zoning concept is one that allows for a gradual blocking of discoloration using two components to maximize the natural characteristics of light. By using the opaquer sparingly, one permits "bare spots" to remain to allow some light transmission through this layer. The remainder of the opaquing is easily achieved by means of the overlying composite. The optical result will be a tooth that has been raised in value, but at the same time has maintained the natural "depth" and appearance we desire.

This concept of using opaquer sparingly on the enamel surface and with an overlying opaque composite has worked successfully in a number of cases and is demonstrated later in this chapter in simplistic diagrams (see Figs. 5-39 and 5-40). The diagrammatic representation of the effect of light rays is an oversimplification; however, it allows for an understanding of the rationale to this approach.

The actual technique of "using opaquer sparingly" may vary. It can be accomplished by using diluted opaquers in two or three layers or by "stippling" of the opaque with a brush as it is applied and quickly polymerizing before it has a chance to coalesce. The "properly" opaqued layer should show a nonuniform blocking of the underlying discoloration. As long as some of the discoloration can be seen "bleeding through" the opaquer, light rays will be able to penetrate beyond this layer, thus promoting some diffuse transmission and diffraction. However, the overlying composite must have some opaquing quality to complete the blocking.

It is recognized that with greater composite depths, the routine concepts of porcelain crown fabrication could be utilized. If stronger dentin bonding agents are made available (Light Cured Scotchbond[4]), a deeper labial preparation (0.75 to 1 mm) could be performed. This would in essence be a labial composite "inlaying" technique. The additional room would allow for complete opaquing, and at the same time, the residual thickness would allow for enough overlying composite to maintain proper "depth" characteristics and natural optical quality.

CONCEPTS IN CREATING NATURAL TEETH

There are several technical "tips" which can assist the practitioner in creating a natural-looking veneer, especially when teeth are to be whitened. Since the whitening of teeth frequently makes them appear more "prominent", we should consider methods to make them less so.

Since all teeth are not monochromatic, the concept of *multiple shading* becomes important (Goldstein, 1976). This "stratifying of shades" is accomplished by using at least two shades of composite: a yellower shade in the gingival and a lighter shade in the body. A third shade can be used as an incisal shade as well. This stratifying technique tends to reduce the intensity of teeth that are whitened with opaquer and opaque composites.

A second method of decreasing the dominance of whitened teeth is by *texturing* the surface of the veneer. In this manner, the reflected light is "broken" into small increments of reflection as opposed to a single flat reflective surface. The inclusion of surface texture not only mimics natural tooth structure more closely, but tends to greatly reduce the dull nature of veneers with high value rankings. Both stratifying and surface texture are demonstrated in included Figures 5-14, 5-62. They are an important aspect in whitening teeth while still maintaining acceptable optical results. These methods can be predictably applied with some practice.

Another effective concept is the idea of *"coupling"* two different types of composite materials in order to achieve the best characteristics of both materials. Some clinicians term this approach the "light on heavy" technique. I prefer the term "sandwiching", which refers to the use of a microfilled composite material in association with a macrofill or hybrid.

For a long time, however, practitioners have had some difficulty establishing a "rule of thumb" for proportioning these composites, i.e., "how much light and how much heavy?" A technique has evolved which successfully simplifies the decision-making process.

First, a basic concept was developed for classifying which composites are light and which are heavy. The classification system is therefore reduced to two groups: microfills and non-microfills. The nonmicrofills include macrofilled and hybrid composite systems (see Chapter 1). With this simple classification, it becomes easy to apply the rule, which is: *All microfill composites are considered as synthetic "enamel". All nonmicrofills are the synthetic "dentin".*

Therefore, when rebuilding a fractured tooth, the dentist would choose the appropriate materials to *anatomically* restructure the tooth. This means that the missing *dentin* portions of the tooth are rebuilt with the *nonmicrofill* and the *enamel* (with one exception) is rebuilt with the *microfill*. Since microfills are basically used for esthetics (polishability), it is not necessary to place them on the lingual surfaces unless desired for possible reduced wear.

This idea of observing a tooth and then deciding simply how much dentin and how much enamel is needed simplifies the decision-making process. Therefore, we would correct a diastema mostly by using a small-particle macrofill (Prismafil;[5] Command[6]) or hybrid (Aurafil[13] or Command Ultrafine[7]) and "glaze" with microfill (Silux;[8] Certain[9]). Owing to the better index of refraction of the nonmicrofills, the possibility of shine-through is reduced. In addition, there is less chance of stress fractures that are so common with microfills. With the "sandwich" technique, shade matching is easier, the restorations are stronger, and they appear more lifelike. This approach is also useful with large class III and V restorations, not only giving a better esthetic result, but also, owing to the sparse use of microfill material, reducing the polymerization shrinkage.

CASE DESCRIPTIONS

Figure 5-1 shows a maxillary left central incisor devitalized as the result of previous trauma in a 24-year-old patient. Owing to the narrow nature of the canal, a retrofill procedure was performed successfully. The tooth, however, remained yellow. Since no endodontic access was available for internal bleaching and to conserve remaining tooth structure, full composite labial veneering was performed using Durafill GO[3] in combination with Estilux Color Modifiers.[10]

Figure 5-2 shows a close-up view of the affected tooth prior to restoration. After enamelplasty (i.e., labial chamfer preparation), the tooth appears as shown in Figure 5-3. A polyethylene strip is used to protect the adjacent teeth from the effects of phosphoric acid etching (Fig. 5-4). A thin layer of bond resin (Durafill Bond[11]) was applied to the etched enamel surface by means of a soft brush (Fig. 5-5), and the bond resin layer was thinned with air (Fig. 5-6). A layer of opaquer (Estilux Color Modifiers[10])(consisting of yellow-red 30% mixed with white 70%) was carefully applied to the labial surface to ensure the absence of "pooling" in the gingival crevice region (Fig. 5-7). The placement of opaquer over the incisal region must be avoided in order to maintain translucency in this area. The microfilled composite material (Durafill GO[3]) was applied in bulk to the labial region (Fig. 5-8) and the proximal areas properly formed using Mylar strips (Fig. 5-9). After proper light cure, the labial composite restoration should demonstrate tight proximal contacts (Fig. 5-10) and, viewed from the incisal (Fig. 5-11), proper bulk. Finish was carried out (Fig. 5-12) by means of the technique previously described (Chapter 3), and Figure 5-13 shows the properly contoured veneer just prior to texturing and final polishing. The finished composite restoration is shown in Figure 5-14. Full face views of the patient before (Fig. 5-15) and after treatment (Fig. 5-16) clearly demonstrate the markedly improved esthetics. In Figure 5-17 the flat emergence profile of the labial restoration is illustrated.

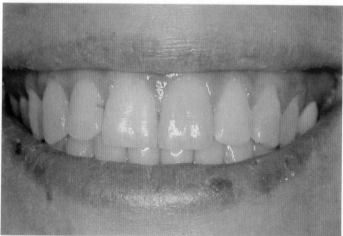

Figure 5-1 A discolored, nonvital maxillary left central incisor.

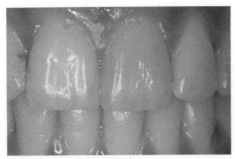

Figure 5-2 Close-up view of the central incisor shown in Figure 5-1 before restoration.

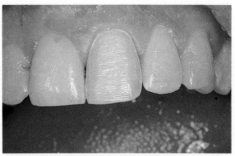

Figure 5-3 The tooth shown in Figures 5-1 and 5-2 after enamelplasty.

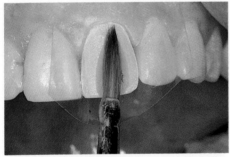

Figure 5-4 A polyethylene strip protects the adjacent teeth during acid etching.

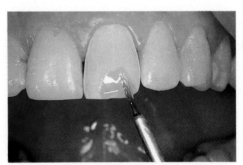

Figure 5-5 Application of bond resin.

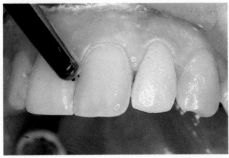

Figure 5-6 Gentle air blowing thins the bond resin layer.

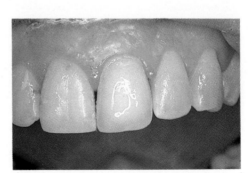

Figure 5-7 A thin layer of opaquer masks the discolored surface.

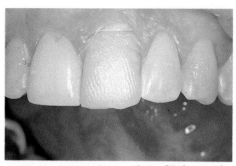

Figure 5-8 Bulk application of microfilled composite material to labial surface.

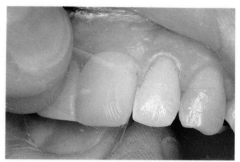

Figure 5-9 Proximal contour of microfilled composite formed with a mylar strip.

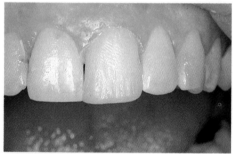

Figure 5-10 The microfilled composite material after light cure, labial view.

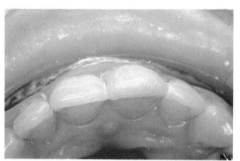

Figure 5-11 Incisal view of composite build-up.

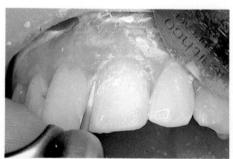

Figure 5-12 Removal of gross excess by means of tapering abrasive instrument.

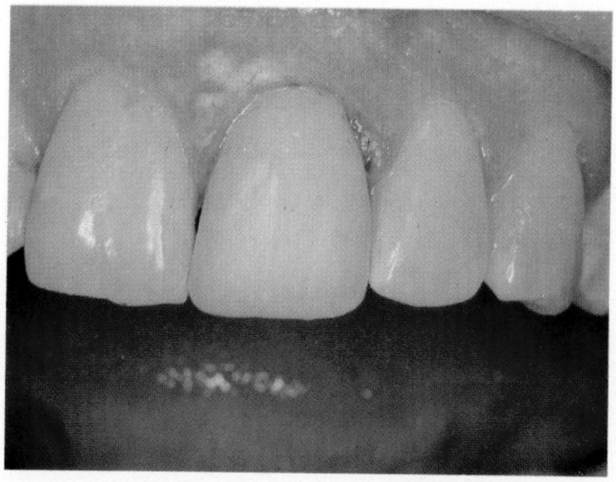

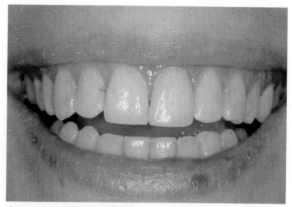

Figure 5-13   Finished labial composite restoration before texturing and final polish.

Figure 5-14   Final microfilled restoration in relation to high lip line.

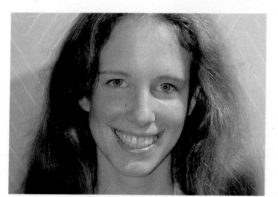

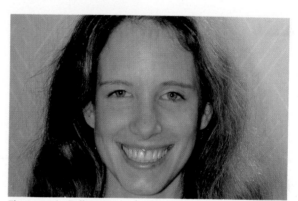

Figure 5-15   Full preoperative face view.

Figure 5-16   Full postoperative face view.

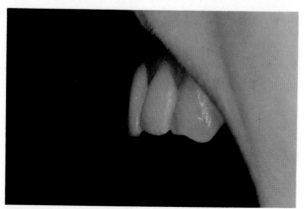

Figure 5-17   Flat emergence profile of labial veneer restoration.

Figure 5-18 shows maxillary central incisors in a 30-year-old patient with hypercalcification and brown fluorosis staining. After the removal of 0.5 mm of labial enamel and acid etching, an opaque shade of light-cured, microfilled composite (Silux UO²) was bulk-packed over the labial surface (Fig. 5-19). This particular material, being of low viscosity, is particularly amenable to a contouring technique using a dry, sable artist's brush (Fig. 5-20), whereby the material may be shaped and formed by means of a delicate manipulation technique so that very little

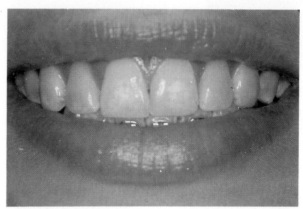

Figure 5-18   Maxillary central incisors with hypercalcification and brown fluorosis stain.

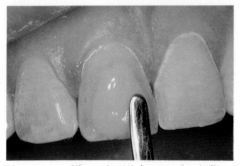

Figure 5-19   Silux microfilled composite bulk-packed over prepared enamel surface.

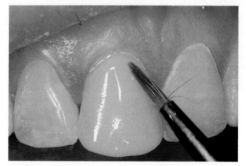

Figure 5-20   Contouring the microfilled composite with dry sable brush.

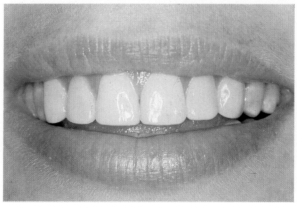

Figure 5-21   Final microfilled composite labial restoration.

gingival finishing is required. The final restorations (Fig. 5-21) demonstrate textured labial surfaces which break up the light, resulting in a lifelike appearance (Fig. 5-22).

Exactly the same technique and material were utilized to restore the central incisors of the patient shown in Figure 5-23. The postoperative result is shown in Figure 5-24.

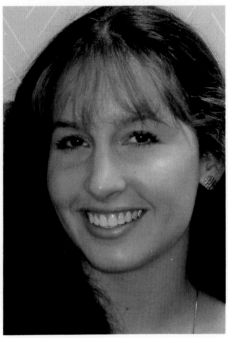

Figure 5-22   Full face view.

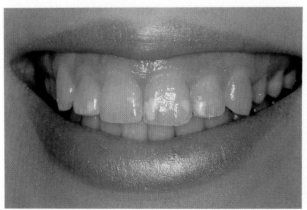

Figure 5-23   Preoperative view of discolored central incisors.

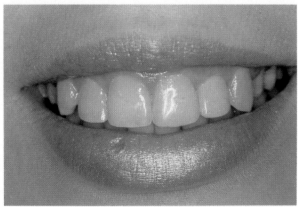

Figure 5-24   Postoperative view of veneered central incisors.

Another case of a nonvital discolored left central incisor (Fig. 5-25) was successfully treated by means of controlled enamelplasty, with Durafill GO[3] veneering in combination with Estilux Color Modifiers.[10]

A profile view of the enamelplasty is shown in Figure 5-26. A labial view of the prepared enamel surface is shown in Figure 5-27. After the labial surface was etched, washed, and dried, opaque (Estilux Color Modifiers[10]) was applied (Fig. 5-28) in the following proportions: 80 percent white / 20 percent yellow-red. A small amount of blue tint (Command Tints[12]) was placed over the incisal region. The finished restoration is shown in Figure 5-29.

Anterior teeth that have darkened with age and years of smoking (Fig. 5-30) may be esthetically veneered by means of enamelplasty in combination with an opaque microfilled material Silux UO[2] (Fig. 5-31).

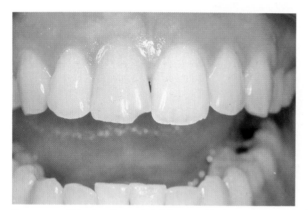

Figure 5-25   Discolored, nonvital right central incisor.

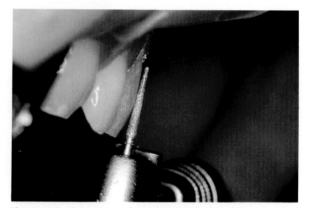

Figure 5-26   Orientation of tapering diamond instru enamelplasty.

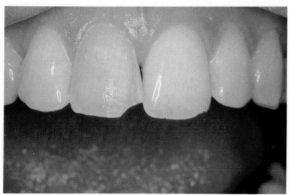

Figure 5-27   Prepared enamel surface.

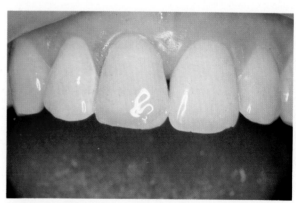

Figure 5-28   Opaquer layer consisting of Estilux Color Modifiers[10].

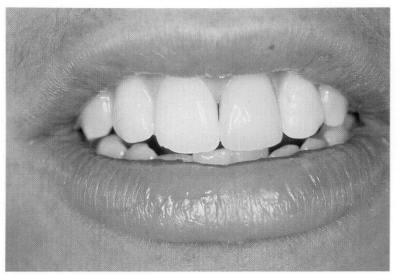

Figure 5-29 Completed labial restoration.

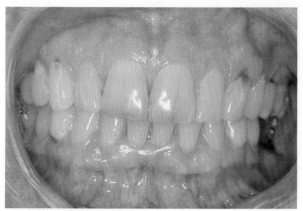

Figure 5-30 Anterior teeth darkened with age and years of smoking.

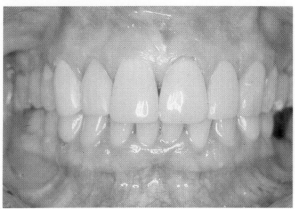

Figure 5-31 The teeth shown in Figure 5-30 after veneering with Silux UO².

Abrasion-erosion involvement of the anterior teeth not only is unsightly (Fig. 5-32 and 5-33), but in addition the associated thermal sensitivity as a result of exposed dentin creates much discomfort for the patient. Direct labial veneer restorations (Fig. 5-34) using a microfilled material (Durafill GO[3]) without opaquer not only provide an excellent esthetic result (Figs. 5-35 and 5-36), but also markedly reduce the sensitivity. Usually there is no need for enamel-plasty in such cases of labial erosion (Figs. 5-37 and 5-38).

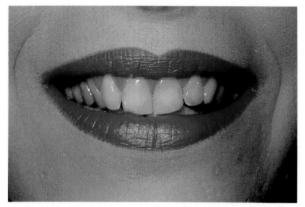

Figure 5-32   Anterior teeth involved with abrasion-erosion.

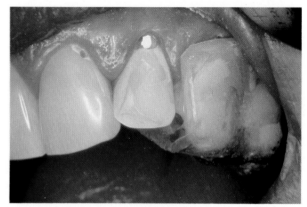

Figure 5-33   Close-up view of the maxillary left lateral incisor.

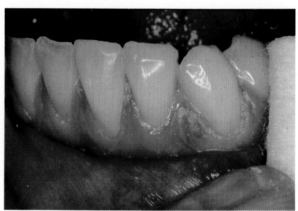

Figure 5-34   Direct labial veneer restorations, mandibular anteriors.

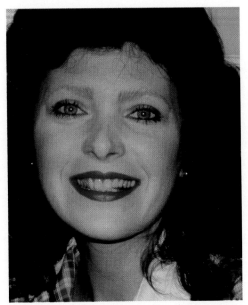

Figure 5-35 Full face view preoperatively.

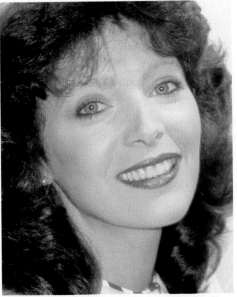

Figure 5-36 Full face view postoperatively after direct veneering.

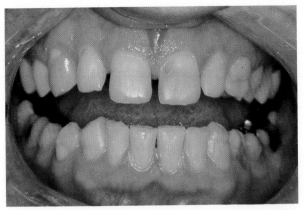

Figure 5-37 Preoperative view of labially eroded anterior teeth.

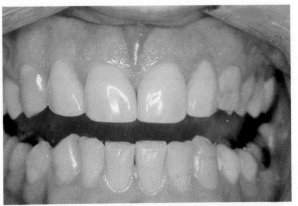

Figure 5-38 Postoperative view of eroded anterior teeth after placement of direct Durafil veneers (without enamelplasty).

The concept of *zone opaquing* involves the use of minimal opaquer together with an overlying opaque composite material, thereby maintaining depth and lifelike quality of the restorations while altering the color significantly. Figure 5-39 shows schematically the effect of large amounts of opaquer applied to a discolored surface. Light rays are fully reflected from the opaqued surface, thereby giving a dull lifeless opaque appearance to the restoration. On the other hand, Figure 5-40 shows schematically the effect of the opaque zone theory. A minimal amount of opaquer covered with an overlying opaque composite masks out the discoloration, but also allows a sufficient amount of light to penetrate the opaqued area, thereby resulting in a lifelike appearance. The practical application of the concept is illustrated in Figure 5-41, which shows a tetracycline-stained maxillary lateral incisor which was treated using a minimal amount of opaquer (Estilux Color Modifiers[10]) with an overlying opaque composite (Durafill GO[3]). The lifelike quality of the veneer restoration is shown in Figure 5-42. A preoperative view of a patient with dark yellow teeth and abraded gingival composite restorations is shown in Figure 5-43. Labial veneer restorations were placed (Fig. 5-44) using Durafill GO[3] in combination with Estilux White Color Modifiers.[10] Too much opaquer was utilized too close to the surface. In addition, the composite shade utilized was too translucent. Figure 5-45 shows a tetracycline case that was properly "whitened" using Silux Shade UO[2] (Shade L on the incisal) without an underlying opaque layer. Using the "zone opaque" concept, it is best to allow some of the discoloration to "bleed through", especially in the gingival region.

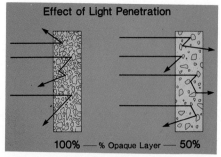

Figure 5–39 Diagrammatic illustration showing the effect of full opaquing (*left*) resulting in total light reflection, whereas partial opaquing (*right*) results in some translucence.

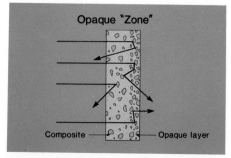

Figure 5–40 "Opaque zoning", i.e., minimal opaquer covered with opaque composite, masks discoloration, but allows some light penetration with resultant "lifelike" appearance.

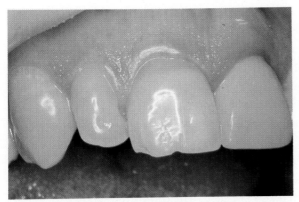

Figure 5–41 Tetracycline-stained maxillary lateral incisor to be zone opaqued.

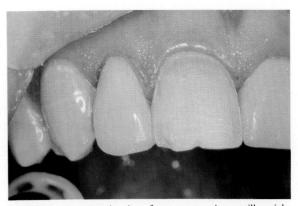

Figure 5–42 Postoperative view of veneer restoration maxillary right lateral incisor.

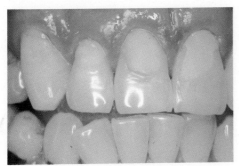

Figure 5–43 Preoperative view of dark yellow teeth with gingival composite restorations.

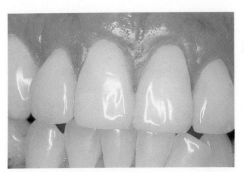

Figure 5–44 Postoperative view of the teeth shown in Figure 5-43 over-opaqued.

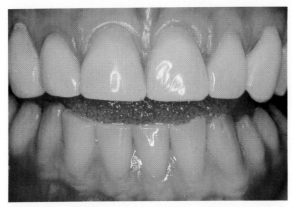

Figure 5–45 Properly "zone-opaqued" maxillary anterior teeth after direct veneering.

Incisal restorations, particularly involving teeth which are relatively thin labiolingually (Fig. 5-46), can be restored with a more natural look using a "sandwich" technique in combination with surface texturing of the resin material. This is particularly helpful when whitening teeth in reducing the harshness of the opacifying materials. In the sandwich technique, a "basic" layer of small-particle macrofilled or hybrid (Aurafil[13]) composite is placed (Fig. 5-47) and then overlaid with microfill (Durafill GO[3])(Fig. 5-48). The resulting "sandwich" restoration with proper surface texture to blend with the surface characteristics of the natural tooth is shown in Figure 5-49. A further illustration of the "sandwich" or "light on heavy" technique is applied to the "peg" lateral incisor shown in Figure 5-50. The crown is partially built up using a "dentin" composite material (Aurafil[13]) (Fig. 5-51) over which "enamel" composite (Silux[8]) was placed and polished. The completed sandwich restoration (Fig. 5-52) will be followed by placement of a resin bonded retainer to replace the maxillary canine (see Chapter 8).

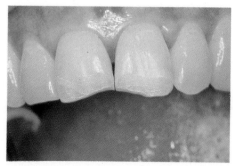

Figure 5–46   Incisal fracture of thin maxillary central incisor.

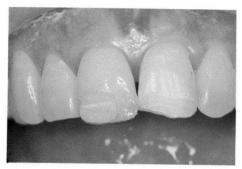

Figure 5–47   Incisal build-up with nonmicrofill composite.

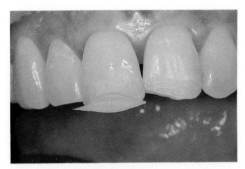

Figure 5-48 Microfill overlay.

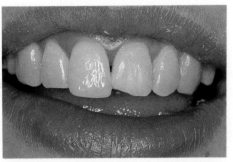

Figure 5-49 Sandwich composite restoration maxillary right central incisor with proper surface texturing.

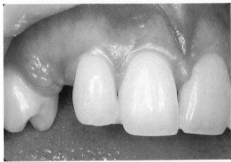

Figure 5-50 A ''peg lateral'' maxillary right incisor bonded to the central incisor after orthodontic treatment.

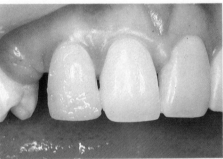

Figure 5-51 Crown build-up using nonmicrofill material (Aurafil⁷).

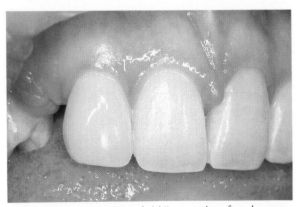

Figure 5-52 Completed ''sandwich'' restoration after placement and finish of microfilled material.

PART TWO
DIRECT COMPOSITE VENEERS
USED WITH OPAQUERS
AND "STRATIFICATION"
TECHNIQUES

The problem in direct composite veneering with stained teeth is that the composite alone cannot always mask out completely the undesirable discoloration. Opaquers are necessary and can be utilized for masking out stained tooth structure. However, once opaquers are used they create several problems. They may (1) result in a "lifeless" veneer, (2) set limitations on the thickness of the composite veneer, and/or (3) affect the color of the final veneer.

The foregoing problems compare to "opaquer" problems found in porcelain-fused-to-metal restorations. However, in preparing a tooth to receive a porcelain-fused-to-metal restoration, labial or buccal reduction is usually 1.5 mm. This reduction allows for a metal coping thickness of 0.3 to 0.4 mm, opaquer 0.1 to 0.2 mm, and up to 1.0 mm of body and incisal porcelain to overcome the opaquer problems and achieve a natural-looking restoration. In direct composite veneer techniques, the operator seldom has the luxury of such extensive space. As a conservative esthetic approach, these restorations have necessarily been performed on enamel, when possible, in order to attain the most retentive bond. Unfortunately, the labial enamel thickness is considerably less than 1.5 mm especially near the cemento-enamel (c-e) junction. With such a limitation of available space, creating an esthetic result constitutes quite a challenge for the dentist.

In a natural tooth, light penetration undergoes reflection, transmission, and absorption by the enamel. Enamel is colorless and the tooth color is derived from the pigments found in the dentin. The color projects through the enamel via a sophisticated network of rods and interprismatic material. A certain thickness of enamel is necessary for a natural tooth to demonstrate vitality. When a translucent composite, such as a microfill, is placed over the labial surface of a tooth, the final color is a combination of natural tooth color and the material. This usually appears very natural. However, once an opaquer is introduced into the system, light penetration terminates at the opaque layer resulting at times in an artificial-looking restoration, i.e., "shine-through". The problem, therefore, relates to how the operator overcomes the discoloration and creates a successful result with direct composite veneers within a limited space. The essential principle is not to overopaque. Opaquing out 50 to 75 percent of the discoloration, then relying on an opaque composite for additional masking, reduces the flatness and artificiality in composite veneers. By not completely opaquing out, light rays are allowed to penetrate into the tooth, resulting in a more vital restoration. For light to mild discolorations, such as yellow to yellow-browns, the entire veneer can be performed and completed on an enamel base. On the other hand, with severe tetracycline discolorations, such as the violets and dark grays, *preparation into the dentin* may be required, especially in the cervical one-third, to attain a natural result.

To increase the natural appearance of the veneer, I advocate the stratification of three or more composites of different colors. The basic three are cervical, body, and incisal, stratified one on top of the other. Additional characterization can be added with the use of tints over the opaquers and under the composite.

The best way to predict the final result is to perform a "test veneer" prior to enamel preparation or isolation with rubber dam. The tooth is pumiced, the opaquer(s) is placed and cured, and then the composite is placed and cured. After allowing rehydration to occur in the mouth for 2 to 3 minutes, carefully evaluate for proper color blend.

CASE DESCRIPTIONS

The following cases illustrate the use of opaquers in conjunction with the stratification of multiple colors of composite.

1. *Case 1, moderate brown discoloration (Fig. 5-53).* After enamelplasty a layer of Silux[14] opaquer was placed followed by composite stratification involving a *gingival* layer of Silux DY[8], a *body* layer of Silux G[8], and an *incisal* layer of Silux U[8] (Fig. 5-54). A marked improvement in appearance followed the placement of the stratified veneer restorations (Figs. 5-55 and 5-56).

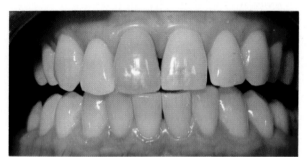

Figure 5-53 Preoperative appearance of moderate brown discoloration of the maxillary anterior dentition.

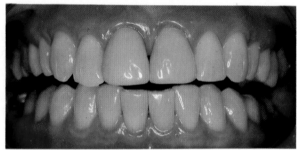

Figure 5-54 The anterior dentition shown in Figure 5-53 after veneering by means of the "stratification" technique.

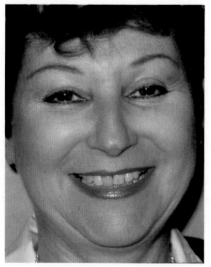

Figure 5-55 Full face view preoperatively.

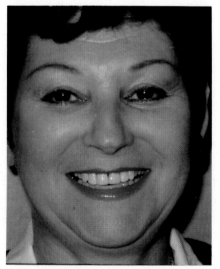

Figure 5-56 Full face view postoperatively.

2 . *Case 2, moderate tetracycline discoloration (Fig. 5-57).* The following stratification was used after two layers of Silux Opaquer[14]: gingival layer, Silux Shade G;[8] body layer, Silux Shade L;[8] and incisal layer, Silux Shade XL[8]. Although the appearance was greatly improved (Fig. 5-58), overopaquing resulted in a somewhat artificial result (Figs. 5-59 and 5-60).

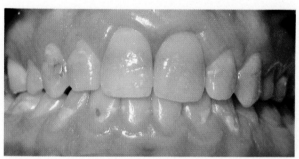

Figure 5-57 Preoperative appearance of moderate tetracycline discoloration.

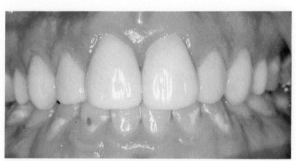

Figure 5-58 Postoperative view of composite veneer restorations.

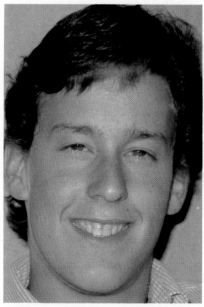

Figure 5-59 Full face view preoperatively.

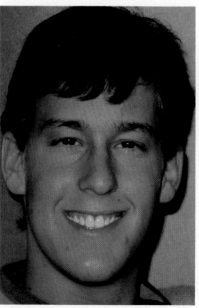

Figure 5-60 Full face view postoperatively.

3. *Case 3, moderate tetracycline discoloration (Fig. 5-61).* Opaquers and tints were utilized in combination with a stratification technique in the following order: (1) a layer of white Estilux Opaquer[10] was placed gingivally followed by a layer of white mixed with yellow-brown; (2) Light Gray Estilux Opaquer[10] was placed toward the incisal; (3) Durafill Tints were then used in the following order: incisal–gray and blue tints; interproximal—yellow-brown tint; and (4) a layer of YO Durafill composite was placed gingivally, a layer of GO (Gray Opaque) Durafill composite was placed on the body, and finally a layer of G (Gray) Durafill composite was placed toward the incisal (Fig. 5-62). A natural appearance of the veneer restorations markedly improved the esthetic result (Figs. 5-63 and 5-64).

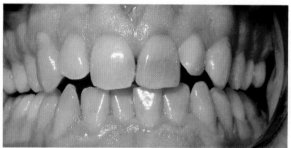

Figure 5-61 Preoperative appearance of moderate tetracycline discoloration.

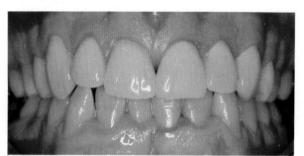

Figure 5-62 Postoperative appearance of the stratified composite veneers.

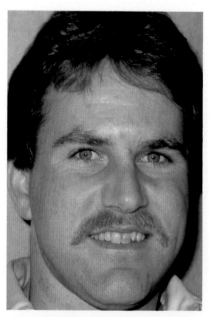

Figure 5-63 Full face view preoperatively.

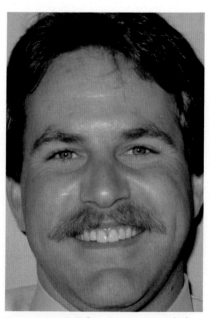

Figure 5-64 Full face view postoperatively.

The basic stratification technique using three composite colors is sequentially illustrated in Figures 5-65 through 5-69 on an extracted natural tooth:

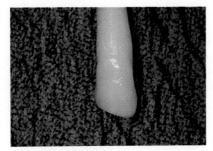

Figure 5-65   Preoperative view.

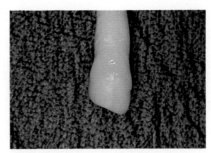

Figure 5-66   Gingival (Silux DY[8]).

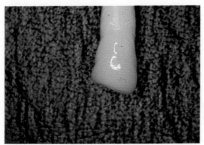

Figure 5-67   Body (Silux Y[8]).

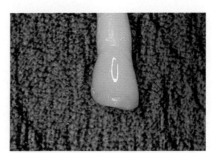

Figure 5-68   Incisal (Durafil L[11]).

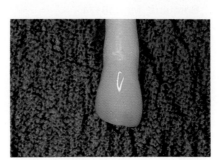

Figure 5-69   Final result of stratification.

References

Goldstein R. Esthetics in Dentistry. Philadelphia: JB Lippincott, 1976.
Kuwata M. Theory and Practise for Ceramomental Restorations. Chicago: Quintessence Co, 1980.
McLean JW. The Science and Art of Dental Ceramics. Chicago: Quintessence Co, 1979.
Preston JD, Bergen SF. Color Science and Dental Art. St. Louis: CV Mosby Co, 1980.

Product Information

Product	Manufacturer/Distributor	Purpose
1. Scotchbond	Dental Products/3M Company 3M Center 270–5N–02 St. Paul, MN 55144	Self-cured, dentin bonding agent
2. Silux UO	Dental Products/3M Company 3M Center 270–5N–02 St. Paul, MN 55144	Opaque microfilled composite
3. Durafill GO	Kulzer Inc. 10015 Muirlands Blvd., Unit G Irvine, CA 92714	Opaque microfilled composite
4. Light Cured Scotchbond	Dental Products/3M Company 3M Center 270–5N–02 St. Paul, MN 55144	Visible-light-cured dentin bonding agent
5. Prismafil	L.D. Caulk Co. P.O. Box 359 Milford, DE 19963	Small-particle, macrofilled composite material
6. Command	Kerr-Sybron Co. P.O. Box 455 Romulus, MI 48174	Small-particle, macrofilled composite material
7. Command Ultrafine	Kerr-Sybron Co. P.O.Box 455 Romulus, MI 48174	Hybrid-type composite material
8. Silux	Dental Products/3M Company 3M Center 270–5N–02 St. Paul, MN 55144	Light-cured, microfilled composite
9. Certain	Johnson and Johnson 20 Lake Drive, CN7060 East Windsor, NJ 08520	Light-cured, microfilled composite
10. Estilux Color Modifiers	Kulzer Inc. 10015 Muirlands Blvd., Unit G Irvine, CA 92714	Opaquer materials for masking discoloration
11. Durafill Bond	Kulzer Inc. 10015 Muirlands Blvd., Unit G Irvine, CA 92714	Light-cured bond resin
12. Command Tints	Kerr-Sybron Co. P.O. Box 455 Romulus, MI 48174	Tint for incisal translucency
13. Aurafil	Johnson and Johnson 20 Lake Drive, CN7060 East Windsor, NJ 08520	Small-particle, macrofilled composite material
14. Silux Opaquer	Dental Products/3M Company 3M Center 270–5N–02 St. Paul, MN 55144	Composite opaquer
15. Durafill L	Kulzer Inc. 10015 Muirlands Blvd., Unit G Irvine, CA 92714	Light-cured, microfilled composite

6

RONALD E. JORDAN

DENTIN BONDING

Dentin bonding differs from enamel bonding in many important respects. In the first instance, enamel may be easily and safely rendered *micromechanically self-retentive* by means of the simple surface application of phosphoric acid. The same is not true of dentin. Although acid treatment of dentin does in fact widen the dentin tubules (Fig. 6-1), thus providing some opportunity for resin tag entry (Fig. 6-2), it must be remembered that such a procedure results in pulp irritation (Eriksen, 1976; Stanley et al, 1975). On the other hand, pulp insult with enamel bonding is virtually unknown, but it presents a real potential problem in dentin bonding. Accordingly, it is imperative that materials be used which chemically bond to dentin without irritation to the underlying pulp. Dentin bonding materials which chemically bond to tooth structure are therefore of a great deal of current clinical interest.

Dentin bonding is of tremendous significance in restorative dentistry. Long-term clinical observations (Jordan et al, 1977) have documented clearly that enamel bonding procedures are ultraconservative, highly reliable, and biologically innocuous. In the event that dentin bonding is eventually rendered equally reliable, the entire conceptual basis of restorative dentistry will undergo significant change (Bowen et al, 1982). The reason for this is that, until recently, the fundamental approach to retention of restorative materials has been almost completely dependent on the resistance retention form of box-type undercut cavity preparation procedures, which invariably result in extensive sacrifice of sound tooth structure. The necessity for this has been dictated by the fact that few if any restorative materials bond reliably to tooth structure. Should materials be developed that in fact bond to both enamel and dentin mechanically and/or chemically, the textbooks relating to restorative dentistry will have to be rewritten since teeth may be restored in the future using infinitely more conservative techniques than have ever been used in the past.

Dentin bonding systems include both *resin* and *glass ionomer* materials.

RESIN DENTIN BONDING AGENTS

Resin dentin bonding is currently in its infancy. Since resin dentin bonding agents have only been used clinically for short periods, long-term clinical recall data relative to their reliability are not yet available.

Typical dentin bonding agents (Scotchbond[1]) are composed of a phosphorus ester of Bis-GMA dissolved in a volatile solvent such as alcohol, which acts as a wetting agent. The resin may be either autopolymerized or light cured. Whichever is used, it must be kept in mind that all dentin bonding agents have limitations. Although some very promising research is currently being conducted relative to the future development of strong dentin bonding materials (Bowen et al, 1982), it is a known fact that the bond of currently available materials to dentin is *a relatively weak one* in comparison to the bond to acid-etched enamel (Table 6-1). A carefully controlled clinical technique therefore must be utilized in order to ensure a predictable level of success.

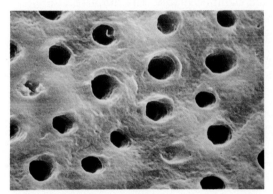

Figure 6–1 Scanning electron micrograph (2000 ×) of widened dentin tubules following phosphoric acid etching. (Courtesy of Dr. A. J. Gwinnett, State University of New York at Stony Brook.)

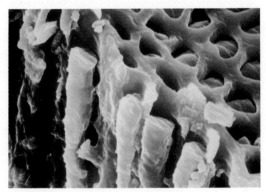

Figure 6–2 Scanning electron micrograph (2000 ×) showing columns of resin entering dentin tubules expanded by phosphoric acid etching. (Courtesy of Dr. A. J. Gwinnett, State University of New York at Stony Brook.)

TABLE 6–1 Adhesion (Shear) Values of Bonding Agents and Composite Materials (kg/cm^2)

	Dentin	Unetched Enamel	Etched Enamel
Concise[21]/Enamel Bond[22]	—	—	125
Concise[21]/Enamel Bond[22]	38.6	70.6	144
Silar[23]/Scotchbond[1]	42.1	89.5	200
Silux[2]/Scotchbond[1]	58.2	66.	218
P-30[11]/Scotchbond[1]	54.2	—	280

Data provided by 3M Co., St. Paul, MN

Conservative Restoration of A Cervical Erosion Lesion Using a Self-Cured Dentin Bonding Agent (Scotchbond[1]) with a Light-Cured Microfilled Composite Material (Silux[2])

A typical cervical erosion is illustrated in Figure 6-3. The occlusal margin is usually located in enamel and the gingival in cementum.

One of the most important considerations in the clinical technique is to secure positive control over the gingival-cemental interface. The free crest of the gingival tissue is usually in close adaptive contact with the cemental margin of the lesion. Because of the hydrophobic nature of the bonding materials, it is mandatory to displace the gingival tissues away from the cemental margin of the lesion, not only to acquire proper access, but also to prevent crevicular fluid contamination of the field of operation. In order to accomplish this goal, there are several clinical approaches that may be taken, such as the use of electrosurgery or gingival retraction cord. Probably the most effective, however, is the use of a properly placed gingival retraction clamp (Fig. 6-4). The gingival retraction clamp gently retracts the gingival tissues away from the field of operation, thereby providing unimpeded access to a clean operative field. There are several types of retraction clamp available. The simplest, a single wing clamp (Brinker B–4[3]), provides excellent results in cases where the gingival margin of the lesion is approximately level with the free crest of the gingival tissues. Situations in which the cervical margin of the lesion is subgingival call for a properly stabilized double-winged retraction clamp (Ivory 212 S.A.[4]) for adequate retraction (Fig. 6-5).

The cervical region should be thoroughly cleaned by use of a pumice slurry and then washed and dried. The cervical area is then swabbed with a cotton pledget soaked in 3 percent hydrogen peroxide for 8 to 10 seconds (Fig. 6-6), and this is followed by a thorough water lavage. Hydrogen peroxide loosens the superficial debris, thereby creating a clean surface for bonding.

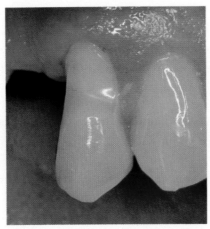

Figure 6-3 Preoperative view of a cervical erosion on the maxillary right first premolar.

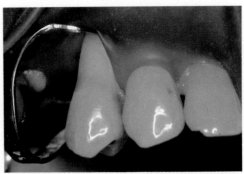

Figure 6-4 Proper isolation of the field by means of rubber dam and gingival retraction clamp application.

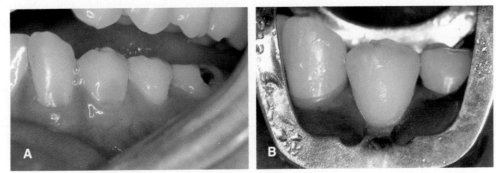

Figure 6-5 *A*, Cervical erosion lesion in the mandibular first premolar. The lesion extends subgingivally by 0.5 millimeter. *B*, After isolation with gingival retraction clamp and restoration.

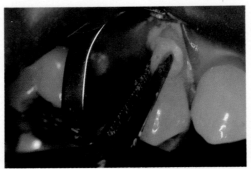

Figure 6-6 Application of hydrogen peroxide.

In the event that the dentin is sclerotic and highly reflective (see Fig. 6-3), it should be lightly stoned (Fig. 6-7) by means of a fine diamond instrument (Douglas, 1982). The "smear" layer thus produced (Fig. 6-8) consists essentially of a gelatinous surface layer of coagulated protein, 0.5 to 15 microns in thickness, which is thought to enhance the efficacy of the dentin bond by creating a "high-energy" surface layer relatively free of dentin fluid contamination. Although the opposite view has also been reported, namely, that the smear layer should be carefully removed prior to bonding (Brannstrom and Johnson, 1974; Brannstrom et al, 1979; Brannstrom et al, 1980), such a procedure is not necessarily applicable to the resin dentin bonding agents (Douglas, 1982).

Considerable doubt currently exists relative to the necessity for further tooth preparation with the resin dentin bonding materials mainly because of the short-term nature of such systems. It should be kept in mind that the bond value of such materials to acid-etched enamel is almost four times the dentin bond value (see Table 6-1). Accordingly, in order to clinically enhance the reliability of the resin bond, a long bevel on the occlusal enamel is strongly recommended (Fig. 6-9). As a further precaution, a shallow undercut slot should be placed in the axiogingival dentin in order to mechanically "lock" the restorative material tightly (Fig. 6-10) to the cervical area.

Pulp protection is normally not required unless the cervical erosion is extremely deep and the remaining dentin thickness overlying the pulp is minimal (Dogon, 1982). Should such be the case, a layer of acid-resistant calcium hydroxide (Prisma VLC Dycal[26]) should be placed over the deepest portion of the dentin in order to protect the pulp. It is mandatory to phosphoric acid-etch the *enamel* periphery, but considerable care must be taken to ensure that the acid does not contact the dentin or severe pulpal irritation may ensue (Aida et al, 1980) and the dentin bond value is decreased (Douglas, 1982). Accordingly, a viscous gel etchant should be carefully applied to the enamel by means of a plastic instrument or a syringe (Fig. 6-11). The high-viscosity nature of the gel prevents flow of the etchant material over the dentinal tissue.

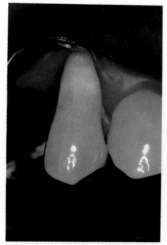

Figure 6-7 Sclerotic dentin surface after light stoning with a diamond instrument.

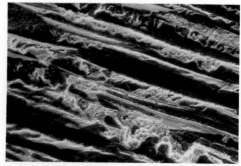

Figure 6-8 Scanning electron micrograph (400 ×) of smear layer resulting from application of diamond instrument to dentin. (Courtesy of Dr. A. J. Gwinnett, State University of New York at Stony Brook.)

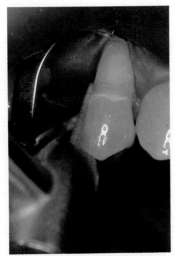

Figure 6-9 Long-bevel preparation on occlusal enamel.

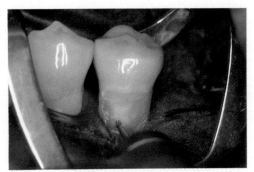

Figure 6-10 Placement of an axiogingival slot.

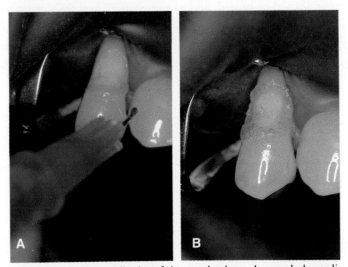

Figure 6-11 Syringe application of viscous gel etchant, *A*, controls the application of phosphoric acid, *B*.

The gel etchant should be left undisturbed on the enamel surface for one minute, after which a copious water lavage, applied for 30 to 45 seconds (Gwinnett, 1978), is used to thoroughly clean the area. After careful air drying, the acid-etched enamel surface should present a frosty white opaque appearance (Fig. 6-12). Care must be taken, particularly at this point, to ensure moisture-free conditions since the enamel-dentin surfaces are most sensitive to contamination from saliva or crevicular fluid.

Dentin bonding materials may be either self-cured (Scotchbond;[1] Creation Bond;[24] J & J Dentin Bond[25]) or visible-light-cured (Light Cured Scotchbond;[5] Bondlite;[20] Prisma Universal Bond[18]). The former are two component systems consisting of "resin A" and "liquid B" (Table 6-2). A drop of each is placed in a well and mixed for 3 to 6 seconds. A small droplet of the mixed bond resin is picked up on the end of a soft fine-tipped brush and carefully "thin-spread" over the enamel (Fig. 6-13), dentin, and cemental surfaces, being careful to avoid "puddling" or gross excess application of the material. Subsequent to initial application with the brush, the bond resin should be gently blown with warm air in order to confirm the thin-spread nature of the application and also to volatilize the alcohol wetting agent within the bonding material. Depending on the particular product used, a minimum of one coat of dentin bond resin should be placed, and two successive coats are usually recommended. Manufacturers' directions should be followed in this regard. Most dentin bond resins are "anaerobically polymerized", that is, after application they do not polymerize until they are covered with composite material (Fig. 6-14). The phenomenon is sometimes referred to as "air inhibition".

TABLE 6-2 Scotchbond Constituents

Resin A	Liquid B
Phosphorus Ester of Bis-GMA	Sodium Benze Sulfinate
Diluent Resin	Aromatic Amine
Benzoyl Peroxide	Ethyl Alcohol

Data provided by 3M Co., St. Paul, MN

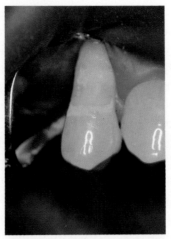

Figure 6-12 Appearance of enamel after phosphoric acid etching.

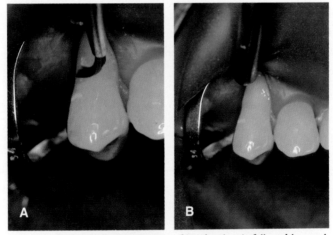

Figure 6-13 Thin spread application of bond resin, *A*, followed by gentle air blowing, *B*.

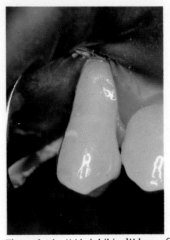

Figure 6-14 ''Air-inhibited'' layer of bonding resin.

In the event that the occlusal margin of the erosion lesion is located in enamel and the gingival margin is in cementum, a two-increment build-up of composite material should be utilized. Should the entire cervical contour be built up with a single increment of composite material, polymerization shrinkage may draw the composite material away from the cemental and dentinal regions, thereby leaving a "contraction gap" (Davidson and de Gee, 1984) in this area (Fig. 6-15). The two-increment technique minimizes this possibility (Dogon, 1982). The first increment of composite should be placed to cover the dentin on the axial wall (Fig. 6-16), then visible-light cured for a 30-second period, after which an air-inhibited layer is observed on the surface (Fig. 6-17). A second increment of composite is then placed over the first, using a suitable composite instrument (Fig. 6-18) to shape and form the material to proper contour. A sable brush is highly useful in further contouring the composite material (Fig. 6-19). During placement of the second composite increment, care should be taken to avoid overfilling the gingival margin (Fig. 6-20). If overfilling occurs, extreme difficulty may be encountered in finishing gross excess in the cervical region, and "ditching" of the cementum commonly results. A final cure is attained by means of a 40-second application of visible light. In some instances, manufacturers recommend delaying the onset of finishing procedures for approximately 5 minutes. Finishing of the composite material should be accomplished by means of tapered multifluted carbide finishing burs (ET–6 or ET–9[6]) to remove gross excess (Fig. 6-21). This is followed by use of 3/8-inch aluminum oxide finishing discs (Soflex Discs[7]),

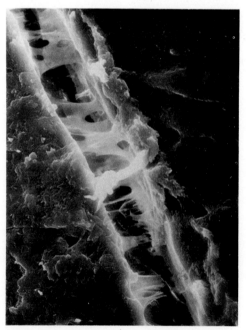

Figure 6–15 Scanning electron micrograph (1,000 ×) of composite dentin interface showing "contraction gap". (Courtesy of Dr. A.J. Gwinnett, State University of New York at Stony Brook.)

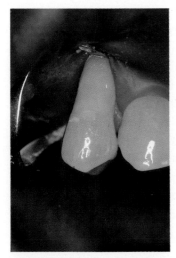

Figure 6-16 First increment of composite is applied to cover the axial dentin.

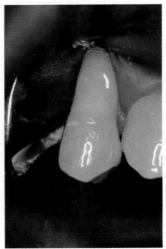

Figure 6-17 The first increment of composite after visible-light cure presents an "air-inhibited" surface layer.

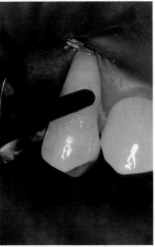

Figure 6-18 The second increment of composite is "bulk-packed" into position to build up full contour.

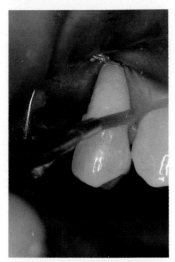

Figure 6-19 A dry sable brush is used to shape and form the composite material.

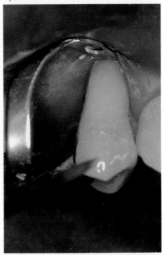

Figure 6-20 Proper contouring of composite material. No gross gingival excess is present.

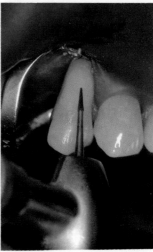

Figure 6-21 Orientation of multifluted tapering carbide bur for removal of gross excess.

beginning with medium and following in order with fine and superfine grit (Fig. 6-22). Particular care must be taken in finishing gingival excess because if the sharply pointed carbide finishing bur inadvertently contacts the cemental root surface, "ditching" of the cementum with associated sensitivity results. Accordingly, best results are obtained when the "pre-marginating" technique is used in the gingival region. A tapering carbide bur (1169L Bur[8]) with a rounded end (Fig. 6-23) is used only long enough to remove gross excess in the cemental region. A thin fin of marginal excess remains (Fig. 6-24) which is finally removed with a carbide hand-finishing composite knife (150-20 Carbide Knife[9]) used in a shaving motion (Fig. 6-25). After final discing, the cervical composite restoration presents a smooth lustrous surface (Fig. 6-26). Thermal sensitivity is not commonly encountered after the use of resin dentin bonding agents combined with microfilled composite materials for the restoration of cervical erosion lesions provided (1) phosphoric acid is not allowed to contact dentin during etching, and (2) ditching of the cementum is avoided during finishing. If either or both occur, prolonged thermal sensitivity is almost inevitable.

Materials. Certain resin dentin bonding agents (Scotchbond[1]) demonstrate best clinical performance when utilized in combination with the same manufacturer's composite materials (Silux;[2] P–10;[10] P–30[11]), whereas others (Adhesit[12]) reportedly, may be used compatibly with a wide variety of composite systems. Should doubt exist, it is clinically prudent to use a particular dentin bonding agent in conjunction with the same manufacturer's composite material.

Early Recall Results

In a sample of over one hundred nonprepared cervical erosion lesions restored using a resin dentin bonding agent (Scotchbond[1]) in combination with a visible-light-cured micro-filled composite material (Silux[2]) and followed for up to 2 years at The University of Western Ontario, the retention was observed to be 96 percent at one-year recall and 84 percent at 2-year recall. The comparatively few losses which have been observed may be attributed to either operator error (i.e., moisture contamination) or possibly dimensional changes (polymerization shrinkage) occurring within the composite material during polymerization. The resin dentin bonding agents currently demonstrate a bond value to acid-etched enamel (Chalkley and Jensen, 1984) which is very high in comparison to the dentin bond value. Furthermore, such materials are known to reduce microleakage of composite materials placed on cemental surfaces (Gillette et al, 1984). There is some concern that polymerization shrinkage occurring in association with the composite material may, under certain clinical conditions, result in a separation of the material from the underlying dentin surface to form a contraction gap (see Fig. 6-15). In clinical circumstances, when there is very little enamel present for bonding and large areas of dentin and/or cementum, the use of a long bevel on the enamel in conjunction with an axiogingival slot is strongly recommended (see Fig. 6-10).

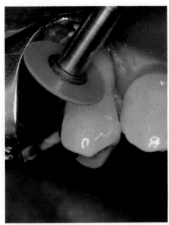

Figure 6-22 Soflex disc applied to composite surface.

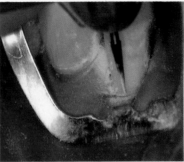

Figure 6–23 The use of a sharply pointed bur for gingival composite finish (*left*) results in cemental ditching. A rounded-end carbide-finishing bur (*right*) is safer.

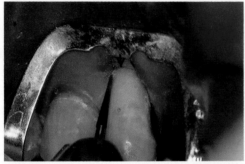

Figure 6-24 Gross gingival excess removal leaves a thin fin of composite material overlying cemental margin (*arrow*).

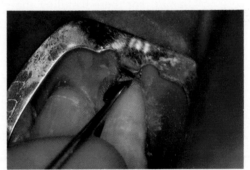

Figure 6-25 Removal of remaining gingival excess using a carbide knife.

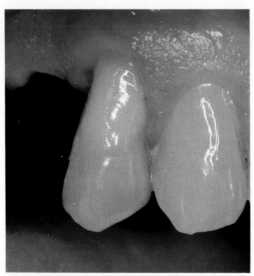

Figure 6-26 Finished cervical composite restoration.

Glass Ionomer Cements

The glass ionomer cements have three major clinical advantages and one major clinical limitation. The major clinical advantages of the glass ionomer cements are as follows:

1. They chemically bond to dentin, cementum, and enamel with a high degree of reliability (Brandau et al, 1984; Mount, 1984; McLean and Wilson, 1977).
2. They are nonirritating to pulp tissues (Kawahara et al, 1979; Tobias et al, 1978).
3. The glass ionomer cements are *anticariogenic* since they have an inherent built-in slow fluoride release mechanism (Forsten, 1977).

The major clinical limitation associated with the glass ionomer cements is that they are often very opaque and do not demonstrate an esthetic acceptability comparable to that of the composite materials. Nevertheless, the glass ionomer cements are dependable materials for dentin-cementum bonding and are indicated for the restoration of root caries or cervical erosion lesions in situations in which there is not a pronounced labial display of restorative material.

Materials. For those handling the glass ionomer cements, a knowledge of their basic chemistry and special setting characteristics is essential. The powder is basically similar to silicate cement since it is made up principally of an alumino-silicate glass powder with fluoride flux. The liquid is polyacrylic acid. When the powder is mixed with the liquid, a calcium polycarboxylate gel is formed, and this provides the initial chemical bond to tooth structure by means of reactive carboxyl groups. Within 24 hours, an aluminium polycarboxylate gel forms, and this provides a stronger physicochemical bond to tooth structure. The bond does not reach its highest level for 24 hours; accordingly, special clinical precautions must be taken during the placement phase in order to protect the integrity of the material. For example, the material is extremely sensitive to both hydration and dehydration during the first hour after placement, and if either occurs, the integrity of the material is considerably compromised. The ionomer cement must not be allowed to undergo initial set in contact with the atmosphere because this would result in severe dehydration and crazing. It is necessary, therefore, to cover the material with a waterproof varnish during the early setting period in order to prevent hydration or dehydration.

The prolonged setting reaction of the glass ionomer cements (i.e., 24 hours) calls for specific manipulative precautions.

Conservation Restoration of a Cervical Erosion Lesion by Means of Glass Ionomer Cement

A typical indication for glass ionomer cement is the cervical erosion lesion (Fig. 6-27) in locations where there is not a prominent labial display of the material. The cervical area is isolated by means of a rubber dam application, and proper gingival retraction is secured by means of a stabilized retraction clamp (Ivory 212 S.A.[4]) (Fig. 6-28). The recessed labial jaw of the clamp (Fig. 6-29) provides effective retraction of the labial gingival tissue away from the site of operation. The cervical region is given a thorough prophylaxis with a flour of pumice slurry followed by cleaning with a 3 percent hydrogen peroxide solution. The cervical surface may be more effectively cleaned by the application of polyacrylic acid (G-C Dentin Conditioner[13]) for 7 to 10 seconds (Fig. 6-30), which enhances bonding of the ionomer material

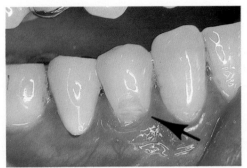

Figure 6-27 A cervical erosion lesion in the mandibular first premolar preoperatively.

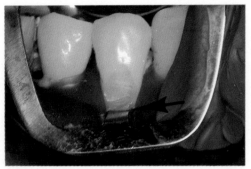

Figure 6-28 After rubber dam application, a gingival retraction clamp is placed.

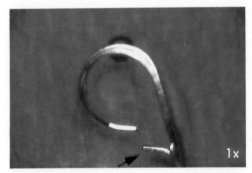

Figure 6-29 Lateral view of gingival retraction clamp showing recessed labial jaw.

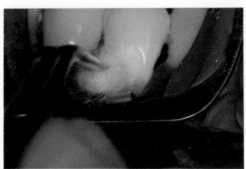

Figure 6-30 Application of polyacrylic acid to the dentinal surface thoroughly cleanses the area prior to bonding.

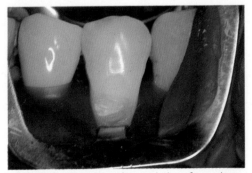

Figure 6-31 The clean dry cervical surface prior to ionomer cement application.

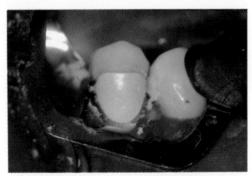

Figure 6-32 Coated metal cervical matrix form applied to labial surface.

(Powis et al, 1982). After washing with water and thorough air-drying, it is important to keep the region free of saliva or blood contamination (Fig. 6-31); accordingly, rubber dam application, together with the proper placement of a gingival retraction clamp, are helpful adjuncts. A metal cervical matrix form (Hawes-Neos[14]) should be properly fitted and formed over the cervical region (Fig. 6-32). Pulp protection, under most circumstances, is unnecessary since the ionomer cements are, for the most part, innocuous materials. However, in the case of a very deep lesion in close proximity to the pulp where the remaining dentin thickness is minimal, calcium hydroxide should be placed. Manufacturers' directions should be closely followed in dispensing powder and liquid since the ratio is critical. Accurately measured precapsulated systems are therefore highly recommended (Ketac Fill[15]). Mixing of the powder and liquid on a glass slab should be carried out rapidly, within 30 seconds, incorporating large amounts of powder with liquid in much the same manner as silicate cements are mixed. After mixing is complete, the surface of the ionomer cement must appear "glossy" (Fig. 6-33); otherwise the material should be discarded.

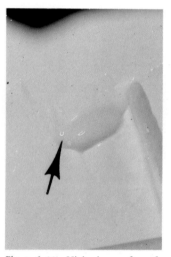

Figure 6-33   High-gloss surface of ionomer cement after mixing.

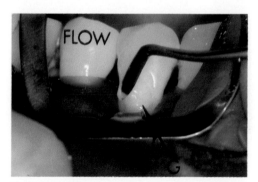

Figure 6-34   The glass ionomer cement is free-flowed over cervical region.

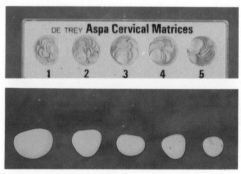

Figure 6-35   Preformed cervical matrix forms (Hawes-Neos[14]).

The mixed cement may be "bulk-packed" with an appropriate plastic instrument (Fig. 6-34) or, preferably, it may be syringed into position. The preformed metal matrix (Fig. 6-35) is now placed into position, thereby providing proper form to the restoration (Fig. 6-36). Gross excess extruding beyond the matrix is removed by means of an explorer before the material sets. Once matrix covered, the ionomer cement should be left undisturbed for a full 4 minutes, after which the matrix is removed, whereupon waterproof varnish (Ketac Varnish[16]) should be applied immediately to the ionomer surface in order to prevent dehydration (Fig. 6-37). Gross excess, if present, may be removed with a sharp scalpel and waterproof varnish reapplied. Ideally, final finishing should be delayed for a 24-hour period.

In finishing, fine diamond instruments are used to remove gross excess; this is followed by final contouring for which progressively finer abrasive discs are used (Fig. 6-38).

The ionomer cements provide a highly dependable bond to tooth structure (Fig. 6-39). However, they characteristically lack the esthetic acceptability of composite materials, particularly at long-term recall, at which time plaque accumulation and discoloration are frequently observed (Fig. 6-40). However, such restorations may be effectively veneered with composite materials, and this produces an excellent esthetic result (Fig. 6-41).

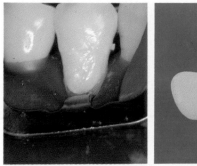
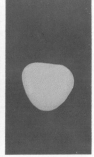

Figure 6–36 After the cervical contour is built up with ionomer cement (*left*), the matrix form (*right*) is placed over the cement surface and left intact for 4 minutes.

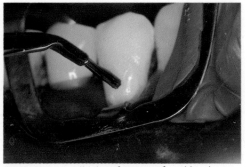

Figure 6-37 Application of waterproof varnish to ionomer surface.

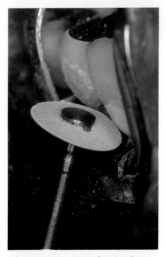

Figure 6–38 Final finish of glass ionomer restoration.

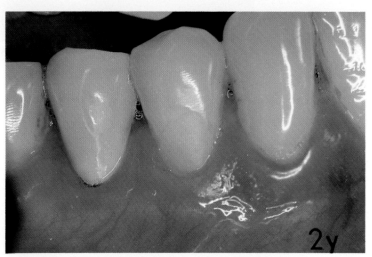

Figure 6-39 Cervical ionomer restoration at 2-year recall.

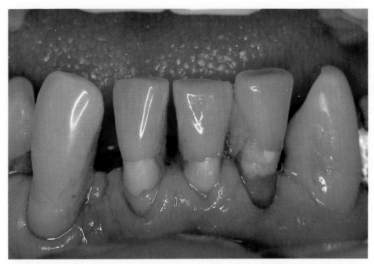

Figure 6-40 Glass ionomer cervical restorations in the mandibular central incisors at 7-year recall.

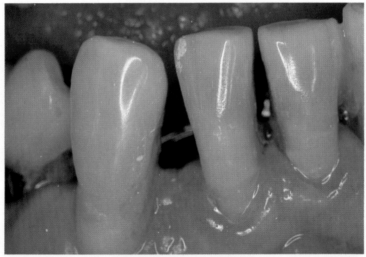

Figure 6-41 The ionomer restorations shown in Figure 6-40 after reveneering with microfill composite.

COMPOSITE-IONOMER LAMINATED RESTORATION

Composite materials may be reliably bonded to ionomer cements (McLean, 1984). The combined composite-ionomer restoration has three clinical advantages: (1) reliable chemical bonding to dentin, (2) pulp compatibility, and (3) esthetic acceptability.

A typical indication for the laminated restoration is shown in Figure 6-42. The cervical erosion lesion is of moderate depth and extremely hypersensitive. No preparation is involved. After isolation (Figure 6-43), the cervical area is cleaned by means of a 10- to 15-second application of polyacrylic acid (Fig. 6-44), washed with water, and thoroughly air-dried (Fig. 6-45). Fast-setting glass ionomer cement (Ketac–Cem[17]) is then flowed over the full extent

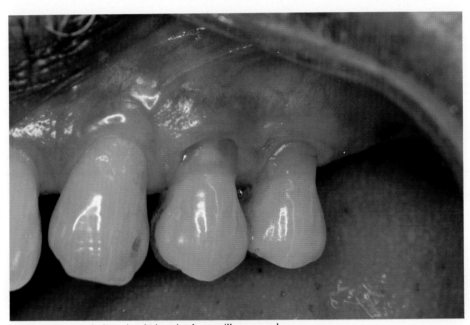

Figure 6–42 Cervical erosion lesions in the maxillary premolars.

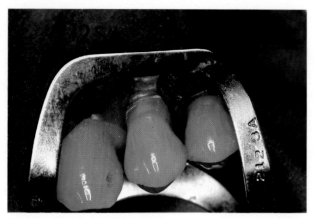

Figure 6–43 Isolation of the field.

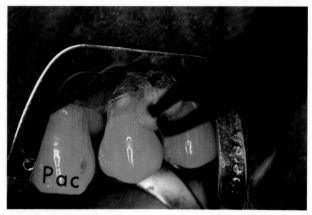

Figure 6–44 Application of polyacrylic acid to dentin surface.

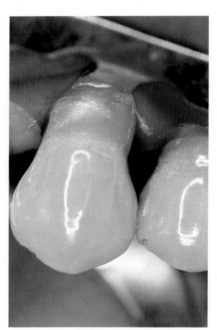

Figure 6–45 Clean dry dentin surface prior to bonding.

of the axial dentinal wall (Fig. 6-46), and at the same time the material is "feathered" to just short of the cavo-surface margins. The ionomer cement is left undisturbed for a period of 4 minutes in order to reach initial set, during which time an enamel bevel is placed by use of a diamond instrument (Fig. 6-47). In applying the ionomer cement, one should not "overbuild" the material in order to avoid a "shine-through" problem. A layer approximately 0.5 mm in thickness is normally placed over the dentin. Should an insufficient thickness be placed, extensive washout may occur. After a 4-minute period of initial set, a gel etchant should be syringed into the cervical region to cover the ionomer cement and the full extent of the enamel and cemental margins (Fig. 6-48). After a one-minute period, the area is washed with a copious water lavage for 30 to 45 seconds and thoroughly air-dried (Fig. 6-49). The acid-etched glass ionomer cement surface presents an extremely porous surface under scanning electron microscopic examination (Fig. 6-50). A micro-mechanical interlocking effect is thus provided on composite insertion. Since the glass ionomer cement undergoes little if any dimensional change (i.e., polymerization shrinkage) during setting, little opportunity exists for the formation of a "contraction gap" at the ionomer-dentin interface.

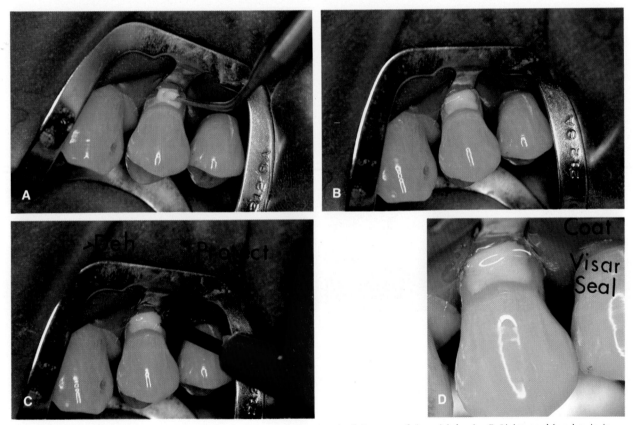

Figure 6-46 Application of free-flow glass ionomer cement, *A*, to cover the full extent of the axial dentin, *B*, Light cured bond resin is applied, *C*, in order to prevent dehydration, *D*.

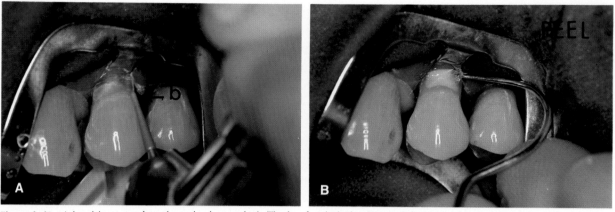

Figure 6-47   A bevel is prepared on the occlusal enamel. *A*, The bond resin is then removed from the ionomer surface, *B*, after a 4 minute period of initial set.

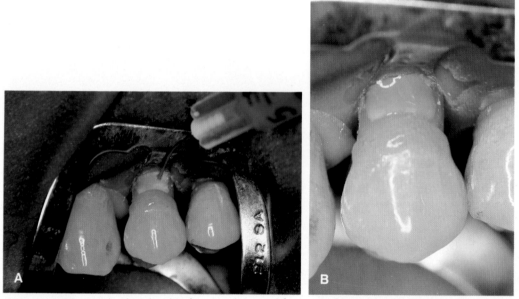

Figure 6-48   Viscous gel etchant is syringed to cover the enamel for 40 seconds, *A*, and then additional gel is placed to cover the ionomer for 20 seconds, *B*.

An Enamel-dentin bonding agent (Creation™ bond 3 in one[1]) is then carefully thin-spread over the ionomer surface as well as the enamel and gingival marginal areas (Fig. 6-51). Gentle air-blowing confirms the thin-spread nature of the application. The bond resin is then light cured for 20 seconds. The air-inhibited nature of the bonding material is self-evident for its surface is glossy in appearance and "tacky" to the touch. A first layer of light-cured microfilled composite (Paste Laminate™[2]) is then bulk-packed into the area by means of a Teflon-coated instrument (Fig. 6-52), and a sable brush is used to contour an initial coat of composite material over the ionomer cement (Fig. 6-53). The first composite layer is then light-cured for 30 seconds (Fig. 6-54), and subsequently the cervical region is built out to full contour by the addition of a second composite layer (Fig. 6-55A). "Contouring" is greatly facilitated by the use of a fine-tipped sable brush. After light-curing for a 30-second period, the composite material is finally contoured and finished by means of instrumentation techniques previously described. The finished ionomer-composite laminated restoration is shown in Figure 6-56.

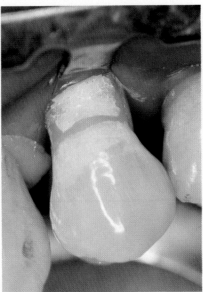

Figure 6–49 Appearance of the enamel and ionomer after erching.

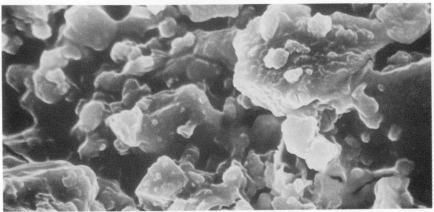

Figure 6–50 Scanning electron micrograph (3500 ×) of the etched ionomer surface demonstrates a highly microporous surface topography.

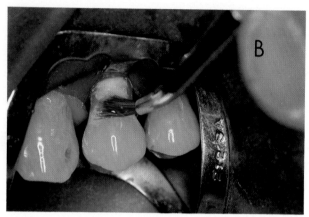

Figure 6-51 Application of bond resin to ionomer, enamel and cementum.

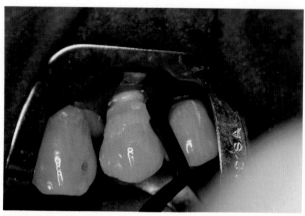

Figure 6-52 The first increment of composite material is "bulk-packed" into position.

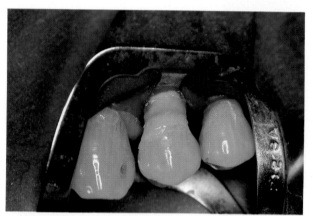

Figure 6-53 First increment of composite as applied to the ionomer surfaces.

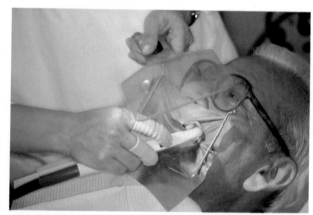

Figure 6-54 Application of visible light for 30 seconds. Note "cure shield"[28] protective.

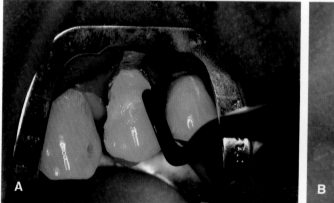

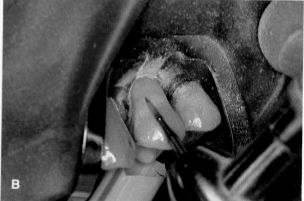

Figure 6-55 The second composite increment is placed to full contour and light cured, *A*. The composite is finally finished, *B*.

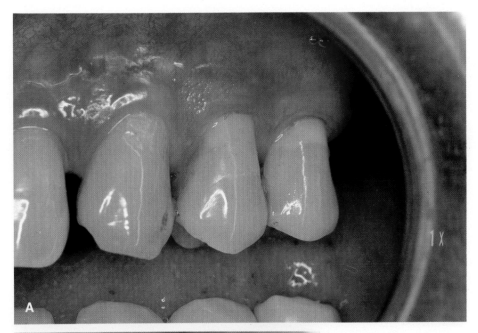

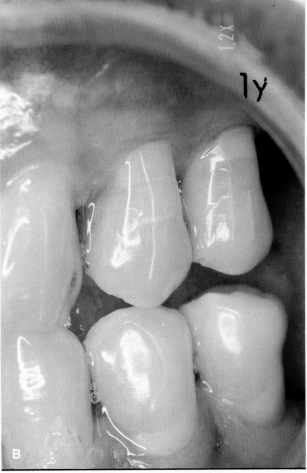

Figure 6-56 The finished ionomer-composite laminated restoration at baseline, *A*, and at one year recall, *B*. Closeup view at one year recall, *C*.

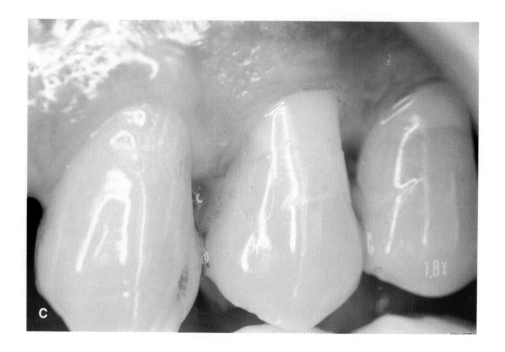

COMPOSITE-IONOMER LAMINATE RESTORATION FOR EXTENSIVE GERIATRIC ROOT CARIES

Deep root caries in geriatric patients present a particular problem to the practitioner since, by their very nature, they are characteristically observed on root surfaces in relatively inaccessible areas where the remaining dentin thickness is minimal (Figs. 6-57 and 6-58). Conventional cavity preparation, with the establishment of box form undercut retention features, almost invariably results in massive pulp exposure.

The first step in the composite-ionomer restoration is to remove all carious dentin by means of an appropriate-sized round bur. No attempt is made to establish "box" form, particularly in the gingival region. In the event that the extent of the caries process approximates the pulp chamber, a small amount of calcium hydroxide is used to cover the thin dentin overlying the pulp chamber. The prepared area is then swabbed with 3 percent hydrogen peroxide, washed, and air-dried.

Fast setting glass ionomer cement (Ketac Bond[19] or G-C Lining Cement[27]) is flowed into the internal areas to cover the full extent of the axial wall as described in the previous section. The ionomer cement is left undisturbed for a 4-minute period. After 4 minutes, the surface of the ionomer cement and the entire enamel cavo-surface periphery are phosphoric acid gel-etched for a one-minute period. After a thorough water lavage and careful air-drying, a bonding resin should be applied. In this particular case, a light-cured dentin bonding resin (Light Cured Scotchbond[5]) was applied thinly to the ionomer-enamel surfaces, air-blown, and light-cured. Composite material was then inserted in two stages and finally light-cured. The final restoration is shown in Figure 6-59.

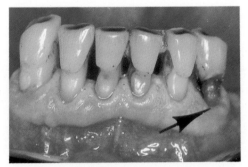

Figure 6-57 Cervical erosion lesions and root caries involving the mandibular incisors of a geriatric patient.

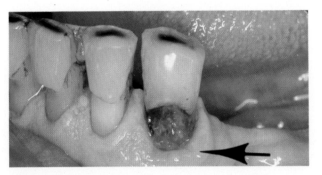

Figure 6-58 Close-up view of root caries on the mandibular canine.

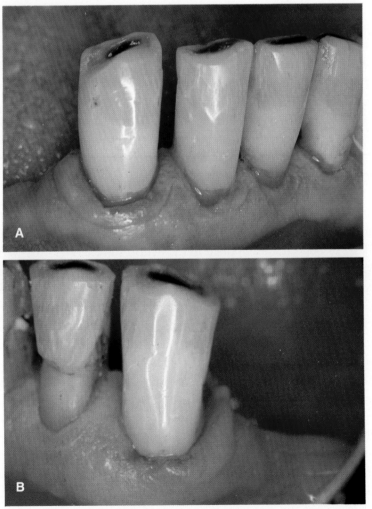

Figure 6-59 Completed cervical restoration of the cervical erosion lesions, *A*, and the mandibular canine, *B*.

LIGHT-CURED RESIN DENTIN BONDING AGENTS

Light cured materials (Light-Cured Scotchbond;[5] Prisma Universal Bond[18] and Bondlite[20]) are the most recently introduced resin dentin bonding agents. Early laboratory testing of one such material (Light Cured Scotchbond[5]) indicates higher dentin bond values than those obtained with comparable self-cured systems (Farah, 1984). Although the clinical performance of such materials remains to be assessed, among the purported advantages of the light curing materials are:

1. More reliable dentin bonding
2. Enhanced pulp protection
3. A more workable clinical surface
4. No delay relative to the onset of finishing

Restoration of a Cervical Erosion Lesion Using Light-Cured Bonding Resin (Light Cured Scotchbond[5]) in Combination With a Light-Cured Microfilled Composite (Silux[2])

Figure 6-60 shows a cervical erosion lesion in maxillary left lateral incisor that is thermally sensitive. After proper gingival retraction and rubber dam isolation, the cervical area is cleansed in the usual fashion by the use of a pumice slurry followed by the application of 3 percent hydrogen peroxide for a 10-second period, washing, and drying (Fig. 6-61). At this point the technique differs markedly from that of the self-cured, dentin bonding agents. Using the latter, a controlled acid-etch technique was used on the enamel prior to the application of the bond resin. Pulp protection was not normally used unless the lesion was very deep. Accordingly, even a small amount of inadvertent acid contact on the adjacent dentin could pose a potentially serious problem of pulp irritation.

With the light-cured dentin bonding agent (Light Cured Scotchbond[5]), a bond/etch/ rebond technique is recommended. After the cervical area is cleaned and dried one drop each of the resin and liquid (Fig. 6-62) are dispersed in a well and carefully mixed (Fig. 6-63). A generous layer of bond resin is applied to the dentin surface (Fig. 6-64), after which it is exposed to visible light for 20 seconds (Fig. 6-65). Unlike the self-cured material, the dentin is now covered by a polymerized "skin" of bonding resin with an air-inhibited surface layer (Fig. 6-66). This layer of bond resin not only bonds to the dentin, but also provides some pulp protection during subsequent acid etching. Unfortunately however, the bond resin may be easily penetrated by phosphoric acid during enamel etching thereby providing the basis for severe pulpal irritation. Accordingly, recent research has shown (Eich, 1986) that the initial layer of bond resin must be covered with a thin layer of acid resistant resin (Silux[2], or Enamel Bond[22] or Com-Plus[28]) properly light-cured before proceeding with enamel etching.

The enamel is now beveled by means of an appropriate diamond instrument (Fig. 6-67), and electively, a shallow slot may be placed axiogingivally (Fig. 6-68). The beveled enamel region is next gel-etched for one minute (Figs. 6-69 and 6-70), washed, and thoroughly dried (Fig. 6-71). Even if some of the phosphoric acid has come into contact with the dentin surface, little harm is done to the pulp tissues since the dentin has been presealed with polymerized bond resin. Such is not the case with the self-cured materials.

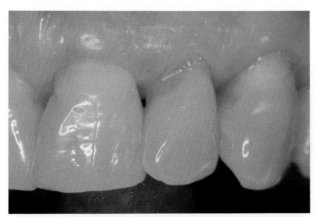

Figure 6-60 Cervical erosion lesion maxillary left lateral incisor.

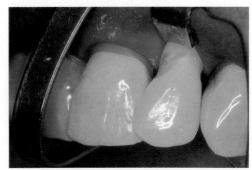

Figure 6-61 The field is isolated and the cervical region is cleaned, washed, and dried.

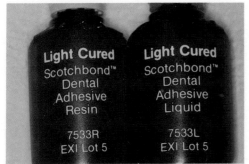

Figure 6-62 Light-cured dentin adhesive (Light Cured Scotchbond⁵) consists of two components, resin and liquid.

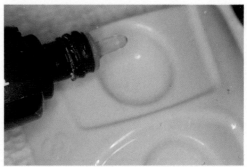

Figure 6-63 A drop of each (resin and liquid) is dispensed and mixed.

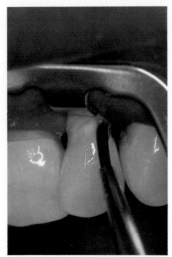

Figure 6-64 A layer of bond resin is applied to the dentin.

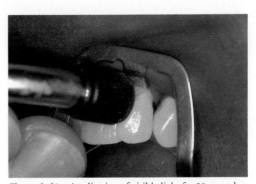

Figure 6–65 Application of visible light for 20 seconds for resin cure.

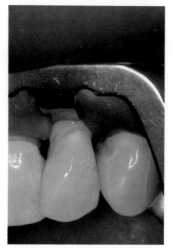

Figure 6-66 Polymerized bond resin demonstrates an "air-inhibited" layer.

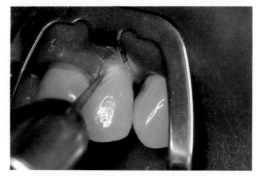

Figure 6-67 Preparation of enamel bevel.

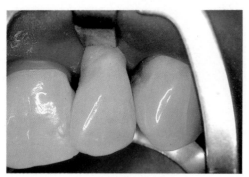

Figure 6-68 The bevelled preparation.

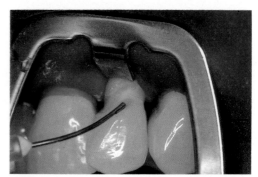

Figure 6-69 Gel etchant is syringed to cover bevelled enamel.

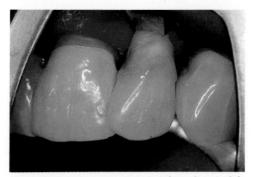

Figure 6-70 The gel etchant is left undisturbed for one minute.

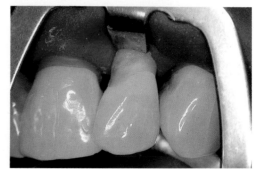

Figure 6-71 The dried cervical region prior to rebonding.

A second layer of light-cured bond resin is now carefully applied to the acid-etched enamel, the resin-coated dentin, and cemental surfaces. This is air-blown and light-cured for 20 seconds (Figs. 6-72 and 6-73). A two-stage composite insertion technique, similar to the "self-cured" format (Figs. 6-74 to 6-76), is now followed. Immediately following visible-light-cure of the final composite layer, finishing is begun without delay, using a multifluted carbide bur (Fig. 6-77) followed by ⅜–inch aluminum oxide discs (Fig. 6-78). The composite restoration is shown on completion in Figure 6-79 and one week later in Figure 6-80, at which time the gingival tissues show excellent adaptation to the cemental-composite interface.

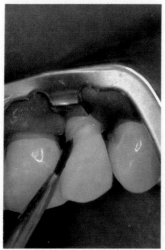

Figure 6–72 The second layer of bond resin is applied to the cervical region.

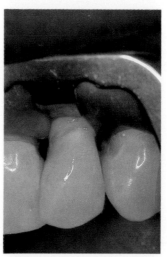

Figure 6–73 Appearance of the second bond resin layer after curing.

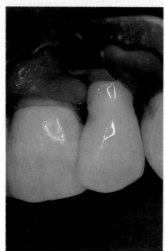

Figure 6–74 The first increment of composite placed to cover the axial wall and cured.

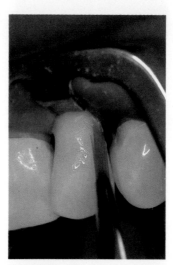

Figure 6–75 The second composite increment is placed and contoured.

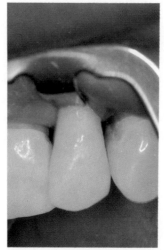

Figure 6-76 The second composite increment fully restores cervical contour.

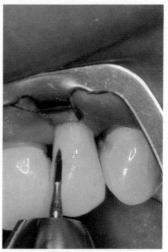

Figure 6-77 Gross finish is accomplished with a multifluted carbide bur.

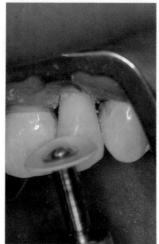

Figure 6-78 Final polish is attained using a ⅜-inch superfine Soflex disc.

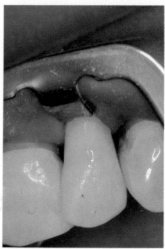

Figure 6-79 Completed composite restoration.

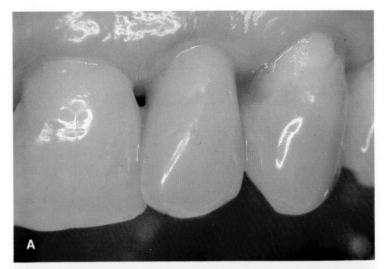

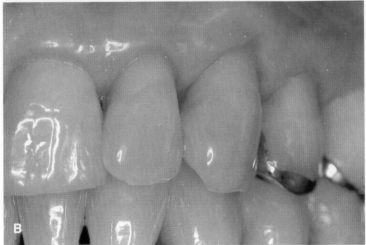

Figure 6-80 Cervical composite restoration one week postoperatively, *A,* and at 18 month recall *B.*

References

Aida S, Matsui K, Hirai Y, Ishikawa T. A Clinicopathological study of pulpal reaction of acid etching with phosphoric acid solution at various concentrations. Bull Tokyo Dent College 1980; 201:163.

Bowen RL, Cobb EN, Rapson JE. Adhesive bonding of various materials to hard tooth tissues: improvement in bond strength to resin. J Dent Res 1982; 61:1070.

Brandau ME, Ziemiecki JL, Charbeneau G. Restoration of cervical contours on nonprepared teeth using glass ionomer cement: a 4½ year report. J Am Dent Assoc 1984; 104:762.

Brannstrom M, Johnson G. Effects of various conditioners and cleaning agents on prepared dentin surfaces: a scanning electron microscopic investigation. J Prosthet Dent 1974; 31:422.

Brannstrom M, Glantz PO, Nordenvall KJ. The effect of some cleaning solutions on the morphology of dentin prepared in different ways: an in vivo study. J Dent Child 1979; 46:19.

Brannstrom M, Nordenvall KJ, Glantz PO. The effect of EDTA containing surface active solutions on the morphology of prepared dentin: an in vivo study. J Dent Res 1980; 59:1127.

Chalkley YM, Jensen ME. Enamel shear bond strengths of a dentinal bonding agent. J Dent Res 1984; 63:320. (Abstract)

Davidson CL, de Gee AJ. Relaxation of polymerization contraction stresses by flow in dental composites. J Dent Res 1984; 63:146.

Dogon L. 3M Symposium on Dental Adhesives. Minaki, Ontario, June, 1982.

Douglas WH. 3M Symposium on Dental Adhesives. Minaki, Ontario, June, 1982.

Erickson HM. Protection against harmful effects of a restorative procedure using an acidic cavity cleanser. J Dent Res 1976; 55:281.

Farah J. Personal Communication. September, 1984.

Forsten L. Fluoride release from a glass ionomer cement. Scand J Dent Res 1977; 85:503.

Gillette BE, Robinson LW, Blank JW, Pelleu GB. A dentin bonding agent and microleakage below the cemento-enamel junction. J Dent Res 1984; 63:179. (Abstract)

Gwinnett AJ. Acid etching for composite resins. Dent Clin North Am 1978; 25:271.

Jordan RE, Suzuki M, Gwinnett AJ. Restoration of fractured and hypoplastic incisors by the acid etch technique: a three-year report. J Am Dent Assoc 1977; 95:795.

Kawahara H, Imanishi Y, Oshima H. Biological evaluation of glass ionomer cement. J Dent Res 1979; 58:1080.

McLean JW, Wilson AD. The clinical development of the glass ionomer cements. Formulation and properties. Aust Dent J 1977; 22:31.

McLean JW. Personal Communication. May, 1984.

Mount GJ. Restoration with glass ionomer cement; requirements for clinical success. Op Dent 1981; 6:59.

Powis DA, Folkras T, Merson SA, Wilson AD. Improved adhesion of a glass ionomer cement to dentin and enamel. J Dent Res 1982; 61:1416.

Stanley HR, Going RE, Chancey HH. Human pulp response to acid pretreatment of dentin and to composite restorations. J Am Dent Assoc 1975; 91:817.

Tobias RS, Browne RN, Plant CG, Ingram DY. Pulpal response to a glass ionomer cement. Br Dent J 1978; 144:345.

Product Information

Product	Manufacturer/Distributor	Purpose
1. Scotchbond	Dental Products/3M Company 3M Center 270-5N-02 St. Paul, MN 55144	Self-cured dentin bonding resin
2. Silux	Dental Products/3M Company 3M Center 270-5N-02 St. Paul, MN 55144	Light-cured, microfilled composite material
3. Brinker B#4	Hygenic Mfg. Co. 1245 Home Ave. Akron, OH 44310	Single-wing gingival retraction clamp
4. Ivory 212 S.A.	Columbus Dental Mfg. Co. 1000 Chouteau Ave., P.O. Box 620 St. Louis, MO 63188	Double-wing gingival retraction clamp
5. Light Cured Scotchbond	Dental Products/3M Company 3M Center 270-5N-02 St. Paul, MN 55144	Light-cured dentin bonding resin
6. ET 6; ET 9 Tapering Carbide Burs	Brasseler USA Inc. 800 King George Blvd. Savannah, GA 31419	Multifluted tapering carbide finishing bur
7. Soflex Discs	Dental Products/3M Company 3M Center 270#5N#02 St. Paul, MN 55144	Aluminum oxide finishing discs
8. 1169L Bur	Ritter/Midwest Co. 901 W. Oakton Des Plaines, IL 60018	Tapering carbide finishing bur with round end
9. 150-20 Carbide Knife	Brasseler USA Inc. 800 King George Blvd. Savannah, GA 31419	Carbide finishing knife

Product Information

Product	Manufacturer/Distributor	Purpose
10. P-10	Dental Products/3M Company 3M Center 270-5N-02 St. Paul, MN 55144	Heavy-filled, self-cured, hybrid composite
11. P-30	Dental Products/3M Company 3M Center 270-5N-02 St. Paul, MN 55144	Heavy-filled, light-cured, hybrid composite
12. Adhesit	Vivadent USA Inc. P.O. Box 304 Tonawanda, NY 14150	Self-cured dentin bonding resin
13. G-C Dentin Conditioner	G-C American Co. LTD Scottsdale, AZ	10% polyacrylic acid for dentin cleaning
14. Hawes-Neos Cervical Matrix Forms	ESPE-Premier Sales Corp. Romano Dr., P.O. Box 111 Norristown, PA 19401	Metal cervical matrix form
15. Ketac Fil	ESPE-Premier Sales Corp. Romano Dr., P.O. Box 111 Norristown, PA 19401	Precapsulated glass ionomer cement
16. Ketac Varnish	ESPE-Premier Sales Corp. Romano Dr., P.O. Box 111 Norristown, PA 19401	Waterproof varnish for coating ionomer cement
17. Ketac-Cem	ESPE-Premier Sales Corp. Romano Dr., P.O. Box 111 Norristown, PA 19401	Fast-setting glass ionomer cement
18. Prisma Universal Bond	L.D. Caulk Co. P.O. Box 359 Milford, DE 19963-0359	Light-cured dentin adhesive
19. Ketac Bond	ESPE-Premier Sales Corp. Romano Dr., P.O. Box 111 Norristown, PA 19401	Fast-setting, glass ionomer cement
20. Bondlite	Kerr-Sybron Co. P.O. Box 455 Romulus, MI 48174	Light-cured dentin adhesive
21. Concise	Dental Products/3M Company 3M Center 270-5N-02 St. Paul, MN 55144	Large-particle, macrofilled, self-cured composite
22. Enamel Bond	Dental Products/3M Company 3M Center 270-5N-02 St. Paul, MN 55144	Enamel bonding agent
23. Silar	Dental Products/3M Company 3M Center 270-5N-02 St. Paul, MN 55144	Self-cured, microfilled composite
24. Creation Bond	Den-Mat Corp. 3130 Skyway Dr., Unit 501 Santa Maria, CA 93456	Self-cured dentin bonding agent
25. J&J Dentin Bond	Johnson and Johnson 20 Lake Drive, CN7060 East Windsor, CT 08520	Self-cured dentin bonding agent
26. Prisma VLC Dycal	L.D. Caulk Co. P.O. Box 359 Milford, DE 19963-0359	Visible light-cured calcium hydroxide for pulp protection
27. G-C Lining Cement	G-C American Co. Scottsdale, AZ	A fast setting lining ionomer cement
28. Com-Plus	Parkell Co. Farmingdale, NY	A light-cured filled glazed resin

7

LEENDERT BOKSMAN
RONALD E. JORDAN

POSTERIOR COMPOSITE
RESTORATIONS

Because of a widespread demand for esthetic dentistry, there is currently a tremendous amount of interest in posterior composite restorations. There are a number of advantages associated with posterior composite materials. Being "tooth-colored", they are highly esthetic; they are also mercury-free and thermally nonconductive. Possibly the most significant advantage, however, is the fact that composite materials are *bondable* to calcified tissues. In this regard, two types of bonding are important. First of all, the physico-mechanical bonding of composite materials to phosphoric acid-etched enamel provides an intimate, deeply penetrative relationship between resin tags and enamel microporosities at the resin-enamel interface. Furthermore, with the advent of dentin bonding materials (Chapter 6), a chemical means of bonding composite and/or glass ionomer materials to dentin has been introduced. Whatever the differential significance of enamel physico-mechanical bonding and dentin chemical bonding, a good deal of evidence exists to indicate that composite materials may well provide the basis for structural support to adjacent cuspal tissues (Morin et al, 1984; Landy and Simonsen, 1984).

Many highly promising posterior composite materials have been recently introduced (P10;[1] P30;[1] Fulfil;[2] Estilux;[3] Visiofil;[4] Status;[5] Marathon;[6] Herculite[7]) which may be used for posterior restorations when esthetics are of prime importance. However, before these composite materials can be recommended as *routine* replacements for silver amalgam, two hurdles must be overcome. The new materials must be subjected to intensive long-term clinical trials. These are under way, but have not yet been completed since only 2- to 3-year observations (Fig. 7-1) currently exist (Wilder et al, 1983; Leinfelder and Roberson, 1983). In addition, techniques specifically "custom-designed" for composite materials must be developed and tested since the composite materials are infinitely more "technique-sensitive" in the posterior region than silver amalgam. What is meant by "technique-sensitive"? Although several examples may be given to illustrate the point, three will suffice: (1) it is much more difficult to restore tight contact relationships posteriorly when composite materials are used (Fig. 7-2); (2) finishing procedures are prolonged and more tedious with composite materials since they do not go through a "carvable" stage; and (3) pulp protection with composite materials is a much more critical factor than with silver amalgam (see Fig. 2-31). In this chapter, an effective clinical technique for posterior class II composite restorations will be presented. In the meantime, indications and materials must be the first considerations.

INDICATIONS AND MATERIALS

Silver amalgam (Fig. 7-3) has been used successfully for decades as a routine posterior restorative material mainly because (1) it is one of the least technique-sensitive long-term restorative materials available and (2) it is "self-sealing". Accordingly, silver amalgam will continue to be used routinely as a reliable posterior restorative material for many years to come. Probably the major clinical pitfall associated with posterior composite restorations is occlusal wear (Phillips et al, 1972; Osborne et al, 1973) and loss of anatomic form (Fig. 7-4). The amount of wear encountered clinically is dictated by many circumstances, including composite material composition, curing method, cavity size, and arch location, to mention only a few (Lutz et al, 1984; Leinfelder and Roberson, 1983). Recent research has shown that wear resistance increases (1) as faciolingual cavity size decreases, (2) with light-cured composite materials, (3) with small-particle composite materials, and (4) the more mesial in the posterior dental arch the material is placed. Accordingly, small-particle-filled, visible-light-cured materials[1-7] may be used posteriorly, primarily in cases in which (1) esthetics are of prime importance, (2) the faciolingual dimension of the cavity preparation is restricted, or (3) the gingival cavo-surface margin is placed in intact enamel. Otherwise, silver amalgam is the material of choice.

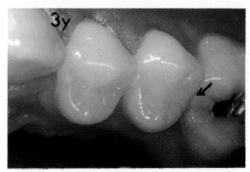

Figure 7-1 A disto-occlusal composite (Fulfil[2]) restoration in the maxillary left second premolar at 3-year recall.

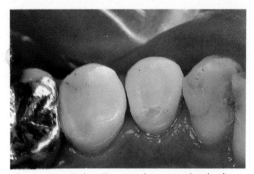

Figure 7-2 A class II composite restoration in the mandibular left first premolar with "open" contact.

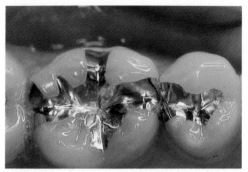

Figure 7-3 Class II silver amalgam restorations in the mandibular second premolar and first molar.

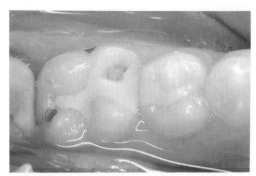

Figure 7-4 Composite restorations in the mandibular left second premolar and first molar at 3-year recall.

Technique of Posterior Composite Restoration

Figure 7-5 shows an occlusal view of the maxillary left quadrant of a young patient with a distal-proximal carious lesion in the first premolar and a mesial lesion in the first molar. Disto-occlusal and mesio-occlusal lingual composite restorations are indicated. After careful quadrant isolation and before any cutting is done, a ''prewedging'' technique is used. Anatomically-contoured wooden wedges (13T,13XT Sycamore Wedges[8]) are lubricated with a small amount of shaving cream and placed to fill the gingival embrasures adjacent to each tooth (Fig. 7-6). Prewedging in such a fashion accomplishes two purposes: (1) it slowly causes sufficient separation of the teeth to allow for the thickness of the matrix band, and (2) the occlusal portion of the wedge provides a guide for the placement of the gingivoproximal floor of the class II cavity preparation (Fig. 7-7). In the event that the gingival wall of a class II preparation approaches the cemento-enamel junction, a composite restoration alone is contraindicated because of the extreme difficulty in securing a positive seal in this critical region. In such cases a glass ionomer cement should be bonded to the cement margin and the remainder of the restoration should be built up in composite.

The cavity preparation for a class II composite restoration should be cut as conservatively as clinical circumstances allow (Fig. 7-8). A ''butt-joint'' clean-cut nonbeveled preparation is preferable to a beveled cavo-surface outline. A beveled preparation results in a thin marginal fin of composite material which is prone to fracture in functional circumstances, thereby leaving a ledge-type defect in the marginal region. Bevels also obscure the cavo-surface finish line, further complicating an already difficult finish situation. A butt-type joint in the cavity preparation, on the other hand, presents a well-delineated marginal periphery to which the composite material may be precisely bulk-finished (Fig. 7-9).

Pulp protection is of primary importance when composite materials are used in posterior preparations because these are among the most toxic materials used in operative dentistry (Leinfelder, 1981; Leinfelder and Roberson, 1983; Goto and Jordan, 1972; Goto and Jordan, 1973). Three precautionary measures in pulp protection are recommended: (1) the use of phosphoric acid washout-resistant pulp protective materials, (2) protection of all dentin from the effects of phosphoric acid etching, and (3) the routine use of a *controlled* phosphoric acid-etching technique.

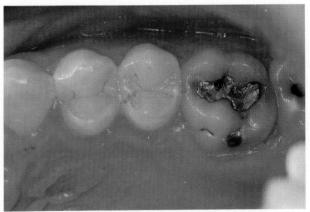

Figure 7-5   Preoperative occlusal view of a maxillary left quadrant.

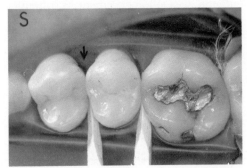

Figure 7-6   Prewedging: placement of anatomically contoured wooden wedges.

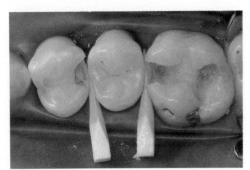

Figure 7-7   Relationship of wooden wedges to gingival proximal floor.

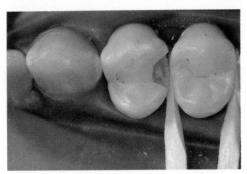

Figure 7-8   DO class II composite cavity preparation in maxillary first premolar.

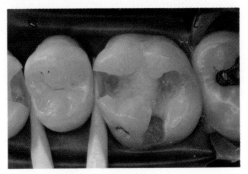

Figure 7-9   MOL class II composite cavity preparation in maxillary first molar.

Calcium hydroxide materials (Dycal Improved;[9] Procal;[10] Renew[11]) are excellent pulp protective materials (Noro and Ishikawa, 1983), but unfortunately are subject to washout after application of phosphoric acid during etching techniques. However, some calcium hydroxide materials are more resistant to phosphoric acid washout than others (Dycal Advanced Formula;[12] Life[13]) (Phillips et al, 1984). The use of biologically acceptable, fast-setting, totally acid-resistant pulp protective glass ionomer materials (Shofu Base Cement,[14] G-C Lining Cement;[34] Zionomer Lining Cement,[15] Gingiva Seal,[16] Ketac-Bond[17]) is becoming increasingly popular. A highly effective, fast-setting, acid-resistant, powder-liquid ionomer cement[34] should be used to cover the pulpal floors and axial walls of the preparations (Fig. 7-10) and should be "lapped" as close to the gingival dentin-enamel junction as possible. Protection of gingival floor dentin is critical since the tubules are usually in close proximity to the pulp. Should the gingival dentin be inadvertently exposed to phosphoric acid during the enamel etching technique, the tubules are considerably opened as a result, thereby providing the basis for direct acid pulp irritation (Goto and Jordan, 1973).

High viscosity gel-type etchants (Scotchbond Gel Etch;[18] Caulk Gel Etchant[19]) are highly recommended for the etching procedure. Owing to their viscous nature, they may be applied on a controlled basis to contact the enamel walls and glass ionomer cement. A convenient method of acid application is as follows:

A viscous gel etchant (Scotchbond Gel Etch[18]) is placed in a tuberculin syringe fitted with a 25-gauge needle. The etchant gel should be syringed over the entire enamel wall periphery of the preparation (Fig. 7-11), and left undisturbed for a one-minute period. Additional gel etchant should be applied to the ionomer surface for a 20-second period.

The preparation must be subsequently washed with a copious water lavage for at least 30 to 45 seconds. Since most gel etchants leave contaminant residues, a prolonged water lavage is necessary to thoroughly clean the etched surfaces. After careful air-drying, the etched enamel should appear frosty white and opaque (Fig. 7-12). Extreme care must be exercised from this point on to maintain thoroughly dry conditions, free of salivary contamination, because the etched enamel surfaces are highly sensitive to salivary contamination. Should salivary contamination inadvertently occur, re-etching with phosphoric acid for 10 to 15 seconds is strongly recommended to thoroughly clean the surface.

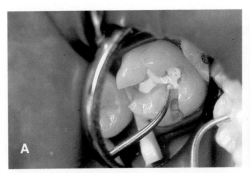 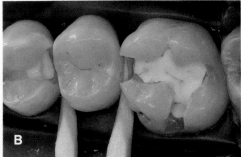

Figure 7-10 *A,* Free-flow application of acid-resistant pulp protective (Dropsin[14]) to pulpal floor of the maxillary first molar preparation. *B,* Occlusal view of the class II preparations after application of the pulp protective material.

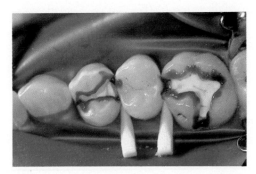

Figure 7-11 Viscous gel etchant applied to enamel walls of preparations for 40 seconds followed by application of get etchant to ionomer surface for 20 seconds.

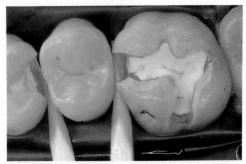

Figure 7-12 Opaque appearance of enamel and ionomer after acid-etching.

A layer phosphonate of bond resin[32] should be carefully thin-spread over the enamel walls and internal details of the preparation by means of a soft fine-tipped brush. The bond resin should then be gently air-blown with an air syringe to ensure a thin film application. "Puddling" of the bond resin should be carefully avoided since "white line margin" may well result.

The matricing technique must be carefully controlled for it is another critical phase in the manipulative technique. A Toffelmire retainer should be used and a precontoured very thin, pliable 0.0010-inch matrix band[35] should be burnished into tight adaptive contact with the adjacent proximal surface by means of a ball burnisher (Fig. 7-13).

The composite material must be inserted in successive laminated increments to ensure proper cure. Further, a controlled condensation technique must be utilized in order to completely seal the marginal areas. An appropriate syringe (Teflon Amalgam Gun;[20] Centrix Syringe;[21]) (Fig. 7-14) should be used to initially place a small amount of the composite material along the gingival wall. The gingival cavo-surface margin is a critical area in the class II composite restoration; if it is improperly condensed "at baseline," automatic failure results (Fig. 7-15). A small, round smooth-faced condenser (Felt Nos. 2, 3, 5, 6[22]) (Fig. 7-16), slightly wetted with bond resin, is used to condense a 1-mm thickness of composite material firmly against the gingival wall. The best posterior composite materials are highly viscous and "condensable" (P10; P30;[1] Fulfil;[2] Status;[5] Herculite[23]) in order to allow positive marginal condensation in critical areas such as the gingivoproximal margin. The condensed composite material is then cured by means of a 40-second application of visible light from the occlusal direction. Additional composite material is then added incrementally to the proximal box region and subsequently cured (40 seconds), making absolutely sure that no thicker a layer than 22 mm is inserted and cured in any given increment. The usual class II preparation requires two to three increments of composite material, each individually cured.

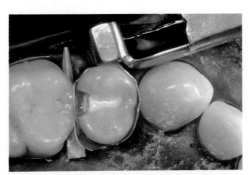

Figure 7-13 A thin precontoured metal matrix properly wedged as seen from occlusal view.

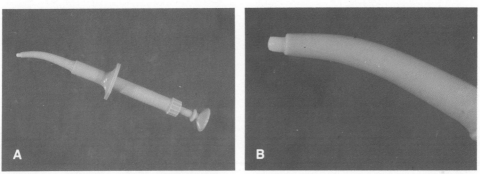

Figure 7-14 *A*, A Teflon carrier suitable for composite insertion. *B*, The composite material does not stick to the Teflon tip.

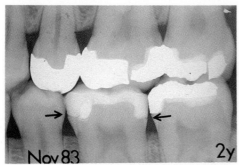

Figure 7-15 Gingival failure of an MOD composite restoration in the mandibular first molar at 2-year recall.

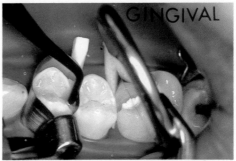

Figure 7-16 A small round condenser is used to positively condense the composite material to the gingival floor.

The final composite material placed over the occlusal cavo-surface region should be carefully controlled during condensation to minimize the amount of gross finishing. To accomplish this purpose, a smooth metallic conical instrument (Mortensen MM[2] Amalgam Condenser;[24] PKT No. 3[25]) (Fig. 7-17), wetted with bond resin, is used to shape and form the occlusal anatomy including the triangular cusp ridges, the marginal ridges, triangular fossae, and pit-groove pattern prior to the cure of the composite material (Fig. 7-18). The anatomically-contoured composite restoration is then cured by means of visible light applied from the occlusal for 40 seconds. Full cure is confirmed by application of visible light from both buccal and lingual directions after the metal matrix retainer and band are removed. Should the composite material be properly contoured before curing, little finishing is necessary (Figs. 7-19 and 7-20).

Finishing of the composite material should be accomplished occlusally by use of multifluted carbide steel finishing burs (T Burs;[26] OS[2] Finishing Bur[27]) to remove gross excess (Fig. 7-21) followed by a sharply tapered, pointed, white polystone (Tapering White Polystone[28]). Aluminum oxide discs (Soflex Discs[29]) may be used for proximal finish.

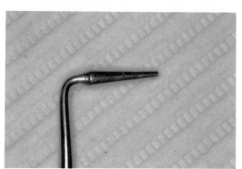

Figure 7–17 Smooth metallic conical instrument (Mortensen MM2 Amalgam Condenser[24]) suitable for shaping composite occlusal detail.

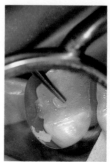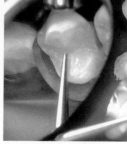

Figure 7–18 The conical instrument is used to shape and form the occlusal surface detail of the composite material prior to curing with visible light.

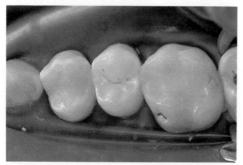

Figure 7–19 Occlusal view of the DO and MOL composite restorations immediately after light cure.

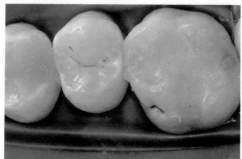

Figure 7–20 Close-up view of the MOL restoration in the maxillary first molar immediately after light cure. Gross excess of composite material is not present.

A smooth reflective surface is finally accomplished using an appropriate fine aluminum oxide paste type abrasive (Command Ultrafine Luster Paste[30]) applied by means of a rubber cup (Fig. 7-22). The completed restorations are shown in Figures 7-23 to 7-25. After careful occlusal adjustment the composite restorations should be recured by means of a 40-second application of visible light applied occlusally in order to ensure complete cure of the function surface.

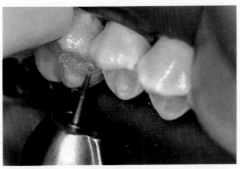

Figure 7–21 Use of tapering multifluted carbide finishing bur for occlusal finish.

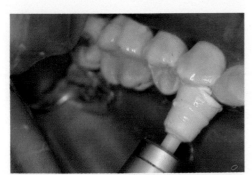

Figure 7–22 Application of polishing paste on a rubber cap.

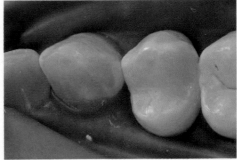

Figure 7–23 Occlusal view of DO composite restoration in the maxillary first premolar.

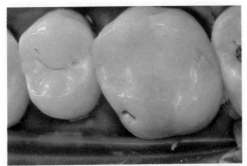

Figure 7–24 Occlusal view of the MOL composite restoration in the maxillary first molar.

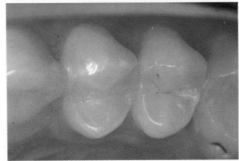

Figure 7–25 Occlusal view of the DO composite restoration in the maxillary first premolar. It is almost undetectable.

COMPOSITE-IONOMER LAMINATED RESTORATIONS

Figure 7-26 shows an occlusal-buccal composite restoration in a mandibular first molar at 3-year recall. The patient experienced the onset of thermal sensitivity approximately 2½ years after the restoration was placed. Since the discomfort persisted for several months without a decrease in severity, the composite restoration was removed and replaced with a reinforced zinc oxide eugenol (Polysyrene Reinforced Zinc Oxide Eugenol[31]) temporary dressing (Fig. 7-27). The thermal sensitivity ceased abruptly within 48 hours after placement of the zinc oxide-eugenol restoration and did not recur over a 2-month waiting period. The zinc oxide-eugenol dressing was removed, and the cavity preparation was thoroughly cleaned (using 3% hydrogen peroxide followed by a water lavage) and dried. A fast-setting glass ionomer cement (Ketac Bond[17]) was placed to cover the pulpal floor of the preparation (Figs. 7-28 and 7-29) as well as the dentin portions of the buccal, lingual, mesial, and distal walls. It was allowed to set undisturbed for 4 minutes, and then the enamel walls of the preparation were lightly stoned with a tapering diamond instrument to ensure a clean enamel periphery.

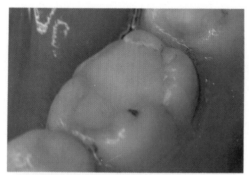

Figure 7-26 An occlusobuccal composite restoration at 3-year recall.

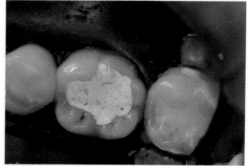

Figure 7-27 Zinc oxide and eugenol anodyne restoration in the tooth shown in Figure 7-26.

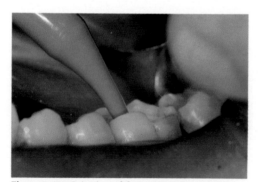

Figure 7-28 Injection of fast-setting glass ionomer cement pulpal protective.

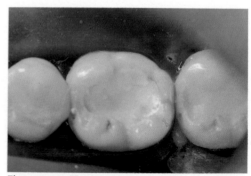

Figure 7-29 The ionomer cement covers the pulp floor and all peripheral dentin.

Phosphoric acid gel was then injected to cover the enamel walls for one minute and the entire extent of the ionomer cement surface for 20 seconds (Figs. 7-30 and 7-31). After a thorough water lavage and careful air-drying, a thin layer of bond resin (Prisma Universal Bond[52]) was placed on the enamel walls and ionomer cement surface and light-cured (Prismalight[33]) for 20 seconds. Composite material (Fulfil[2]) was then placed, contoured, and cured. The finished, completed laminated restoration is shown in Figures 7-32 and 7-33.

Rationale of Ionomer-Composite Treatment

In my experience, thermal sensitivity after composite restoration is a sure clinical symptom of pulp irritation. When thermal sensitivity persists (i.e., beyond 4 weeks), the composite restoration should be replaced with a zinc oxide-eugenol dressing to sedate the pulp. Following this, extreme care must be taken to place a final restoration which is totally nonirritating. The ionomer cement layer provides a chemical bond to dentin and is, for the most part,

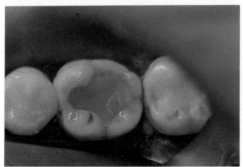

Figure 7-30 Gel etchant applied to enamel walls and ionomer cement surface.

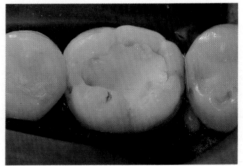

Figure 7-31 The enamel and ionomer surfaces after acid etching.

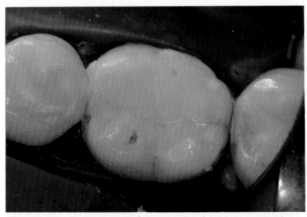

Figure 7-32 Occlusal view of the completed ionomer-composite restoration.

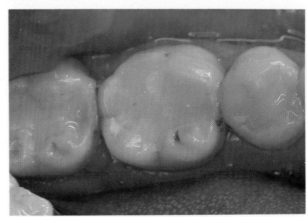

Figure 7-33 Occlusal view of the completed ionomer-composite restoration.

nonirritating to pulp tissue (Kawahara et al, 1979; Tobias et al, 1978). Furthermore, after acid etching of the glass ionomer surface, the basis for micromechanical bonding of the overlying composite material is provided (see Fig. 6-50). The ''dual-bonded'' restoration thus provides pulp protection in addition to effective dentin and enamel bonding.

Postoperative sensitivity with posterior composite restorations:

There are innumerable potential causes of postoperative sensitivity with posterior composite restorations. Probably the most common are:

1. Inadvertently subjecting dentin to phosphoric acid etching. This may be minimized by means of the careful application of fast setting glass ionomer cement[14-17] to all dentin surfaces prior to acid etching.
2. Polymerization contraction shrinkage with resultant "cuspal tension." This may be minimized by a "layering" insertion technique.
3. Maryinal leakage, particularly at the proximo-gingival margin. This may be reduced by means of a carefully controlled bonding and condensation technique.

CURRENT STATUS OF POSTERIOR COMPOSITE MATERIALS

Although patients universally demonstrate tremendous enthusiasm relative to the new ''tooth-colored'' posterior restorative materials, their routine use at the present time must be regarded as experimental. Although 3-year recall results (Wilder et al, 1983) relative to wear resistance appear promising (see Fig. 7-1), particularly regarding light-cured composite materials, an acceptable substitute for silver amalgam in the posterior region has not yet been found (ADA Status Report, 1983). Until longer-term clinical observations relative to the durability of composite materials in the posterior region are available, posterior composite materials should only be planned under the following circumstances:

1. Where esthetic requirements are primarily essential, i.e., in maxillary and mandibular canines and premolars.
2. In situations in which the buccolingual width of the cavity preparation can be restricted.
3. When the patient is fully informed as to the experimental nature of the posterior materials.
4. When the dentist is prepared to minimize the technique-sensitivity of the materials by means of a meticulously controlled clinical procedure involving (a) conservative cavity design, (b) ''prewedging'' and customized matricing techniques, (c) controlled pulp protection, and (d) a controlled insertion technique which minimizes the need for extensive finishing procedures.

LONG-TERM RECALL OBSERVATIONS

Long-term follow-up observations on direct placed light cured composite materials[1-7] indicate that when such materials are placed in conservative class I and II cavity preparations in the premolar and molar regions, the restorations are durable and highly wear resistant over prolonged periods (see Fig. 7-1). However, when placed in very large cavity preparations in the molar region, sufficient wear may occur over a 5-year period so as to compromise the integrity of the posterior occlusion (Fig. 7-34). With such restorations, either a *direct hybrid composite inlay technique* or an *indirect porcelain inlay technique* is recommended because wear resistance and marginal integrity with both are considerably improved.

Direct Hybrid Composite Inlay Technique:
(Coltene Brilliant Direct Inlay System[36], Patent Pending)

A brief description of highlights of the technique follows. For more details, manufacturer's directions should be followed closely.

A large MOD amalgam restoration in the maxillary first molar and a failed mesioocclusal composite restoration in the maxillary first premolar are shown in Figure 7-35. The restorations are removed and preparations are made that draw occlusally with a taper of approximately 7 to 10° (particularly on the axial walls), Figure 7-36. The axial wall convergence is necessary since, upon polymerization, the composite material shrinks towards the midcentral region of the occlusal surface.

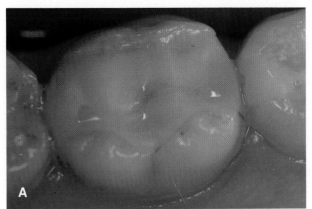
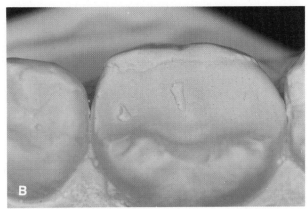

Figure 7-34 *A*, An MOD direct placed light-cured, composite restoration in the mandibular first molar at 5-year recall, and *B*, the diestone cast of the same restoration, which shows both generalized wear in addition to localized wear on the buccal margin.

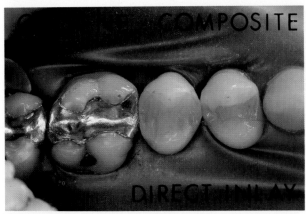
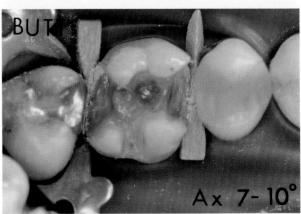

Figure 7-35 Occlusal view of an MOD amalgam restoration in the first molar and an MO composite restoration in the first premolar.

Figure 7-36 MODL cavity preparation of first molar. Note the taper of the axial walls.

The entire dentinal surfaces of the preparations are lined with a fast setting glass ionomer cement[17,34] (Fig. 7-37). Clear polyethylene matrix bands[37] are placed in addition to reflective gingival wedges[38] (Fig. 7-38), and an agar alcohol separating medium[38] (DI Separator[39]) is then painted over the ionomer surfaces and the enamel walls of the cavity preparations (Fig. 7-39A) after which warm air is applied for 15 seconds. A high viscosity light cured hybrid composite (Brilliant DI composite[40]) is then condensed into the preparations, and the composite material is formed to anatomic detail. The composite restorations are then light cured for 40 to 60 seconds both from a gingival direction (Fig. 7-40) and occlusally (Fig. 7-41). After gross finish (Fig. 7-42), the composite patterns are removed from the preparations using a spoon excavator (Fig. 7-43). The axial walls of the composite patterns are then relieved using a multifluted carbide finishing bur (Fig. 7-44), and anatomic details of the occlusal surface are clarified. Proximal contours and contact may be added by lightly abrading the proximal surface, which is followed by the placement of a thin film of bond resin on the composite surface. Then directly, new composite is added to the proximal surface, followed by proper contouring and finally visible light cure. The patterns are then reseated into the preparations in order to reaffirm that correct proximal contours and contacts exist. The patterns are inserted into an oven at 110 °C for 5 minutes of heat treatment (Fig. 7-45). It has been shown that the degree of polymerization of composite materials increases from self cured to light cured to heat cured systems. Accordingly, the heat treatment procedure significantly enhances all physical properties including hardness and wear resistance.

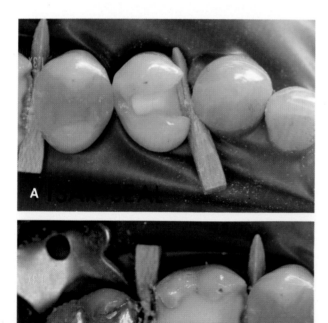

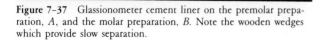

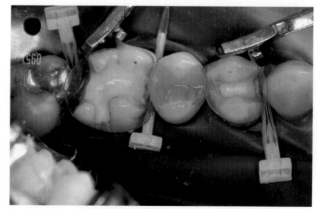

Figure 7–37   Glassionometer cement liner on the premolar preparation, *A*, and the molar preparation, *B*. Note the wooden wedges which provide slow separation.

Figure 7–38   Clear matrix bands and "cure through" gingival wedges.

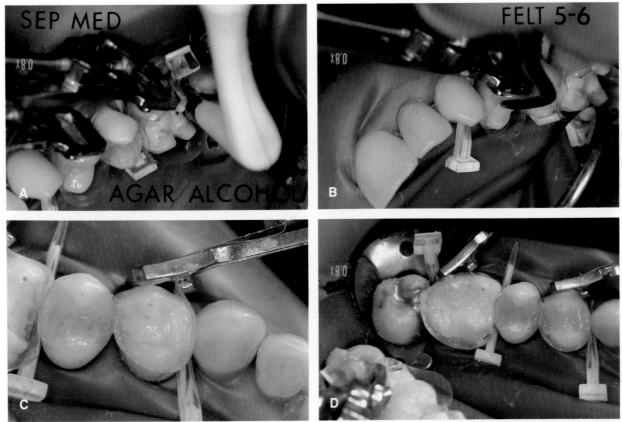

Figure 7-39 *A,* DI Separator is applied to the walls of the cavity preparations and the ionomer cement lining. *B,* Condensation of the composite material into all details of the cavity preparations. *C,* The composite material is shaped and formed into the premolar preparation. *D,* The composite material is shaped and formed into the molar preparation.

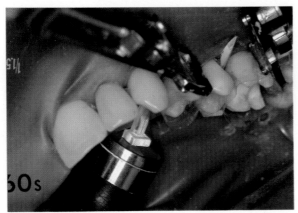

Figure 7-40 Application of light to the reflective wedge gingivally.

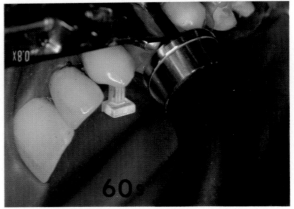

Figure 7-41 Application of light from the occlusal direction.

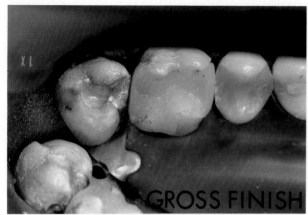

Figure 7-42 The composite pattern after gross finish.

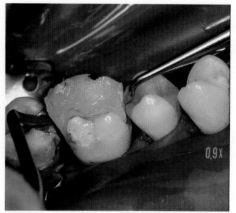

Figure 7-43 The composite pattern is removed by means of a spoon excavator.

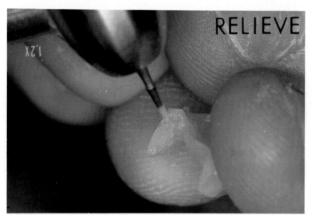

Figure 7-44 Relief of axial walls.

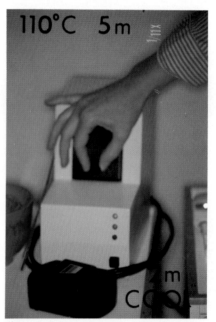

Figure 7-45 An appropriate oven for heat treatment of the composite patterns.

In preparation for insertion, polyethylene bands and reflective wedges are placed (Fig. 7-46), and the enamel walls of the preparations and the ionomer cement linings are phosphoric acid etched for a 30-second period, followed by washing and drying. A layer of bond resin is applied to the internal composite surfaces as well as to the enamel walls and ionomer liners of the preparations (Fig. 7-47). A low viscosity, dual initiated (i.e., both light- and self-cured) composite luting material[41], DI Duo Cement, is now mixed and placed on the internal surfaces of the hybrid composite patterns (Fig. 7-48), which are then seated and held under firm pressure while light curing is carried out from both the occlusal and gingival directions for 60 seconds. (Fig. 7-49). The composite restorations are now finished using the same technique as described previously (Fig. 7-50). Careful occlusal adjustment follows.

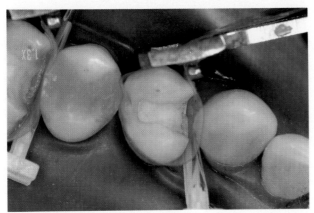

Figure 7-46 Clear matrix bands and reflective wedges in place preparatory to insertion.

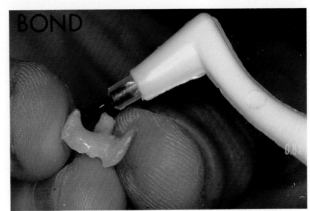

Figure 7-47 Application of bond resin to the composite pattern.

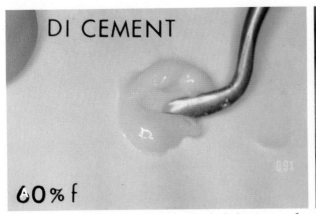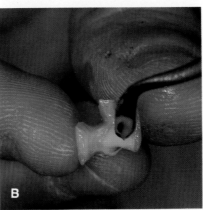

Figure 7-48 *A,* Appearance of the low viscosity luting cement after mixing. *B,* Application of the luting composite to the pattern.

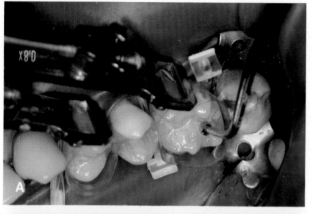

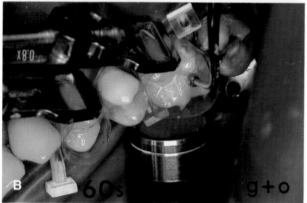

Figure 7-49 *A*, Placement of composite pattern under pressure. *B*, Application of visible light.

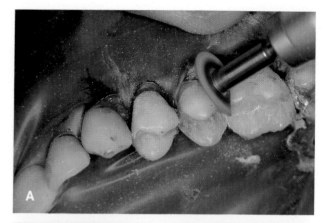

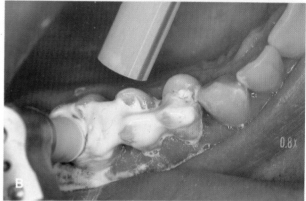

Figure 7-50 *A* and *B*, Finish of the composite restorations is accomplished in the usual manner.

The completed restorations are shown in Figures 7-51 to 7-53.

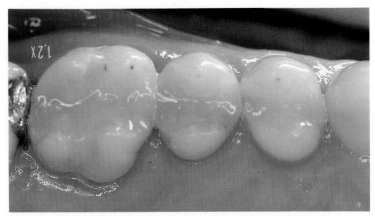

Figure 7–51   Completed direct hybrid inlay restorations in the maxillary first premolar and first molar.

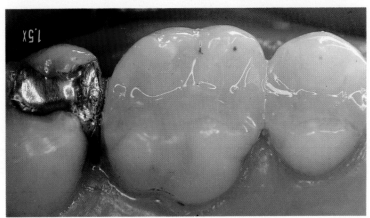

Figure 7–52   Closeup view of the finished molar restoration.

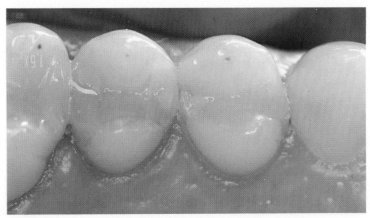

Figure 7–53   Closeup view of the finished first premolar restoration.

Advantages of the direct composite hybrid inlay restorations are as follows:

1. Since all physical properties are enhanced, it is expected that durability and wear resistance will be considerably improved (Figs. 7-54 to 7-56) over direct placed light cured systems.
2. The limited depth of cure of direct placed composite restorations is not a problem with the hybrid inlay.
3. Marginal adaptation is excellent since the luting composite material completely fills any marginal contraction gaps that exist (Fig. 7-54).
4. Polymerization contraction shrinkage is virtually nonexistent since the only shrinkage possible is with the luting composite which is present in a very thin layer (100 microns).
5. Postoperative sensitivity is not commonly encountered due primarily to the pulpal protective effect of the glass ionomer liner.

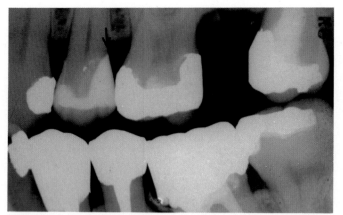

Figure 7-54   Postoperative radiograph of a class 2 hybrid inlay showing the excellent seal at the proximogingival margin (arrow).

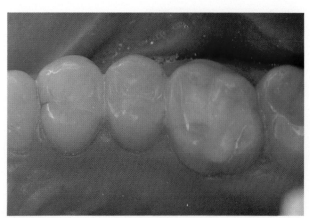

Figure 7-55   A quadrant of direct hybrid composite inlays at 6-month recall.

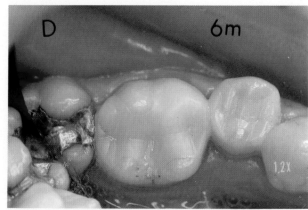

Figure 7-56   A direct hybrid onlay in the mandibular first molar at 6-month recall.

Porcelain Inlay (Cerinate[41]) Technique

An additional method of effectively restoring a stable posterior occlusion esthetically is by means of the Cerinate inlay technique. Figure 7-57 shows a maxillary quadrant of large silver amalgam restorations. Before cavity preparations are started, an alginate impression of the arch is taken in order to facilitate the fabrication of temporary restorations. The amalgam restorations are removed, and cavity preparations are made with some degree of occlusal draught (Figs. 7-58 and 7-59). The occlusal enamel cavo-surface margins should not be bevelled, since if this is done, a thin fin of porcelain results at the occlusal margin, which is prone to fracture under function.

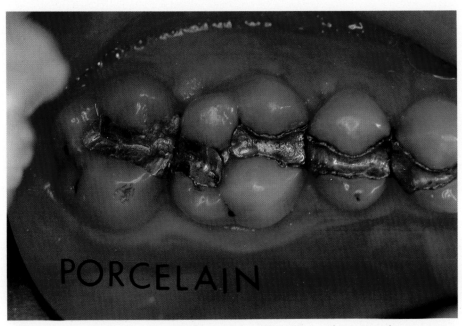

Figure 7–57 Preoperative view of a maxillary quadrant of large silver amalgam restorations.

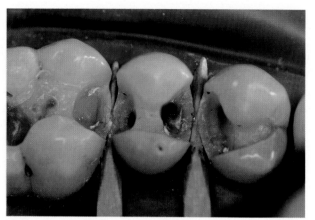

Figure 7-58   Roughed out cavity preparations for porcelain inlays.

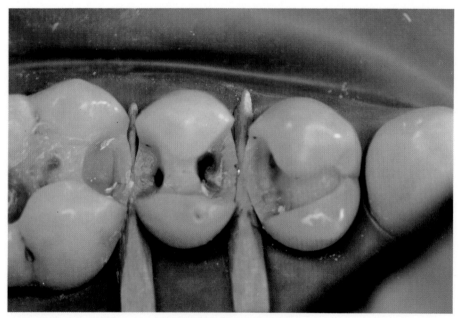

Figure 7-59   Closeup view of cavity preparation for porcelain inlays.

A fast setting glass ionomer cement[43] is then placed to cover all dentin on the pulpal and gingival floors and the axial walls (Fig. 7-60). The glass ionomer cement not only protects the underlying pulp, but in addition, constitutes a "bonded base" to the dentinal surfaces. The cavity preparations are now refined and finally finished (Fig. 7-61).

A full arch impression is taken (Fig. 7-62) using either thiokol rubber base or a polyvinyl siloxane material[44,45]. The polyvinyl siloxane (addition silicone) is preferred because of the accuracy and extreme dimensional stability of the material. An additional silicone bite registration index[46] is taken (Fig. 7-63) in order to facilitate mounting of the maxillary and mandibular casts (Fig. 7-64). Temporary restorations are then fabricated and luted in the usual manner (Fig. 7-65), preferably by use of noneugenol containing temporary luting material.

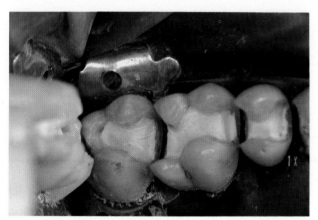

Figure 7-60 The ionomer lining cement covers all dentin on the pulpal floor axial walls and gingival walls.

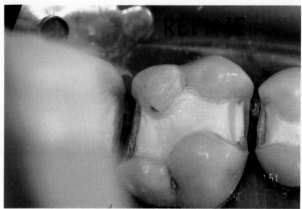

Figure 7-61 Completed MOD cavity preparation for porcelain inlay restoration.

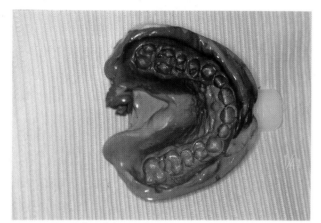

Figure 7–62   Full arch impression.

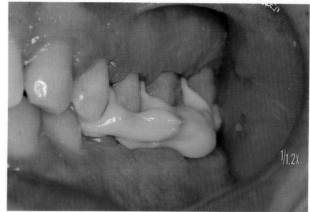

Figure 7–63   A bit registration is made using a polyvinyl siloxane paste, Ramitec[46].

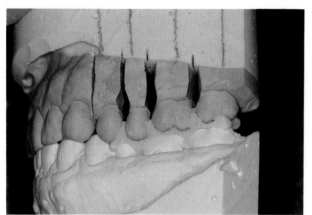

Figure 7–64   Mounted maxillary and mandibular casts.

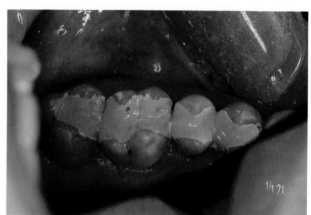

Figure 7–65   Temporary restorations in the maxillary quadrant.

Following standardized laboratory procedures, the porcelain inlays are fired and glazed in the usual manner (Fig. 7-66). The internal surfaces of the inlays are treated by means of a 3 minute application of hydrofluoric acid that effectively etches the porcelain surfaces (Fig. 7-67), thereby creating deep microporosities (Fig. 7-68). The treated porcelain surfaces are now "micromechanically self retentive" for the composite luting material.

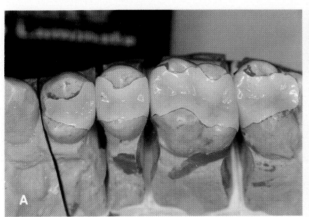 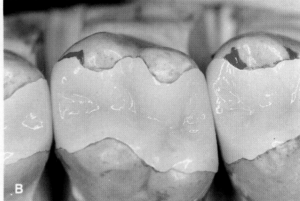

Figure 7-66 *A,* Cerinate inlay restorations on the master model. *B,* Closeup view.

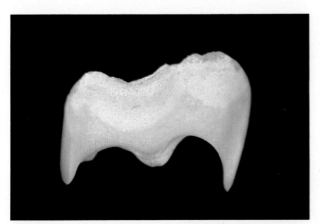 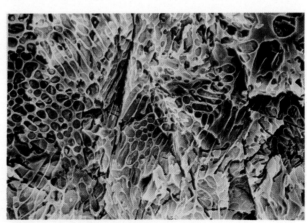

Figure 7-67 Internal porcelain surfaces after hydrofluoric acid etching.

Figure 7-68 Scanning electron micrograph of hydrofluoric etched porcelain surface.

The porcelain inlays are now seated into position (Fig. 7-69). Marginal fit is rarely exact due to the inevitable shrinkage of the porcelain during the firing procedure (Fig. 7-70). This does not constitute a problem since the luting composite material more than adequately seals the marginal region. The occlusion should not be checked until after the porcelain inlays are luted because, if any attempt is made to check the occlusion before the inlays are luted, fracture may well occur.

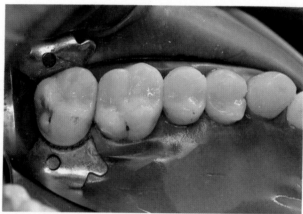

Figure 7-69 Porcelain inlays seated into position.

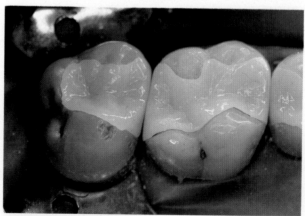

Figure 7-70 Closeup view of the MOD porcelain inlay showing lack of precise marginal adaptation.

Prior to bonding, porcelain conditioner[47] (Fig. 7-71) (citric acid) is applied to the internal porcelain surfaces (Fig. 7-72) for a 20 second period (in order to clean the porcelain), and the inlays are washed with water and thoroughly dried. A silane primer (Cerinate Prime[TM][48]) is then painted on the internal porcelian surfaces and air dried (Fig. 7-73). A gell etchant is applied to the enamel walls and the ionomer surfaces by means of two stages application technique (Fig. 7-74). After washing and thorough drying, a bond resin (Creation Bond 3 in one[49]) is applied to the enamel walls and ionomer surfaces (Fig. 7-75), using a fine tipped brush. The bond resin is then gently air blown. A thin layer of bond resin is also applied to the internal porcelain inlay surfaces. a low viscosity dual initiated hybrid composite (Ultrabond[50]) is now applied to the internal porcelain surfaces, and the inlays are seated individually and light cured from both occlusal and gingival directions (Fig. 7-76). clear matrix strips, applied to the individual teeth prior to luting, facilitates the process (Fig 7-77). Excess luting composite is now removed using diamond or carbide finishing stones, and the occlusion is carefully adjusted (Figs. 7-78 and 7-79). Final finishing is facilitated by means of appropriate finishing points (Fig. 7-80) and a fine polishing paste[51]. The completed restorations are shown in figures 7-81 to 7-84.

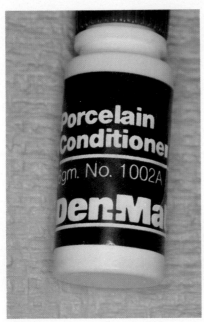

Figure 7–71 Porcelain condition (citric acid).

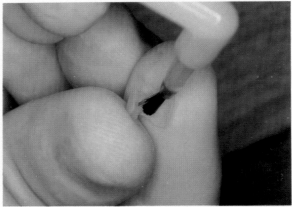

Figure 7–72 Application of porcelain conditioner to porcelain internal surfaces.

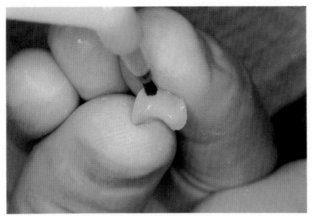

Figure 7–73 Application of silane primer to internal porcelain surfaces.

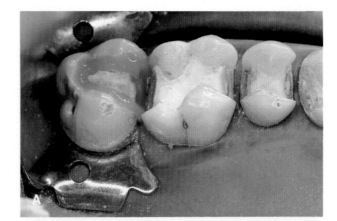

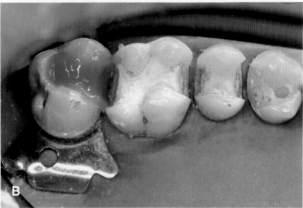

Figure 7–74 Prior to luting the porcelain inlay, a two stage application of phosphoric acid gel is applied to the preparations. Acid gel is injected to cover the enamel walls for 40 seconds, *A*, and additional gel is then injected to cover the ionomer surfaces for 20 seconds, *B.*

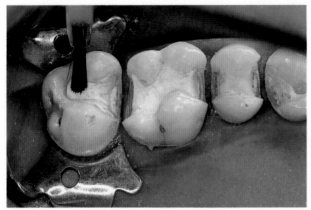

Figure 7–75 Application of bond resin to cavity preparation.

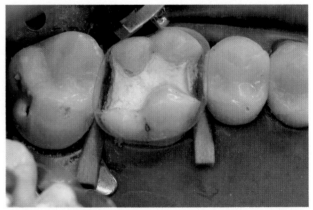

Figure 7–76 The MO porcelain inlay on the maxillary second molar seated and cured, following which a clear matrix strip is applied to the first molar prior to luting.

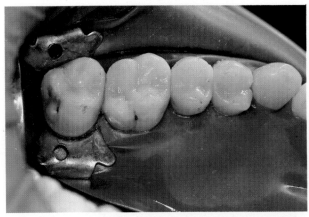

Figure 7-77 The porcelain inlays immediately subsequent to luting with composite material.

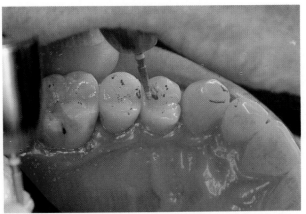

Figure 7-78 After luting, the occlusion can be checked and adjusted without danger of porcelain fracture.

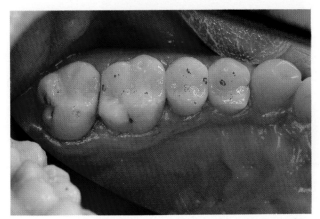

Figure 7-79 "High" spots on the occlusal surfaces require careful adjustment.

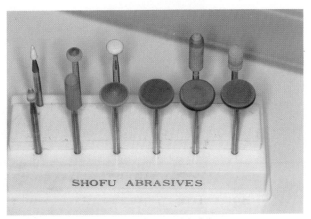

Figure 7-80 Finishing points for porcelain inlays.

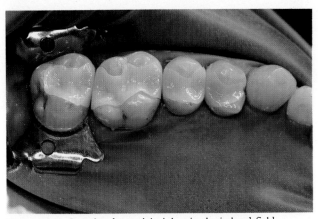

Figure 7-81 Completed porcelain inlays in the isolated field.

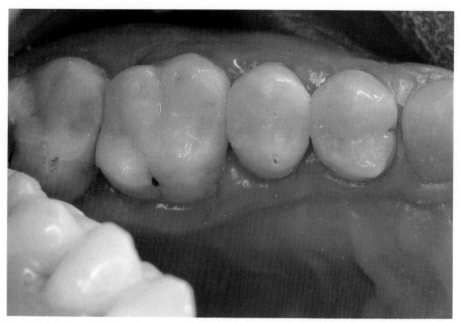

Figure 7–82   Porcelain inlays after removal of rubber dam.

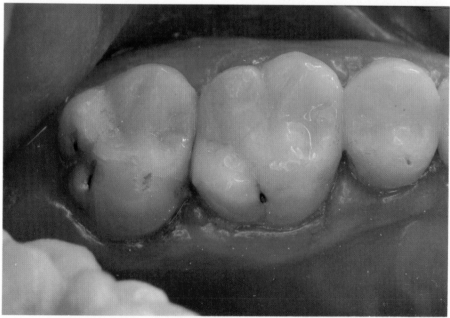

Figure 7–83   Closeup view of porcelain inlays in maxillary molars.

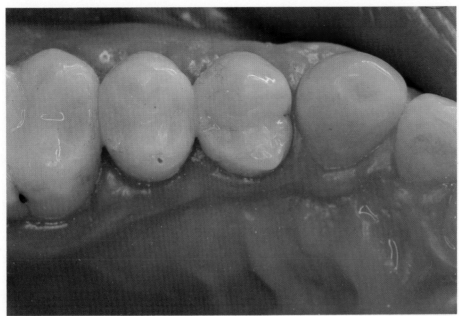

Figure 7-84 Closeup view of porcelain inlays in maxillary premolars.

The advantages associated with porcelain inlays are as follows:

1. The porcelain inlays are not only highly esthetic but, in addition, are virtually totally wear resistant.
2. The bonded restorations significantly strengthen adjacent tooth structure.
3. Polymerization contraction shrinkage is negligible.
4. Marginal adaptation is excellent.
5. Postoperative sensitivity is rarely encountered.

References

Goto G, Jordan RE. Pulpal response to composite resin materials. J Prosthet Dent 1972; 28:601.

Goto G, Jordan RE. Pulpal effects of concentred phosphoric acid. Bull Tokyo Dent C 1973; 14:105.

Kawahara H, Imanishi Y, Oshina H. Biological evaluation of glass ionomer cements. J Dent Res 1979; 58:1080.

Landy NA, Simonsen RJ. Cusp fracture strength in class II composite resin restorations. J Dent Res 1984; 63:175. (Abstract 40)

Leinfelder KF. Composite resins in posterior teeth. Dent Clin North Am 1981; 25:357.

Leinfelder KF, Roberson TM. Clinical evaluation of posterior composite resins. Gen Dent 1983; 31:276.

Lutz F, Phillips RW, Roulet JF, Setcos JC. In vitro and in vivo wear of potential posterior composites. J Dent Res 1984; 63:914.

Morin D, Delong R, Douglas WH. Reinforcement by the acid etch technique. J Dent Res 1984; 63:1075.

Noro A, Ishikawa K. A clinicopathological study of pulp response of a restoration system with ultra violet light polymerized resin and the effectiveness of several lining materials. Bull Tokyo Dent C 1983; 24:61.

Osborne JW, Gale EN, Ferguson GW. One-year and two-year clinical evaluation of a composite resin vs amalgam. J Prosthet Dent 1973; 30:795.

Phillips RW, et al. Observations on a composite resin for class II restorations. Two-year report. J Prosthet Dent 1972; 28:164.

Phillips RW, Crim G, Swartz ML, Clark HE. Resistance of calcium hydroxide preparational to solubility in phosphoric acid. J Am Dent Assoc 1984; 52:358.

Status Report on Posterior Composites. J Am Dent Assoc 1983; 107:74.

Tobias RS, Browne RM, Plant CG, Ingram DY. Pulpal response to a glass ionomer cement. Br Dent J 1978; 144:345.

Wilder AD, May KN, Leinfelder KF. Three-year clinical study of UV-cured composite resins in posterior teeth. J Prosthet Dent 1983; 50:26.

PRODUCT INFORMATION

Product	Manufacturer/Distributor	Purpose
1. P10; P30	Dental Products/3M Company 3M Center 270–5N–02 St. Paul, MN 55144	Posterior composite materials; P10, self-cured; P30, light-cured
2. Fulfil	L.D. Caulk Co. P.O. Box 359 Milford, DE 19963–0359	Light-cured posterior composite
3. Estilux	Kulzer Inc. 10015 Muirlands Blvd., Unit G Irvine, CA 92714	Light-cured posterior composite
4. Adaptic II	Johnson & Johnson 20 Lake Drive CN 7060 East Windsor, NJ 08520	Light-cured posterior composite
5. Status	Healthco 25 Stuart St. Boston, MA 02116	Posterior composite material
6. Marathon	Den-Mat Inc. 3130 Skyway Dr., Unit 501	Light-cured posterior composite
7. Herculite (Condensable)	Kerr-Sybron Co. P.O. Box 455 Romulus, MI 48174	Light-cured posterior composite
8. 13T, 13XT Sycamore Wedges	ESPE-Premier Sales Corp. Romano Dr., P.O. Box 111 Norristown, PA 19401	For "prewedging" technique
9. Dycal Improved	L.D. Caulk Co. P.O. Box 359 Milford, DE 19963–0359	Calcium hydroxide pulp protective
10. Procal	Dental Products/3M Company 3M Center 270–5N–02 St. Paul, MN 55144	Calcium hydroxide pulp protective
11. Renew	S.S. White Co. Three Parkway Philadelphia, PA 19102	Calcium hydroxide pulp protective
12. Dycal Advanced Formula	L.D. Caulk Co. P.O. Box 359 Milford, DE 19963–0359	Calcium hydroxide pulp protective
13. Life	Kerr-Sybron Co. P.O. Box 455 Romulus, MI 48174	Acid-resistant, calcium hydroxide pulp protective
14. Shofu Base Cement	Shofu Company 420 Bohannon Drive Menlo Park, CA 94025	Fast setting glass ionomer cement
15. Zionomer Lining	Den-Mat Corp. 3130 Skyway Dr., Unit 501 Santa Maria, CA 93456	Fast-setting glass ionomer cement
16. Gingiva Seal	Parkell Co. Farmingdale NY	Fast-setting, glass ionomer pulp protective
17. Ketac Bond	ESPE-Premier Sales Corp. Romano Dr., P.O. Box 111 Norristown, PA 19401	Fast-setting, glass ionomer pulp protective
18. Scotchbond Gel Etch	Dental Products/3M Company 3M Center 270–5N–02 St. Paul, MN 55144	Viscous gel etchant

PRODUCT INFORMATION

Product	Manufacturer/Distributor	Purpose
19. Caulk Gel Etchant	L.D. Caulk Co. P.O. Box 359 Milford, DE 199963-0359	Viscous gel etchant
20. Teflon Amalgam Gun	ESPE-Premier Sales Corp. Romano Dr., P.O. Box 111 Norristown, PA 19401	Carrier for insertion of composite material
21. Centrix Syringe	Centrix Inc. 480 Sniffens Lane Stamford, CT 06497	Syringe for insertion of composite material
22. Felt Nos. 2,3,5,6	American Dental Instrument Manufacturing Co. 2800 Reserve St., P.O. Box 4546 Missoula, MT 59801	Teflon-coated condensation instruments
23. Herculite (Condensable)	Kerr-Sybron Co. P.O. Box 455 Romulus, MI 48174	Condensable posterior composite
24. Mortenson MM2 Amalgam Condenser	Star Dental Co. P.O. Box 896 Valley Forge, PA 19482	For shaping and forming occlusal anatomic detail
25. PKT No. 3	American Dental Instrument Manufacturing Co.	For shaping and forming occlusal anatomic detail
26. T Burs	Ritter/Midwest Co. 901 W. Oakton Des Moines, IL 60018	Tapering multifluted finishing bur
27. OS^2 Finishing Bur	Brasseler USA Inc. 800 King George Blvd. Savannah, GA 31419	Tapering multifluted finishing bur
28. Tapering White Polystone	Shofu Co. 420 Bohannon Dr. Menlo Park, CA 94025	For occlusal composite finishing
29. Soflex Discs	Dental Products/3M Company 3M Center 270–5N–02 St. Paul, MN 55144	For interproximal composite finishing
30. Command Ultra-fine Luster Paste	Kerr-Sybron Co. P.O. Box 455 Romulus, MI 48174	For final surface smoothing
31. Polysyrene Reinforced Zinc Oxide Eugenol	Anodyne Products Box 1144 Guelph, Ontario N1H 6N3	Anodyne zinc oxide eugenol cement
32. Bond lite	Kerr-Sybron Co. P.O. Box 455 Romulus, MI 48174	Light-cured enamel-dentin phosphonate bond resin
33. Prismalight	L.D. Caulk Co. P.O. Box 359 Milford, DE 19963–0359	Visible light-curing unit
34. G–C Lining Cement	G.C. International Corp. 7830 East Redfield Rd. Scottsdale, AZ 85260	Fast-setting, glass ionomer cement for pulp protection
35. Ho Matrix Band	Ho Dental Co. 966 Embarcadero Del Mar Goleta, CA 93117	Thin (.001 inch) matrix band for Class 2 composite restorations

PRODUCT INFORMATION

Product	Manufacturer/Distributor	Purpose
36. Coltene Brilliant Direct Inlay System	Coltene USA Inc. 5205 Avenida Encinas, Ste. L Carlsbad, CA 92008	Direct hybrid composite inlay restorations
37. Clear Matrix Bands	Hawes Neos Dental Dr. H.V. Weissenfluh A.G. CH–6925 Gentilino Switzerland	Clear matrix bands for Class 2 composite restorations
38. Cure Through Wedges	Hawes Neos Dental Dr. H.V. Weissenfluh A.G. CH–6925 Gentilino Switzerland	Clear gingival wedges with internal reflector for positive cure of proximogingival composite
39. DI Separator	Coltene USA Inc. 5205 Avenida Encinas, Ste. L Carlsbad, CA 92008	An agar-alcohol separating medium
40. Brilliant DI Composite	Coltene USA Inc. 5205 Avenida Encinas, Ste. L Carlsbad, CA 92008	A high viscosity hybrid composite material
41. DI Duo Cement	Coltene USA Inc. 5205 Avenida Encinas, Ste. L Carlsbad, CA 92008	A low viscosity dual initiating luting composite
42. Cerinate Porcelain Inlay	Den-Mat Corp. 3130 Skyway Dr., Unit 501 Santa Maria, CA 93456	Porcelain inlays for large posterior esthetic restorations
43. Zionomer Lining Cement	Den-Mat Corp. 3130 Skyway Dr., Unit 501 Santa Maria, CA 93456	Fast setting ionomer cement used as a bonded base.
44. Cerinate Vinyl Polysiloxane	Den-Mat Corp. 3130 Skyway Dr., Unit 501 Santa Maria, CA 93456	Vinyl polysiloxane (addition silicone) impression material
45. President	Coltene USA Inc. 5205 Avenida Encinas, Ste. L Carlsbad, CA 92008	Vinyl polysiloxane (addition silicone) impression material
46. Ramitec	ESPE-Premier Sales Corp. Romano Dr., P.O. Box 111 Norristown, PA 19401	Polyvinyl siloxane bite registration material
47. Porcelain Conditioner	Den-Mat Corp. 3130 Skyway Dr., Unit 501 Santa Maria, CA 93456	Citric acid for cleaning the internal porcelain surfaces
48. Cerinate Prime	Den-Mat Corp. 3130 Skyway Dr., Unit 501 Santa Maria, CA 93456	A silane porcelain primer
49. Creation Bond 3-in-1	Den-Mat Corp. 3130 Skyway Dr., Unit 501 Santa Maria, CA 93456	A light-cured enamel-dentin resin
50. Ultrabond	Den-Mat Corp. 3130 Skyway Dr., Unit 501 Santa Maria, CA 93456	A powder-liquid hybrid composite for luting porcelain inlays
51. Cerinate Polishing Paste	Den-Mat Corp. 3130 Skyway Dr., Unit 501 Santa Maria, CA 93456	A fine aluminum oxide polishing paste for final Cerinate inlay polish
52. Prisma Universal Bond	L.D. Caulk Co. P.O. Box 359 Milford, DE 19963-0359	A phosphonate light cured enamel-dentin bond resin

8

DONALD R. GRATTON

ESTHETIC COMPOSITE BONDING AND FIXED PROSTHODONTICS

Esthetic composite bonding techniques have made a dramatic impact in the area of fixed prosthodontics. Other chapters describe ultraconservative techniques that are proving highly successful in the restoration of single teeth in situations that formerly demanded full-crown coverage. This chapter will describe the application of composite bonding techniques to the replacement of missing teeth.

Clinical and research activity in this area has developed along two distinct avenues. Parallel but differing concepts, both first reported in 1973, will be presented under the general headings of *All-Resin Bonded Bridges* (i.e., resin-resin bonding) and *Cast-Metal Bonded Bridges* (i.e., resin-metal bonding). Examples of each type are shown in Figures 8-1 to 8-4.

ALL-RESIN BONDED BRIDGES

Development

Some of the pioneers of the enamel-etching / resin-bonding era were among those who first began testing the potential of the system in the replacement of missing anterior teeth (Buonocore, 1975; Ibsen, 1973). In the techniques they and others described, pontics were bonded with auto-curing or ultraviolet light-curing unfilled and filled resins directly to the etched enamel of adjacent teeth. *Acrylic resin denture teeth* were most frequently used as pontics although *natural teeth*, immediately after extraction, as well as custom-made pontics, fabricated from a variety of resin materials, were also utilized. Single and multiple missing anterior teeth were replaced in this way (Portnoy, 1973; Stolpa, 1975; Jenkins, 1978; Simonsen, 1978).

Further developments included efforts to increase the resistance of the bonding materials to cohesive fracture by the use of class III type preparations or threaded pins (see Figs. 8-19 and 8-20) in the proximal surfaces of abutment teeth (Jordan et al, 1978; Sweeney et al, 1980). With the current availability of visible-light-cured composite materials, these can be used efficiently to fabricate any of the all-resin bonded prostheses.

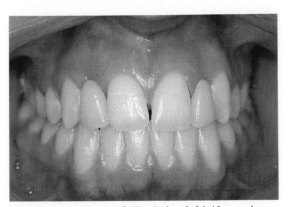

Figure 8–1 Labial view of all-resin bonded bridges replacing the right and left maxillary lateral incisors.

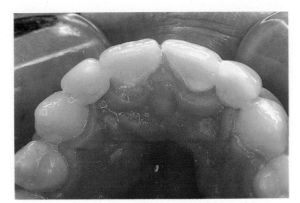

Figure 8-2 Lingual view of the all-resin bonded bridges.

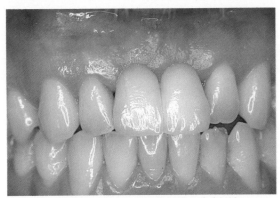

Figure 8–3 Labial view of a cast-metal bonded bridge replacing the maxillary central incisors.

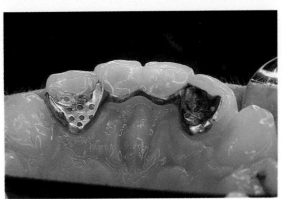

Figure 8–4 Lingual view of the cast-metal bonded bridge (shown in Figure 8-3).

Performance Considerations

Clinical Findings

Clinical investigators have all reported a similar problem. Loosening of the pontics was very common although reported periods of service varied from days to 3 years or more (Kochavi et al, 1977; Jenkins, 1978; Jordan et al, 1978). More predictable performance was obtained when greater bulk of composite material was used in class III preparations in abutment teeth or when pins were placed in the proximal surfaces of the abutments.

The most common mode of fracture involved cohesive breakdown of the bonding material itself. A less common problem occurred when composite and acrylic resins separated at the pontic interface. This led to the use of custom-made *composite* pontics as a potential means of eliminating interfacial failure. The impressive performance of the enamel-resin bond, on the other hand, was reinforced by reports of enamel being separated from its underlying dentin when bonded pontics were forcibly lost or removed. Investigators have suggested that factors involved in pontic loosening included lack of patient cooperation (particularly relative to incisive function), technique problems (bonding contamination or hyperocclusion), and pontic location (longest serviceability was observed in the lower anterior region).

Research Information

In reported in vitro studies, Lambert et al (1976), Kochavi et al (1977), and Sweeney et al (1980) assessed the amount of force required to dislodge pontics bonded with enamel etching alone, proximal class III abutment preparations, and proximal preparations reinforced with a continuous wire bonded within the pontic and into each of the abutment preparations. Greatest strength was obtained with the proximal class III abutment preparation, seemingly from sheer bulk of material, whereas lowest values occurred with the "reinforcing wire", which apparently disrupted the continuity of the composite material. In comparing the mean load values required to dislodge the pontics with reported in vivo biting forces, observations were made that these bonded restorations have sufficient retention to function adequately when properly placed in indicated clinical situations. Other clinical investigators point out, however, that inadvertent extremes of force occurring clinically, as well as horizontal movements of natural teeth, are complicating oral factors (Kochavi, 1977; Jenkins, 1978), so that what seems adequate "on the bench" may not fare nearly so well in the mouth. Such would seem to be the case with these bonded pontics since eventual loosening appears likely or perhaps inevitable. Careful case selection and precise clinical techniques are required for successful use of these restorations. Jordan and others (1978) have suggested, as a general guideline, that for *longevity requirements of up to 9 months, the acid-etch resin technique alone may be used, whereas for requirements of a year or more, supplemental retention in the form of pins or proximal preparations is recommended.*

Case Selection

Indications

Although lack of strength on the part of the composite bonding materials continues to be a major shortcoming of the all-resin bonded bridge, there are many advantages which make familiarity with and use of this technique extremely valuable. Bearing in mind the previously mentioned guidelines and with an appreciation of the fact that a loosened pontic (generally occurring at only one connector site as in Fig. 8-22) is easily repaired by techniques detailed in a following section (Maintenance), the clinician will find a variety of situations which lend themselves ideally to this ultraconservative approach.

As an interim or *short-term restoration*, the all-resin bonded bridge has tremendous potential in the immediate placement of anterior teeth which have been lost through accident or planned extraction (Figs. 8-5 to 8-8). Because the restoration does not require dental laboratory service, it can be completed on an "as required" basis, providing "instant" esthetic replacement, intra- and inter-arch stability, and a degree of functional efficiency.

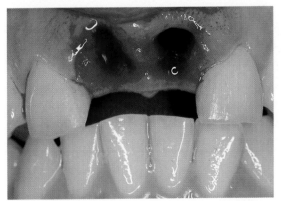

Figure 8-5 A young female patient whose severe localized periodontal disease precipitated the loss of the maxillary central incisors.

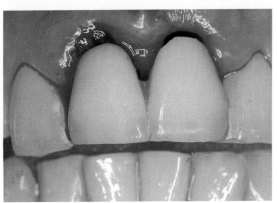

Figure 8-6 Immediate replacement of the extracted teeth with an all-resin bonded bridge.

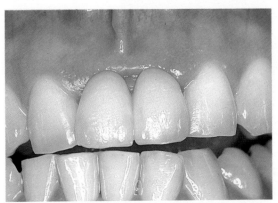

Figure 8-7 Following a 12-month healing period, a cast-metal bonded bridge was inserted to replace the missing incisors, as seen from the labial.

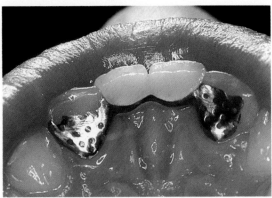

Figure 8-8 A lingual view of the same prosthesis.

Tissue remodeling subsequent to extraction or accidental tooth loss can be given the time it requires. Assessment and restoration of remaining diseased or damaged teeth can proceed unhurriedly. Treatment plans can be methodically established and then systematically implemented. All of these are possible while the interim restoration with its bonded pontic(s) performs in a positive fashion in contrast to the deleterious effects so often associated with traditional removable interim prostheses.

For patients being retreated with "fixed" prostheses whose tissues have responded negatively to a removable appliance, the bonded pontic(s) offer an opportunity for abused tissues to "regroup", unquestionably permitting a higher-quality final restoration (Figs. 8-9 to 8-11).

For the very young patients with congenitally missing teeth, including those treated orthodontically, the all-resin bonded bridge is possibly the treatment of choice, even when a somewhat longer service period is required. Abutment teeth, probably with large pulps, perhaps not fully erupted and possibly requiring a period of postorthodontic stabilization can support a resin bonded pontic without suffering any "side effects". The economy of these prostheses permits them to be used as a preliminary appliance (to a conventional fixed prosthesis or to a cast-metal bonded bridge) while a greater degree of maturity and stability is achieved in the young dentition (Figs. 8-12 and 8-13). From an esthetic point of view, the opportunity afforded the clinician of customizing the pontic(s) in respect to size, shape, and color, all at chairside, in addition to the lack of cutting and therefore esthetic change incurred by the abutments, can make these restorations truly superior (Fig. 8-14).

The serviceability of resin-bonded pontics has, on many occasions, surpassed expectations (Fig. 8-15). In such situations, the all-resin restoration can justifiably be considered a "permanent" prosthesis. Experience with such long-term success has led to the intentional use of similar restorations as final or permanent treatment (Figs. 8-16 to 8-18).

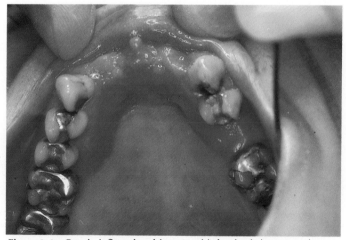

Figure 8-9   Grossly inflamed and hypertrophied palatal tissues associated with a removable prosthesis. (Note outline of the acrylic coverage.)

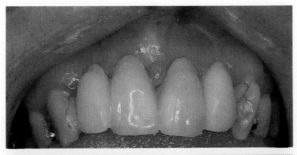

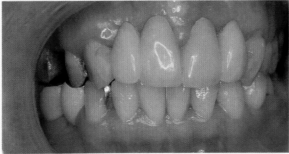

Figure 8–10 Upper panel shows the removable prosthesis in place. The all resin bonded bridge, as seen in the lower panel, uses composite in the class III lesions on both canine abutments to supplement the retention for the pontics.

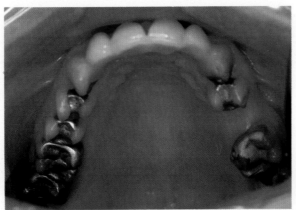

Figure 8–11 Within 6 weeks a favorable tissue response was observed. This interim all-resin bridge served the patient for a 2-year period before a conventional fixed bridge was inserted.

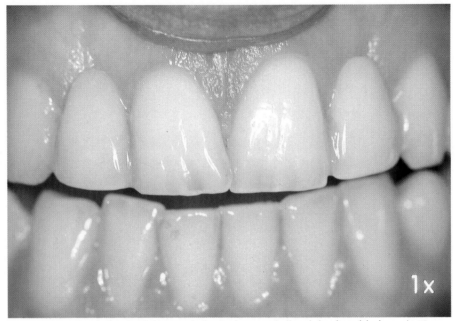

Figure 8–12 All-resin bonded bridges replacing both congenitally missing lateral incisors. At 12 years of age, the abutment teeth were virgin with very large pulps.

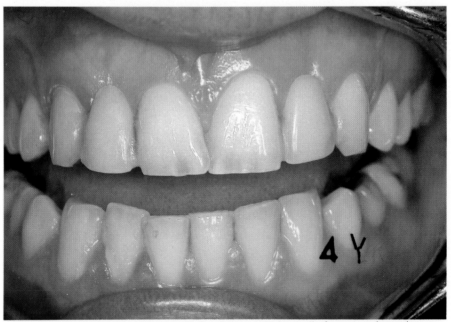

Figure 8–13 At 16 years, the patient is still functioning with the acrylic denture tooth pontics. (These were eventually replaced by cast-metal prostheses at age 18.)

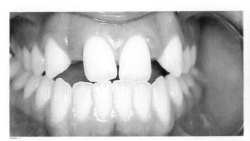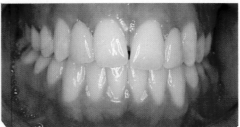

Figure 8–14 The before and after panels show the highly esthetic results that can be achieved with the all-resin bonded bridge approach.

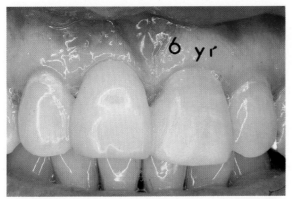

Figure 8-15 This figure shows an all-resin bonded bridge at 6 years. An acrylic denture tooth replacing 11 was luted to the adjacent incisors to permit the soft tissues to recover from the effects of a "flipper". A variety of personal problems has made treatment with a conventional bridge impossible, and so, after 8 years, the same prostheses continues to function satisfactorily. It has been dislodged twice by trauma and simply repaired.

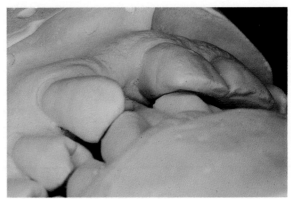

Figure 8-16 Treatment with a conventional bridge was unacceptable to this patient. An all resin bonded bridge was the treatment selected because of the horizontal and vertical overlap relationships shown here on the study models.

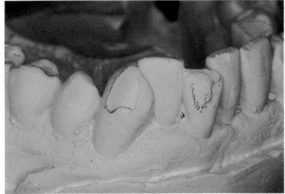

Figure 8-17 Extensive facial wear facets seen on the lower model, along with thin lingual enamel on the opposing maxillary teeth, contraindicated further enamel modification.

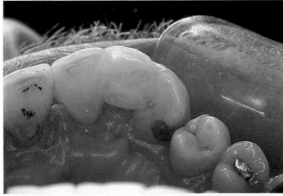

Figure 8-18 The long proximal surface available for bonding made permanent treatment with an all-resin bonded bridge a viable alternative.

Clinical Requirements

To use a bonded pontic in any of these applications, a number of conditions must be met. First, the patient *must understand the limitations* of the restoration, namely, its lack of strength and therefore its inability to perform as a natural tooth, particularly in regard to incisive function. It is hoped that the patient's appreciation of the qualities of the restoration will permit him to accept the somewhat unpredictable life expectancy and, particularly in the case of long-term restorations, view the repair of a loosened pontic as a normal "maintenance" procedure. Second, the patient's occlusion must be favorable. There should be *positive posterior occlusal support*, absence of parafunctional habits, and an eccentric pattern of movement that permits the sharing of guidance responsibility by teeth not involved in the bridge. This is particularly important in respect to protrusive and lateral protrusive mandibular movements.

Finally, regarding individual abutments, better results are obtained with *longer clinical crowns*. Considering the importance of composite bulk, a longer proximal surface permits a larger incisal-gingival connector area, providing a better bonding zone without encroaching on the gingival papilla area (see Fig. 8-18).

Fabrication Techniques

The materials and techniques required to prepare and insert an all-resin bonded bridge have been well-described and illustrated (Jordan et al, 1981; Simonsen et al, 1983). A brief overview of the procedure is given in steps 1 to 12.

1. In the case of a single-unit prosthesis, an acrylic-resin denture tooth of suitable shade and mold is fitted and aligned into proper position, either directly in the mouth or on the study model.
2. In the case of multiple units, such as the four maxillary or mandibular incisors, the acrylic resin denture teeth are properly aligned on a study model, then luted together utilizing cold-cure acrylic. Custom-made pontics are best fabricated with the aid of a study model using appropriate crown forms.
3. Class III box-type lingual approach preparations are made in the proximal surfaces of the pontic(s) adjacent to the abutment teeth. The preparations are made self-retentive by means of undercut grooves placed in the axiogingival and axioincisal line angles.
4. The abutment teeth are thoroughly cleaned by means of flour of pumice slurry.
5. The anterior arch segment is carefully isolated by means of cotton rolls or rubber dam, and the proximal surfaces of both abutment teeth adjacent to the space are acid-etched for a one-minute period utilizing a 37 percent aqueous or gel solution of phosphoric acid. The abutment teeth are then washed with a copious water lavage for 15 seconds and subsequently thoroughly dried with an air syringe. The acid-etched enamel should appear frosty and opaque.
6. A thin layer of Bis-GMA bonding resin (Adaptic; Concise; Prismafil; Command Ultrafine[1]) is then applied to the acid-etched enamel on the proximal surfaces of the abutment teeth and allowed to polymerize, or it is polymerized with visible light. A thin layer of bonding agent is similarly applied to the proximal class III slot preparations previously made in the pontic(s).
7. The pontic(s) is aligned carefully in correct relationship to the abutment teeth. It is then preliminarily luted to the abutment teeth in proper position by means of a drop of the bonding resin (auto- or light-polymerized) placed just labial to the mesial and distal contact points between the pontic and abutment teeth.

8. Composite materials (Adaptic; Concise; Prismafil; Command Ultrafine[1]), properly "diluted", are used to bond the pontics to the abutment teeth. "Dilution" of the composite materials is accomplished by means of the careful addition of their corresponding bonding agents to the composite pastes in order to provide a free-flowing mix of composite material.

9. The diluted mix of the composite material is injected into the class III proximal slot preparations in the pontic by means of a composite syringe (Centrix Syringe[2]). The diluted composite thus fills the class III preparations in the pontic and overflows to adapt to the bonding resin previously placed on the proximal surfaces of the abutment teeth.

10. After a five to ten minute auto-polymerization period or visible-light polymerization for 40 seconds the excess luting resin is removed using standard composite finishing instruments (#7902; Esthetic Trimming Kit; Soflex Discs[3]). Extreme care is taken to ensure that the luting resin does not impinge on the interdental papillae of the abutment teeth.

11. The occlusion is carefully adjusted in centric, protrusive and lateral protrusive positions to give light contact during function.

12. Patients are advised to use extreme care during mastication and they are particularly cautioned not to incise brittle substances with the prosthesis.

When supplemental retention is required and is readily available, as in the existence of class III proximal lesions or restorations, exactly the same technique as previously described is utilized to lute the prosthesis to the abutment teeth, with the following exceptions. The existing proximal restoration material and/or the carious and demineralized tooth structure is removed to establish, as closely as possible, an ideal class III proximal preparation.

A composite material is used, according to its manipulative instructions, to restore the proximal surfaces and establish ideal contours. If the pontic is to be bonded immediately, the technique beginning with step 5 above is then followed. If the pontic is to be bonded at a separate appointment, the technique beginning with step 4 (above) should be followed.

When supplemental retention is provided by proximal pins, the following technique is suggested. After prophylaxis of the abutment teeth, and before acid etching of the proximal surfaces, a No. 33½ inverted cone bur is used to establish a shallow gingival seat located at the level of the contact areas of the proximal surfaces of the abutment teeth. The gingival seat is placed just within the dentin-enamel junction. A 0.017-inch spiral drill (TMS Minikin[4]) is used to prepare a 1.5 mm deep channel aligned in such a direction as to avoid either undermining the proximal enamel or exposing the pulp. Alignment of the pin directly on the radiographs of the abutment teeth is helpful in this regard. A 0.017-inch self-threading pin (TMS Minikin[4]) is then placed in the proximal surface of each abutment tooth and subsequently bent slightly to protrude into the space (Fig. 8-19). A luting technique identical to the one previously presented, beginning with step 5, is then carefully followed (Fig. 8-20).

In selecting a composite material to bond a pontic(s) to adjacent enamel, preference should be given to the macrofilled materials (see Chapter 1). The additional strength gained appears to be significant relative to the performance of the restorations. The increased color stability available with the visible-light-cured materials, especially when a long-term restoration is being placed, is an important consideration (Fig. 8-21; see also Fig. 1-44).

Maintenance

As has been described, cohesive fracture of the bonding composite is not uncommon. The usual problem involves linear fracture through one of the connector areas and can be repaired by the following technique (Fig. 8-22):

1. Isolate the area with cotton rolls or, preferably, rubber dam.
2. With a thin-tapered diamond bur, slice through the fracture zone more at the expense of the proximal surface of the pontic than involving the enamel of the abutment.
3. Carefully clean the area with flour of pumice.
4. Acid-etch the connector area as previously described. It is recognized that little enamel may be available for etching in this repair technique. However, the freshening effect of the phosphoric acid on the existing composite material will enhance the chemical bond expected as new composite is added to it.
5. Following the rinse-dry cycle, the bonding sequence, as already described, is carefully followed, with the diluted composite being pressure-injected into the slice preparation between the pontic and the abutment.
6. Finishing is carried out after polymerization is complete.

When a pontic(s) is totally dislodged, residual composite materials are removed from both the abutments and the pontic(s) by means of carbide-tipped hand instruments (Carbide Finishing Knives[5]) and diamond or composite finishing burs (#7902; Esthetic Trimming Kit; Soflex Discs[3]). The class III type preparation in the pontics may have to be recut, and the supplemental retention in the abutments (if present) may also need refining.

The reinsertion steps then follow the bonding technique already outlined. Experience has proved that all-resin bonded bridges continue to serve for extended time periods after undergoing such repair procedures.

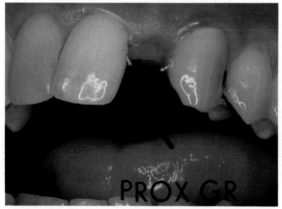

Figure 8–19 Supplemental retention being provided by TMS pins placed just into the dentin and projecting into the pontic space.

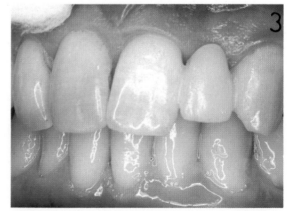

Figure 8–20 The pontic is bonded over the pins shown in Figure 8-19. It is positioned so that the pins project into the proximal boxes cut into the acrylic pontic material.

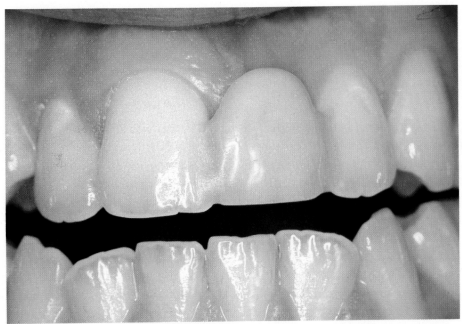

Figure 8–21 Note the discolored bonding resin in the connector areas, typical of long-term auto-polymerized materials.

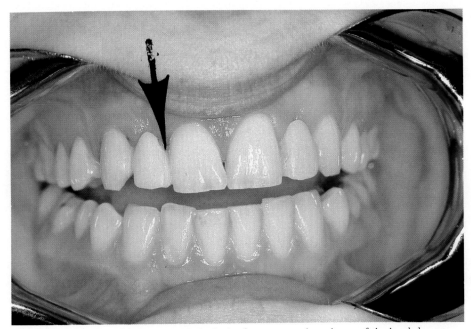

Figure 8–22 The arrow indicates a typical cohesive fracture zone through one of the bonded connectors. The other intact connector is not disturbed in the repair activity.

CAST-METAL BONDED PROSTHESES

Development

Perforated Metal Retention Type (Rochette Type)

While others were bonding pontics directly to natural abutments, Rochette, a French dentist, was experimenting with cast-metal frameworks fitted and bonded to periodontally compromised lower anteriors. For retention, these castings relied on resin extrusion through small perforations in the framework surface. The resin was compressed between the framework and the etched tooth enamel during framework insertion and, as a result, squeezed out through the holes. Ceramo metals were used, and when teeth were missing, porcelain was fused to the framework to create an esthetic pontic. Unfilled resin was used, and the clinical insertion steps, as reported, were precise and demanding (Rochette, 1972, 3).

Further use of this technique to replace missing maxillary and mandibular anteriors was described in 1977 by Howe and Denehy. A ceramic nonprecious metal was used, and casting thickness of 1 to 1.5 mm was recommended. Margins were supragingival and feathered, and the retentive holes were 0.5 mm in diameter and as numerous as possible. An autopolymerizing composite system, with first an unfilled and then a filled composite, was used for cementation. The majority of these early cases were apparently in open-bite situations and no tooth reduction was required to compensate for the thickness of the casting. Later reports (Denehy and Howe, 1979; Jordan et al, 1981) described tooth preparation techniques designed to create sufficient clearance between maxillary and mandibular anterior teeth, but beyond this, tooth modification was not emphasized. The retainers basically sat on the lingual surfaces of the abutments, obviously relying heavily on the composite bonding material for retention (Fig. 8-23). Casting thicknesses were reduced to a minimum of 0.5 mm and pontic materials included, in addition to porcelain, acrylic denture teeth.

The use of cast-metal bonded retainers for posterior teeth was first reported by Livaditis in 1980. These retainers were perforated for retention, but in addition, the role of three very distinct design segments was described. These were the occlusal rest, the proximal segment, and the lingual segment. Each of these required some enamel modification, and together they provided substantial improvement in the stability and retention of the prosthesis. Their value lay in the fact that a very definite ''path of insertion'' was created for the prosthesis, so that forces attempting to dislodge a fully-seated restoration in directions other than along this path were resisted, not only by the composite bonding material, but also by the physical design of the prosthesis itself (Fig. 8-24). These design features are now considered essential for the survival of metal-bonded restorations in stress-bearing areas (posterior tooth replacement and functioning anterior occlusions). Posterior teeth lend themselves readily to the provision of these modifications. For obvious reasons, their inclusion is much more difficult on smaller, more esthetically demanding, anterior teeth, but their role is no less important and methods of providing them will be described in detail when clinical techniques are presented.

While the role of design in retention was being reassessed, the efficiency of the perforations as a retentive mechanism was also being appraised, and as a result at least three concerns were identified:

1. The stress concentration in the composite at each perforation site predisposes the composite to fracture.
2. The exposure of composite to the oral environment produces the potential for wear and leakage at each perforation site.
3. An overall weakening effect results from the numerous perforations in the framework itself, even when stronger base metal alloys were utilized.

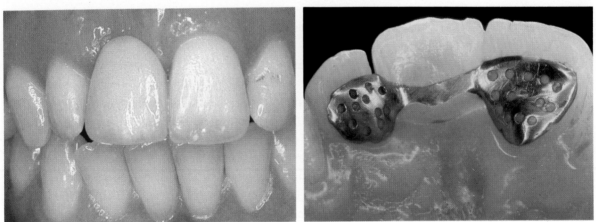

Figure 8-23   A perforated metal bonded bridge placed without tooth modification using a lingual path of insertion.

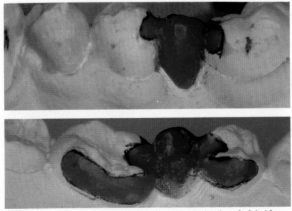

Figure 8-24   A waxed-up design for a posterior bonded bridge showing the extensions on the lingual, proximal, and facial which create resistance-retention form.

Etched-Metal Retention Type (Maryland Type)

A search for an alternative retentive mechanism resulted in the introduction of an etched-metal retention design (Livaditis, 1981; Livaditis and Thompson, 1982; McLaughlin, 1981). Electrolytic etching of base metal frameworks produces a microscopically porous surface providing for resin tag retention not unlike that available at the etched enamel surface (Fig. 8-25). A sandwich of composite between the etched metal and the etched enamel served as an internal retentive mechanism, leaving the outer retainer surface intact and smooth (Fig. 8-26).

This new retention mechanism, coupled with resistance and retention design features drawn from traditional crown and bridge techniques, appeared to offer tremendous potential, and given the frustrations frequently encountered with conventional treatment forms (Figs. 8-27 to 8-30), widespread interest within the dental profession was predictable. Activity was sparked not only by the apparently effective conservative and economical aspects of the etched-metal retainer, but also by extensive promotion on the part of both dental laboratories and lecturing clinicians. While those developing and working with the concept freely acknowledged a lack of long-term performance data, practitioners placed these protheses in very large numbers, in some cases at least, viewing the restorations as primarily a cheaper and easier shortcut to fixed-bridge performance.

Clinical use coupled with research observations identified some concerns with the etched-metal approach. Aside from the application of the concept in some questionable clinical situations and ignoring for the moment that many protheses failed to evidence a resistance-retention component in their design (problems not restricted to etched-metal restorations), the predictability of the metal-etching process as a routine procedure in the dental laboratory came under question. Closely related to this was the real danger of contamination of the etched surface before it is placed in the mouth. Complicating these concerns was the fact that evaluation of the retentive surface of an etched-metal restoration was difficult without high magnification, something not often available in the dental office or even the dental laboratory (Fig. 8-31).

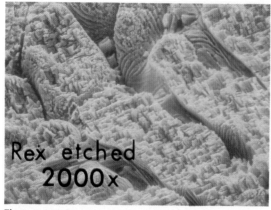

Figure 8-25 Scanning electron micrograph (2000 ×) showing the micro-mechanical retention potential of an electrolytically etched metal surface.

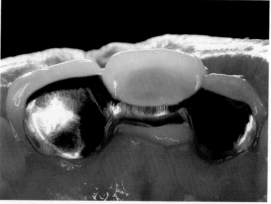

Figure 8-26 An etched-metal retained prosthesis. (Note maximum surface coverage with extension of the framework over the proximal marginal ridges.)

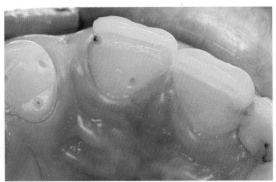

Figure 8-27 A lingual view of a conventional three-quarter crown preparation on the central incisor and a pinledge preparation on the canine illustrates the high degree of technical precision necessary for successful use of these retainer designs.

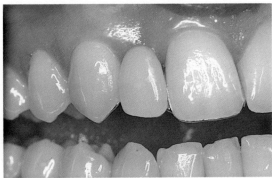

Figure 8-28 Even with the expertise evident in the preparations shown in Figure 8-27, the metal display incisally and proximally with the prostheses in place is objectionable to many patients.

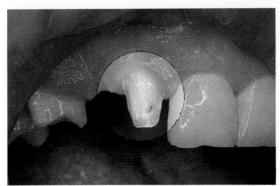

Figure 8-29 A constant concern with porcelain-fused-to-metal retainer designs is the radical tooth reduction required. Reduction of a small tooth with a large pulp has in this case resulted in exposure of the pulp.

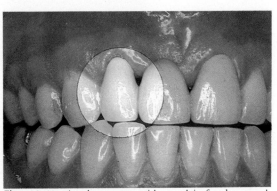

Figure 8-30 Another concern with porcelain fused to metal is the maintenance of gingival tissues at retainer margins. Many factors are involved in a gingival response, as illustrated here, but similar results are by no means rare.

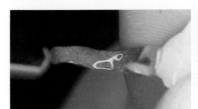 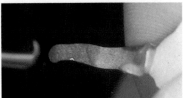

Figure 8-31 The etched surface of this molar retainer has been thoroughly sprayed with water and is then, as shown *left*, dried with air (tip of air/water syringe seen at the left of each panel). As the air is directed along the retainer away from the pontic, the drying affect can be seen as a distinct line of color change, *right*. While by no means proof of a well-etched surface, the slow, deliberate drying does indicate that the water had penetrated into the metal surface, giving some evidence of a potentially retentive surface.

Macrosurface Retention Type

Primarily to provide a predictable, readily cleansable, and more easily visualized retentive surface, investigators introduced a number of retention mechanisms which may be described as macrosurface retention designs. Mesh patterns, resin beads, and dissolvable crystals (Dura-lingual; Micro Retention Beads; Cubic Salt Crystals; Crystal Bond[6]) were utilized to produce a macroscopically rough or porous inner surface on the cast-metal retainer (Figs. 8-32 and 8-33) (Forbes and Horn, 1984; LaBarre and Ward, 1984; Moon, 1984).

In summary, in the broad classification of cast-metal bonded bridge designs, there are at present three basic restoration types based on a description of their retention mechanism. These are the perforated-metal, the etched-metal, and the macrosurface retention types.

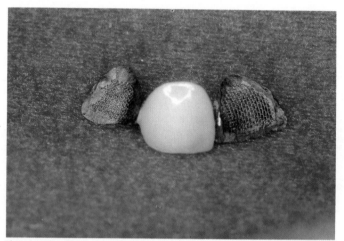

Figure 8-32 The internal surfaces of these retainers with their mesh pattern retention design can be readily inspected prior to bonding.

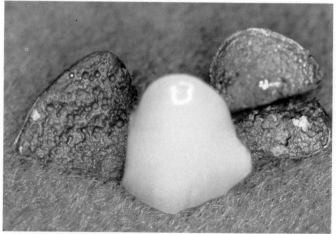

Figure 8-33 Similarly, the presence of the macroretention beads on these retainers can be verified and examined by the clinician. The clinical effectiveness of these types of retention is in an early stage of evaluation.

Performance Considerations

Research Information

Although the clinical performance of these various cast-metal bonded bridge designs is currently being monitored, periods of evaluation are, for the most part, short and results are somewhat varied. Longest in service are the perforated anterior bridges. Williams and others (1984) have reported on the performance of 63 perforated metal bridges which had been placed over a 7-year period. The majority of the restorations were maxillary anterior three-unit prostheses. Ten restorations (15.5%) were reported as having lost attachment, with many variables making it difficult to determine cause. Caries on retainer teeth were almost nonexistent and periodontal tissues were not adversely affected. There was no association between the loss of attachment and erosion of composite from retainer holes. Other reports of perforated bridge service give loss of attachment (''debonding'') rates at 15 to 30 percent (Bergendal et al, 1983; Eshleman et al, 1984; Gratton et al, 1983). These reports identified trauma as a significant cause of debonding, with patient selection (based on age, sex, and occlusal function or habits), prosthesis size, abutment size, and bonding technique cited as additional factors in attachment loss. Information from these studies as well as from in vitro investigation is not conclusive in respect to the weak link in the bonding chain. Williams and others (1982), in studying various perforated retainer designs, state that all of the designs investigated ''may be retentive enough for anterior forces of occlusion''. Others (Eshleman et al, 1981; Bergendal et al, 1983) report a problem with composite fracture at the metal interface, while yet another study found the majority of separations to occur at the enamel surface (Eshleman et al, 1984). In any event it appears that the majority of perforated cases reported as having loosened can continue to function acceptably following reinsertion procedures.

In vitro testing of the retentive potential of the etched-metal surface and then comparison with perforated-metal retention seem to establish the former's superiority, at least under research laboratory conditions. In one series of tests, the in vitro tensile stress-testing values were found to range from 1198 ± 603 psi to 1593 ± 617 psi for etched-metal castings, depending on metal used, whereas for perforated-metal castings, values ranged from 651 to 1315 psi (Sloan et al, 1983). Similar testing of some of the macrosurface retention (Duralingual[6]) has given values of 1220 ± 302 psi to 1565 ± 208 psi, again depending on metal type. The highest readings in this study were given by a mesh surface additionally, electrolytically-etched and ranged from 2024 ± 784 psi to 2154 ± 382 psi (Nykamp and Lorey, 1984) Others have determined the resin-to-alloy tensile bond strengths of properly-etched nonprecious alloys to be greater than 2900 psi and point to at least a 2–1 differential when comparing these etched metal values to average resin-to-enamel tensile strengths of 1160 to 1450 psi (Thompson and

Livaditis, 1982). The same investigators give a range of cohesive bond strengths for composite resin at 4800 to 8700 psi (Livaditis and Thompson, 1982). Large numbers of prostheses of the etched-metal type are being assessed in several clinical studies, and for the most part, their performance is impressive. In December 1983, Thompson and co-workers reported a sample of over 350 etched prostheses at the University of Maryland. Performance information is not given, but in a previous reference (Thompson and Livaditis, 1982), presumably to the same sample then numbering 140 bridges, a total of four "debonds" (3 posterior and 1 anterior) were acknowledged. From very preliminary data at the University of Western Ontario, "debond" rates are considerably higher (at 6 months, 7 of 24 etched-metal prostheses had loosened). Trauma was involved in approximately one-half of the "debonds", and in addition, the relationship of prostheses design and of laboratory and clinical technique to the loosening of these prostheses is being very carefully studied (Gratton et al, 1983).

Clinical research data on the performance of macrosurface retention prostheses is at this time largely unavailable.

In the absence of clear, conclusive, long-term clinical data and with the ever-present difficulty of relating in vitro testing to the in vivo oral environment, clinicians are understandably concerned as to the appropriate use of these prosthesis types.

Clinical Use

Certain performance characteristics have been related to the clinical management of these various restorations and may influence the choice in particular cases. Although metal perfora tions as a means of retention appear to be less efficient than an etched-metal surface, their very design permits a simpler clinical procedure. A perforated bridge can be tried-in, adjusted, and then, after simple cleaning, luted on the same appointment. However, because of contamination of the etched-metal surface, during try-in procedures, either re-etching or very careful cleansing of the metal surface (at least 3 mins. in ultrasonic cleaner) is required prior to bonding. The perforated type also allows easy elimination of the retention (by drilling composite from the framework holes), permitting removal in the event of partial "debonding". After simple cleaning at chairside, a perforated prosthesis can be ready for reattachment. An etched-metal bridge, on the other hand, can be difficult or even impossible to remove and reuse if that, for any reason, is required (see Figs. 8-158 to 8-162). Even if it is successfully removed, the etched-metal surface requires laboratory service before it can be reattached (see Figs. 8-150 and 8-151).

Among the advantages attributed to the macrosurface retention designs, in addition to a more readily identified, less easily contaminated retention pattern, is the potential of casting the framework in a gold-colored and possibly less abrasive alloy.

Base metal alloys are to date the only alloys successfully electrolytically etched. Unfortunately, they turn dark in the process, creating a potentially "hard to manage" greyish "shine-through" on thin abutment teeth (Fig. 8-34). The use of a yellow semiprecious alloy, possible with macrosurface retention techniques, can provide a more predictable esthetic result. As regards wear potential, the relative hardness of base metal alloys has long been a matter of concern based on experiences with removable partial denture frameworks. Use of macrosurface retention permits metal-bonded bridges to be cast from potentially less abrasive alloys. On the negative side, the macrosurface retention techniques tend to produce a thicker retainer, a particularly significant problem in tight anterior occlusions.

Whatever reasons are considered in choosing a particular cast-metal bonded bridge type, especially while researchers are in the process of evaluating their comparative performances, it must be emphasized that prosthesis success can be dramatically optimized by careful patient selection as well as by adequate regard for those requirements which govern all successful crown and bridge treatment. The importance of thorough diagnosis and treatment planning, careful clinical technique, quality laboratory service, and enthusiastic patient cooperation cannot be overstated.

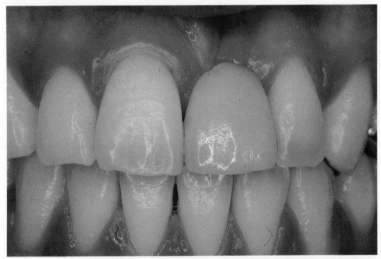

Figure 8-34 A comparison of the incisal edges of the right and left lateral incisors will show the degree of incisal greying produced by the cementation of a metal-resin bonded bridge from Figure 8-11 to 8-22.

Case Selection

Advantages

The advantages of the cast-metal bonded prosthesis are appealing for any patient requiring the replacement of a missing tooth or teeth or the stabilization of the dentition for periodontal or orthodontic reasons. Obvious advantages include minimal tooth preparation; no anesthesia is required, dentin is not involved, and pulps, especially younger ones, are therefore spared; supragingival margins, soft tissues are not disturbed and impression procedures are simplified; there is reduced laboratory involvement and complex procedures are minimized; the patient saves money, time commitments of both dentist and technician are somewhat reduced; and finally the treatment is essentially reversible. Many examples can be shown to illustrate the potential of these restorations in all areas of the mouth (Figs. 8-35 to 8-41).

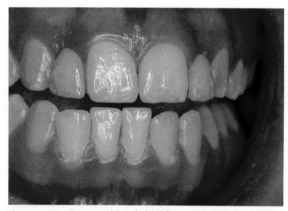

Figure 8-35   Cast-metal bonded bridges, replacing the congenitally missing maxillary lateral incisors.

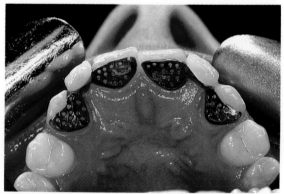

Figure 8–36   A lingual view of the bridges shown in Figure 8-35. (Note perforated retention mechanism and the degree of coverage of the lingual enamel surfaces.)

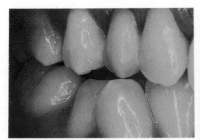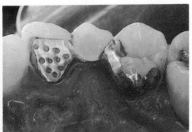

Figure 8-37 A perforated cast-metal bonded bridge with the pontic in the canine position, shown at 4-year recall. The mesial abutment is the canine which has been orthodontically moved into the lateral incisor position. Occlusion is favorable, and again maximum lingual coverage is utilized.

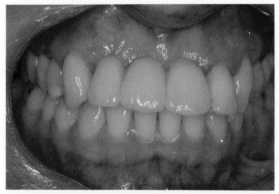

Figure 8-38 Two central incisors plus the right lateral incisor have been replaced with porcelain pontics retained by etched metal retainers on the right canine and left lateral incisor. The prognathic tendency of the lower incisors necessitated the labial inclination of the pontics.

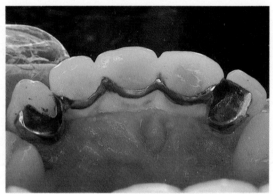

Figure 8-39 The eccentric occlusal contacts between the canines restricted the surface area of the canine retainer. A very distinct path of insertion is largely credited for a successful 3-year service period.

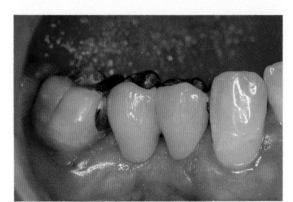

Figure 8-40 A buccal view of an etched metal bridge replacing both right mandibular premolars. (Note the facial extension on the mesial of the molar to achieve a "wrap-around" retention design.)

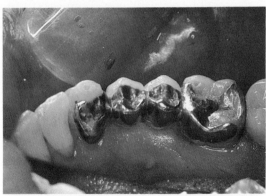

Figure 8-41 Note the lingual extension of the framework on both abutments. The occlusal rest on the molar has been placed on an existing amalgam. Various methods of handling existing restorations are discussed in *Clinical and Laboratory Techniques.*

Limitations

With so many attractive features, the temptation to apply the concept universally must be resisted. As an ultraconservative approach, its potential should be considered for all patients requiring fixed prosthodontic treatment, but it should be obvious that many cases will not be suitable for treatment with metal-bonded prostheses. Among the more apparent contra-indications are cases with unesthetic abutments or abutments with little sound enamel, whether due to disease or to existing restorations. Small crown size may not provide sufficient bonding area (Figs. 8-42 and 8-43), and tooth position can militate against the use of a metal-bonded bridge when an insertion path for the prosthesis would involve tooth preparation through the enamel layer (Fig. 8-44).

Span length is another limitation. Some early results indicate a higher ''debond'' rate for prostheses with multiple pontics or multiple abutments (Gratton et al, 1983) (Figs. 8-45 and 8-46). The amount of retention required in relation to the number of missing teeth is even more difficult to determine than with conventional crown and bridge designs. Bonded retainers utilize only a portion of each abutment and tend to cover a limited amount of the abutment's occluding surface. What a long span cast-metal bonded prosthesis involving multiple abutments and pontics must do is tie a number of natural teeth *rigidly* together so that they function as a unit even though each of the abutments has its own physiologic predisposition for normal movement. The prosthesis must accomplish this while, as has been stated, a substantial portion of each abutment is left uncovered and is therefore subject to individual occlusal loading during the patient's normal function. This situation is not unlike the condition that develops when cast inlays are used as bridge retainers in conventional crown and bridge designs. These sometimes break loose because biting force applied to some portion of the occlusal surface of the abutment tooth does not load the inlay within the abutment to the same degree. The abutment tooth is able to move in its periodontal space and may begin to do so, while the inlay, which is rigidly attached to other components of the bridge and cannot move, must attempt to prevent any such movement. Under these conditions, the cement bond between the casting and the tooth frequently breaks down because of extremes of tensile stress. Comparatively, then, the more natural teeth involved in a cast-metal bonded framework, the greater the difficulty encountered by the framework, preventing individual tooth movement and literally keeping the abutments bonded to itself. Clinical experience should eventually provide answers as to the predictability of larger bonded prostheses; in the meantime, multiple abutments combined in a rigid framework may not necessarily solve the problem of the longer edentulous span.

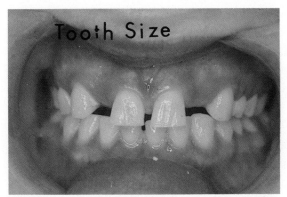

Figure 8-42 The short teeth pictured here did not provide sufficient surface area for successful bonding.

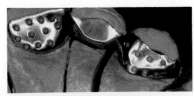

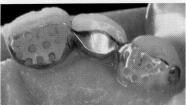

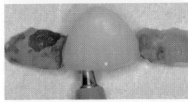

Figure 8-43 One of the bridges that was made for the mouth shown in Figure 8-42 is seen on the dies and then bonded in the mouth. Every effort was made to cover all available enamel surface, but debonding at the composite enamel interface, as seen in the lower panel, repeatedly occurred and conventional bridges were fabricated.

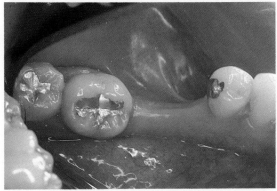

Figure 8-44 The mesial and lingual tipping of the potential molar abutment contraindicates treatment with a cast-metal bonded bridge.

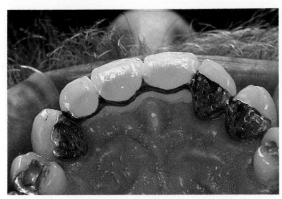

Figure 8-45 A post-insertion view of the lingual surfaces of an extenisve perforated design metal bonded bridge.

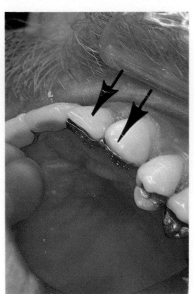

Figure 8-46 At 11 months, note the space between the retainers on both the lateral incisor and canine abutments. "Debonding" was unilateral, and although the bridge was removed and reinserted, it has to date loosened on two more occasions (4½-year service period).

Complicating Factors

For patients who require anterior tooth replacement, several factors must be considered as complications if not definite limitations to the use of cast-metal bonded prostheses. Although the data are minimal and early, there is some evidence that the debond rate may be highest for maxillary anterior restorations (Gratton et al, 1984). This may relate to the nature of occlusal stresses directed on these restorations (Figs. 8-47 and 8-48). If posterior bonded prostheses enjoy a higher success rate it may be partly because the abutments are loaded primarily in a vertical direction, especially if steps have been taken to minimize or eliminate eccentric posterior tooth contact. Aside from the problem of differential loading, as already discussed, posterior function then would tend to seat the posterior prosthesis in its abutments. An anterior restoration, on the other hand, placed in an occlusion with eccentric guidance provided by the anterior (including abutment) teeth is likely to have a much harder task "hanging on" to its abutments. Remembering the labial inclination of most maxillary teeth and recognizing that incisal stress through a food bolus or in guidance activity may move off a bonded retainer and on to natural tooth structure, it is not hard to envision a rotating potential on the part of an abutment, away from its lingually bonded retainer (Fig. 8-49). As was earlier stated, the resistance-retention form incorporated into the prosthesis design must play a key role in absorbing this rotation tendency if loosening of the restoration is to be avoided. Given the minimal size and the esthetic concerns common to anterior teeth, the provision of such a design is far from easy. Thus a patient with heavy anterior function and obvious guidance wear facets may not be a good candidate for a cast-metal bonded prosthesis (Figs. 8-50 to 8-52).

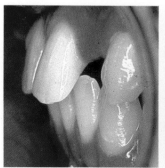
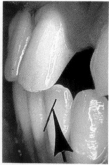

Figure 8–47 The contact relationship between maxillary and mandibular incisors in both centric and eccentric positions clearly produces horizontal or rotating forces against the maxillary teeth and their supporting tissues.

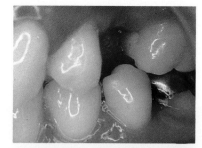
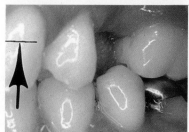

Figure 8–48 In contrast, occlusal forces involving potential posterior abutments are primarily vertical, assuming eccentric contacts are nonexistent or can be eliminated.

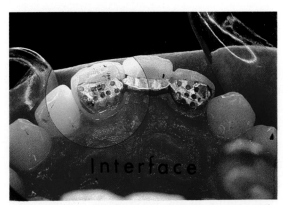

Figure 8-49   The articulating paper marking on the central incisor abutment, as highlighted in the circle, illustrates how a problem can arise as incisal forces are transferred from the metal framework out onto the lingual surface of the abutment.

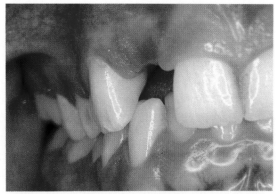

Figure 8-50   Although the patient is young and the teeth are virgin, the horizontal and vertical overlap relationships are such that a cast-metal resin bonded bridge is probably contraindicated.

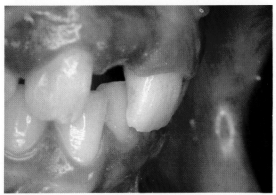

Figure 8-51   This view shows that there is no available space between the lingual surfaces of these maxillary teeth and the facial surfaces of the lower incisors.

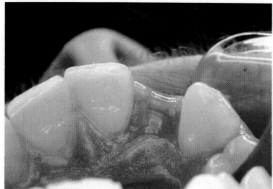

Figure 8-52   Lingual faceting indicates heavy occlusal function in the dentition, pictured in the previous two figures.

A further complication in patients with intimate and extensive anterior contacts in both centric and eccentric jaw positions relates to the simple question of "room". To place a metal framework on the lingual surface of maxillary incisors without tooth reduction inevitably makes the abutment more bulky, and if the lower incisors touch the abutment in any jaw position, the mandible is required to adapt to a new position or movement pathway. The significance of this is realized when one considers that the lack or disruption of incisal guidance can be a factor in TMJ disorder (Figs. 8-53 to 8-55). Reduction of tooth structure is advocated to preserve the integrity of the maxillary-lingual concavity, such reductions to be carried out within the lingual enamel of the maxillary abutments and perhaps by the reshaping of the lower incisal edges. The lack of enamel thickness on the lingual of maxillary anteriors (Table 8-1) may preclude adequate reduction. Arbitrary reshaping of the lower incisors could conceivably alter mandibular movement pathways. To judge when to forgo treatment of patients whose anterior tooth relationships will be iatrogenically altered or when to predictably alter the existing natural tooth surfaces so that the relationships of upper and lower teeth after insertion of a metal-bonded prosthesis remain physiologically acceptable demands a degree of preliminary study which *at least* parallels that required by a conventional anterior fixed bridge.

TABLE 8-1 Maxillary and Mandibular Anterior Teeth: Mean Lingual Enamel Thickness (mm)

	Incisal third	Middle third	Gingival third
Maxillary central	.65	.6	.4
Maxillary lateral	.7	.6	.4
Mandibular incisors	.55	.45	.3

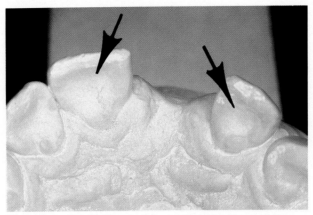

Figure 8-53 The likelihood of altering both the shape and the dimension of the lingual concavity by bonding a metal framework to the enamel surface is underscored by this view of these delicately curved surfaces.

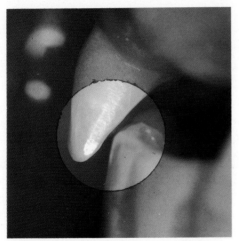

Figure 8-54 Space appears to be available for a bonded framework with the teeth in the centric occlusion relationship shown here.

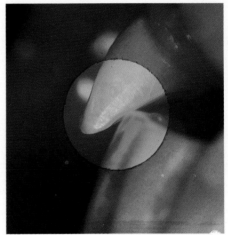

Figure 8-55 The space seen in Figure 8-54 disappears as the mandibular moves forward into a protrusive position. A framework simply bonded into this apparent space will obviously force the mandible into a different and perhaps unacceptable eccentric pathway.

Preliminary Clinical Procedures

Diagnosis and Treatment Planning

It is recognized that a considerable amount of diagnostic information must be gathered before a patient is treated with a conventional fixed prosthesis, and this activity is no less important with a cast-metal bonded prosthesis. On the basis of a thorough history, careful clinical examination, and quality radiographs, the clinician begins to determine the patient's suitability for a fixed prosthodontic restoration. Further steps in the planning of this restoration involve the preparation of study models to help in framework design and occlusal analysis.

Study Models: Framework Design and Tooth Modification. By surveying the study models, determining a path of insertion, completing tooth preparations on the stone abutment teeth, outlining the retainers, and perhaps waxing up the retainers and pontics, one can ascertain the feasibility of a metal-bonded bridge (see Figs. 8-62, 8-63, 8-68 to 8-71, and 8-79 to 8-81). Because ideal design demands tooth modification and because the modification must be executed within the enamel thickness, these preliminary activities on the study model are particularly valuable.

Generally, in designing a framework, efforts are made to cover the maximum amount of the lingual surface on each abutment tooth. Occlusal or incisal extension may be limited by opposing occlusal contacts or, in the anterior, by the tendency for an abutment to change shade as the framework approaches the incisal edge (extensions closer than 1.5 mm to the incisal are likely to alter shade) (see Figs. 8-107 and 8-108). Gingival extension should terminate a minimum of 1 mm from the gingival tissue crest. On a posterior abutment, the framework should extend to the lingual-proximal line angle distant to the edentulous area; on an anterior abutment, the framework achieves a greater resistance form if the marginal ridge farthest from the pontic area is covered by the framework (Figs. 8-56 to 8-58). Posterior teeth require enamel modification so that with the framework in place (0.3 to 0.5 mm thick and thinning to a feather or very slight chamfer gingivally), the lingual height of contour remains unchanged (Figs. 8-59 to 8-61).

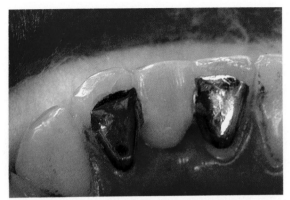

Figure 8-56 Note the retainer coverage stopping approximately 1 mm above the gingival crest, 2 mm from the incisal edges, and extending over the marginal ridges farthest from the pontic.

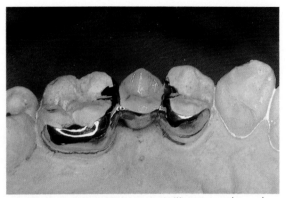

Figure 8-57 This posterior prosthesis illustrates again maximum lingual coverage by the retainers on both abutments.

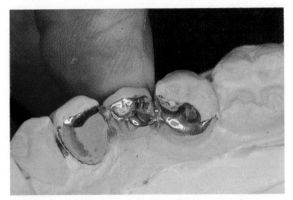

Figure 8-58 Occlusion permitted extension of this framework over a portion of the lingual cusp on the premolar abutment while the facial lingual dimension of the canine abutment allowed significant incisal extension, both design features increasing the retentive potential.

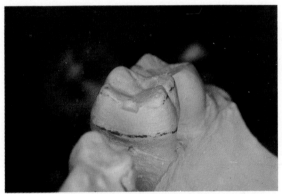

Figure 8-59 The lingual surface of this maxillary molar abutment displays conservative yet important tooth reduction in the mid and occlusal third.

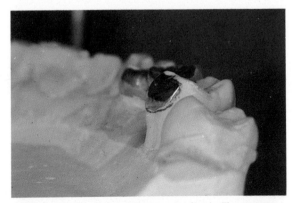

Figure 8-60 Prosthesis in place on the dies in Figure 8-59 showing the maintenance of ideal tooth contour by the metal framework.

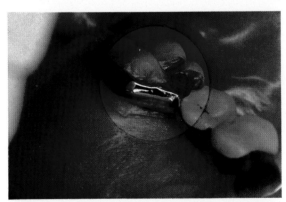

Figure 8-61 A potentially harmful situation is seen in the circle where insufficient tooth modification and poor framework design have produced a serious plaque "trap".

Adjacent to the pontic area, the proximal surfaces of both anterior and posterior abutments require careful preparation. Posteriorly, the proximal height of contour is lowered to within 1 mm of the gingival tissue or at least enough to provide an occlusal-gingival dimension for the framework of 2 mm (Fig. 8-62). The facial-lingual curvature is maintained during the tooth modification so that as the framework extends beyond the facial-proximal line angle, as far as esthetics will permit, it should achieve a 180° coverage of the tooth circumference and also develop a definite path of insertion (Figs. 8-63 to 8-65). The framework, of necessity, thickens to perhaps 1 mm as it goes into the connector area, obviously to provide adequate strength in this high-stress zone (Fig. 8-66). In the case of anterior abutments, esthetic considerations sharply limit the facial extension of the retainer. This, coupled with minimal facial-lingual tooth dimension, will result in proximal modification that is subtle, primarily an effort to move the proximal height of contour (as viewed in the facial-lingual plane) toward the lingual.

The goal is to develop sufficient resistance form so that the proximal area engaged by the framework, together with its extension into the proximal areas of the other abutment(s), will create a distinct insertion path. The exercise of preparing these surfaces on the study model and inspecting them on a surveyor should be routine (Figs. 8-67 to 8-71).

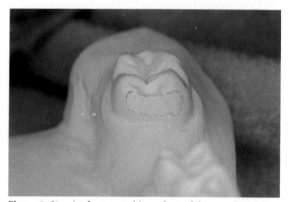

Figure 8-62   As drawn on this study model, posterior proximal contours are modified to produce a broad area for bonding and sufficient dimension for framework rigidity.

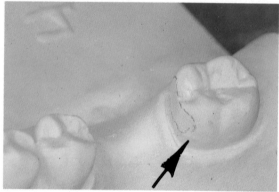

Figure 8-63   The proximal modification allows the framework to "wrap" out to the facial.

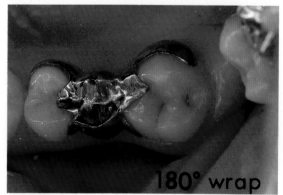

Figure 8-64   Viewing the abutments from the occlusal, the framework should extend at least 180° around the tooth circumference.

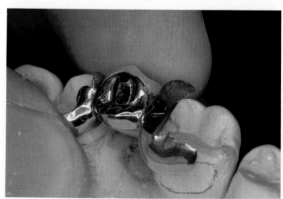

Figure 8-65   Note bridge being seated on its dies following a precise insertion pathway.

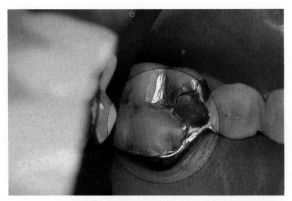

Figure 8-66 Note thicker dimension of the metal framework at the junction of the proximal and lingual sections of the retainer.

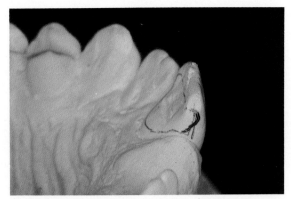

Figure 8-67 The outline for a proposed retainer on the proximal surface of the abutment illustrates the problem of achieving retention while maintaining esthetic requirements.

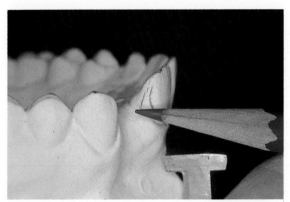

Figure 8-68 The distal facial line angle of the incisor abutment is outlined followed by the proximal height of contour in the facial lingual plane.

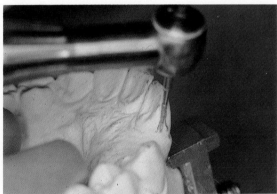

Figure 8-69 A thin diamond is used in an effort to prepare an area for "proximal wrap" facial to the height of contour and lingual to the distal facial line angle.

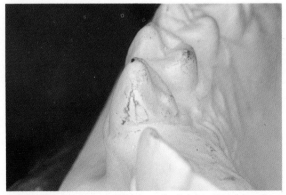

Figure 8-70 In the modification, the height of contour (facial lingual plane) is sharpened and moved toward the lingual.

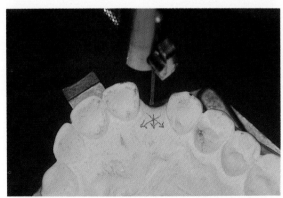

Figure 8-71 With the study model on a surveyor, it is verified that the modification of the proximal surfaces provides for a framework design that cannot be displaced in any direction other than along its "path of insertion".

The final element of design is the occlusal or cingulum rest (Fig. 8-72). The common location of the posterior rest in the proximal marginal ridge permits the preparation of a substantial rest area approximately 1.5 to 2 mm in width and length by 1 mm in depth. Its greatest depth should be farthest from the marginal ridge to positively key the framework into the abutment tooth (Fig. 8-73). A lack of enamel thickness requires a conservative groove or notch-type preparation in the cingulum area of anterior teeth. Nonetheless, even as a delicate element of the framework design, it serves an important function in assuring precise seating of the restoration initially and then in transfer of occlusal stress to the abutment tooth (Fig. 8-74).

Study Models: Occlusal Analysis. When a proposed metal-bonded bridge is expected to play a significant role in a patient's occlusion, particularly an anterior occlusion, preliminary analysis of study models mounted in centric relation position on a semiadjustable articulator (Whip Mix[7]) is essential. The existing occlusal relationship can be assessed on the articulator and a decision made as to the advisability of occlusal adjustment of natural teeth in advance of the prosthodontic treatment (e.g., CR prematurities or eccentric balancing contacts). The mounted models also provide an excellent opportunity to visualize the impact of the proposed metal-bonded bridge on the patient's occlusion as well as the possible effects of the occlusion on the prosthesis (Figs. 8-75 to 8-77). Some of the complexities of anterior occlusion have been discussed in a preceding section. At this stage, it may even become apparent that, because of the anterior tooth relationships, a bonded prosthesis is not indicated. When it is obvious that substantial tooth modification is required, involving the lower incisal edges, the technique shown in Figures 8-78 to 8-93 can (1) assist in determining whether the degree of reduction necessary can be safely completed, and (2) provide an adjustment template to facilitate the occlusal reduction of the lower incisors *after* the prosthesis has been luted.

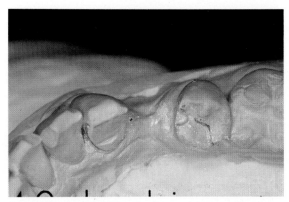

Figure 8-72 Note mesial occlusal rest on the premolar abutment and the cingulum notch or rest on the canine.

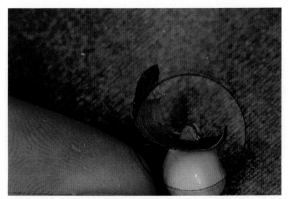

Figure 8-73 The posterior occlusal rest is prepared precisely within the marginal ridge enamel as seen by the casting detail pictured in the circle.

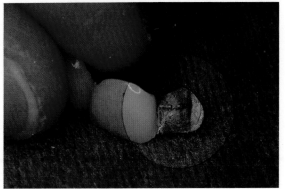

Figure 8-74 Rests are of necessity much more delicate in the cingulum area of anterior teeth. Offsets (not shown) prepared in the marginal ridge areas where the enamel is thicker may provide additonal stability.

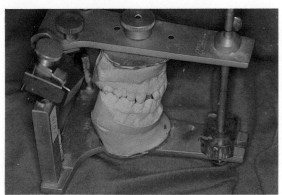

Figure 8-75 Study models mounted on a semiadjustable articulator in an effort to determine the feasibility of a cast-metal bonded bridge.

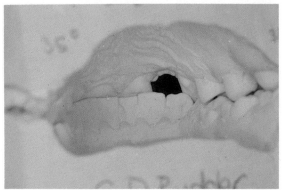

Figure 8-76 Study models permit inspection of the relationship of the potential abutments as viewed from the lingual.

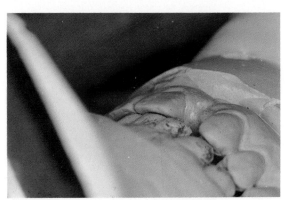

Figure 8-77 Important eccentric movements can be simulated and assessed as the models are moved on the articulator.

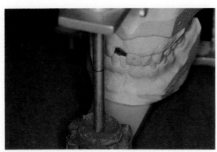

Figure 8–78 A custom incisal guidance is made from methylmethacrylate (Duralay Kit[8]) (Kaiser, 1981) to capture the relationships between the anterior teeth.

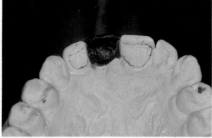

Figure 8–79 With the articulator programmed to reproduce the patient's incisal relationships, the prosthesis is designed and waxed up on the study models. This figure shows the "waxed-up" pontic and the outlines drawn for the retainers.

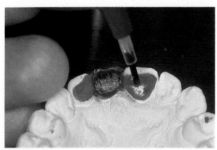

Figure 8–80 Methylmethacrylate (Duralay Kit[8]) is being applied to the study model to simulate the extent and thickness of the metal retainers.

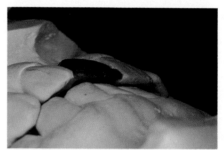

Figure 8–81 As the articulator is now closed, the lower incisors contact the simulated bridge.

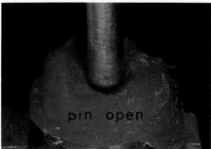

Figure 8–82 As a result of this contact between the lower incisors and the bridge components, the incisal pin of the articulator will not contact the incisal table.

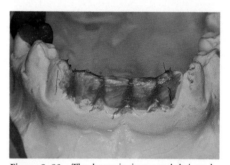

Figure 8–83 The lower incisors are lubricated (Duralay Kit[8]).

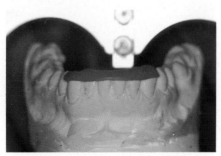

Figure 8–84 A template (Duralay Kit[8]) is molded along the incisal edges of these teeth.

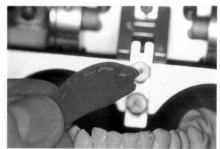

Figure 8–85 Following polymerization, the template is removed as shown.

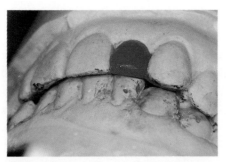

Figure 8–86 The areas of contact on the lower incisors as they close on the simulated bridge are assessed visually.

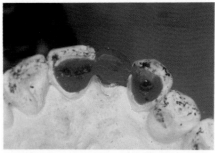

Figure 8–87 Articulating paper (MDS Truspot[9]) is also used to determine the centric and eccentric contacts.

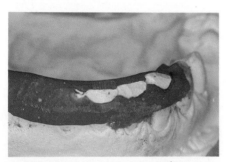

Figure 8–88 The acrylic template is repositioned on the mandibular anteriors and the incisal edges are reduced by first cutting through the template and then into the study model.

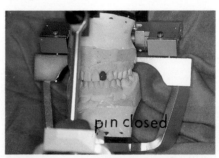

Figure 8–89 The adjustment sequence is continued until the articulator pin closes into contact with and follows the contours of the custom incisal guidance, with the modified lower incisors occluding with the simulated bridge.

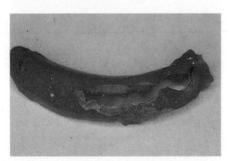

Figure 8–90 The template is preserved to be used orally.

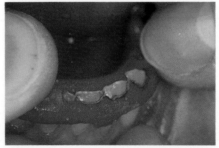

Figure 8–91 The template is placed on the patient's incisors to determine whether the modification required to make room for the bonded bridge is indeed feasible.

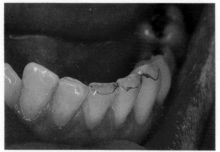

Figure 8–92 The amount of tooth reduction, as indicated by the template, has been traced on the incisors.

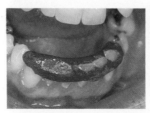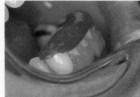

Figure 8–93 The decision was made to proceed with the bridge in this instance, and the template is shown here as a guide for accurate reduction of the patient's incisal edges. This modification is not done until the bridge insertion appointment to avoid eruption of the mandibular incisors.

Periodontal Therapy

Periodontal therapy as a preliminary procedure should be routine to ensure optimal health of supporting tissue, but also may be considered a practical means of increasing retentive area through clinical crown-lengthening techniques. This is especially significant for patients whose lingual tissues have proliferated or are hyperemic owing to effects of a previously worn removable appliance (Figs. 8-94 to 8-97).

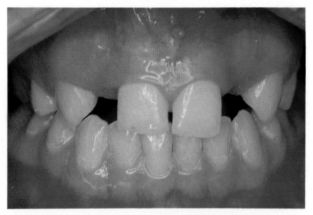

Figure 8-94 Gingivectomy was chosen to elongate the crowns so that metal bonded bridges could be inserted to replace a removable partial denture.

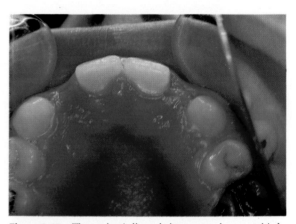

Figure 8-95 The patient's lingual tissues were hypertrophied and inflamed from the effects of the removable appliance.

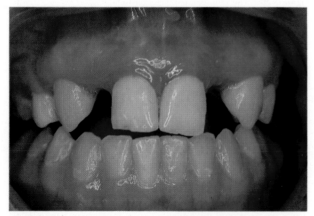

Figure 8-96 A facial view of the abutments following periodontal surgery.

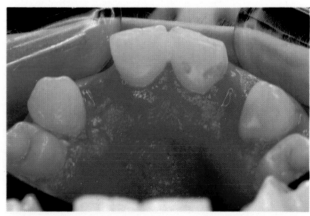

Figure 8-97 A substantial increase in available bonding surface has been achieved on the lingual.

Orthodontic Considerations

Orthodontic procedures also can greatly increase the potential of a metal-bonded prosthesis. As regards esthetics, the mesial and distal dimensions and relative alignment of abutments and pontics cannot be improved by a lingually bonded framework to the extent possible with full crown coverage. Thus some prealignment permits a much improved result (Figs. 8-98 to 8-101). Composite proximal additions following techniques addressed in Chapter 2 can, alone or in combination with orthodontic procedures, solve tooth size-space problems in esthetic areas of the mouth prior to the insertion of a metal-bonded prosthesis (Figs. 8-102 to 8-104).

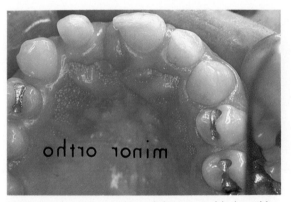

Figure 8-98 A young patient missing a central incisor with the lateral incisor drifting into the space.

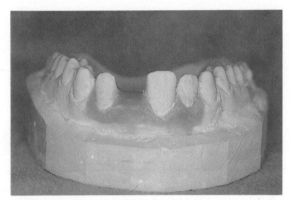

Figure 8-99 The remaining incisors have been sectioned from the study cast and waxed into a favorable abutment position. The potential of orthodontic treatment can be assessed.

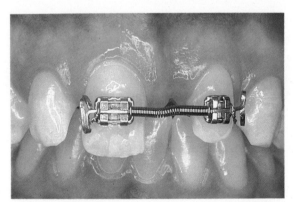

Figure 8-100 Minor orthodontic movement is in progress.

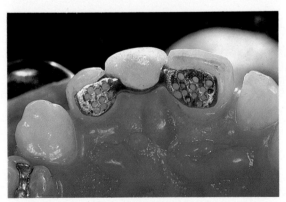

Figure 8-101 A perforated metal bonded bridge was inserted after sufficient space had been gained for an esthetic pontic (early design, minimal extension).

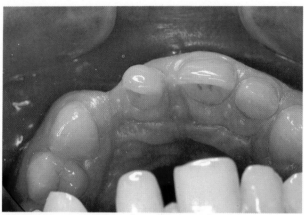

Figure 8-102 A poorly formed central incisor and a missing lateral incisor present a difficult esthetic problem.

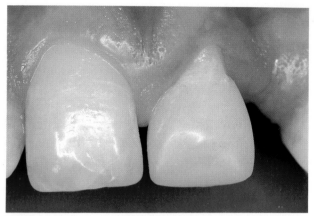

Figure 8-103 The central incisor has been recontoured by composite addition to the proximal and facial surface.

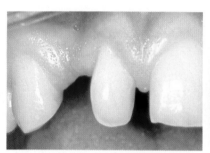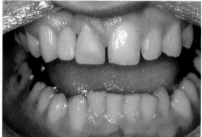

Figure 8-104 Before and after views with the right panel showing the recontoured incisor serving as the mesial abutment for a cast-metal bonded bridge replacing the right lateral incisor. The retainer utilizes the lingual enamel as well as the lingual surface of the mesial and distal composite "build-ups" to secure adequate bonding areas.

Esthetic Preevaluation

One further step may prove worthwhile when dealing with thin, delicate, anterior abutments. The problem of retainer "shine-through" has already been mentioned. The seriousness of the problem and possible methods of dealing with it may, to a degree at least, be predetermined by adapting metallic foil as closely as possible to the lingual of an abutment and observing the shade change. Some composite material must be used between the foil and the enamel to complete the "optical circuit". Simply holding the foil against the teeth does not produce the degree of "shine-through" that will occur once the composite is in place and acts as an intermediary layer.

Experimentation with opaque composite materials (Comspan Opaque; Conclude; Retain[10]) specifically designed to minimize the color change should give some indication as to the likely success of this approach (Figs. 8-105 and 8-106). In addition, the distance that the retainer margins should be kept from the incisal edges may also be determined with this technique (Figs. 8-107 and 8-108).

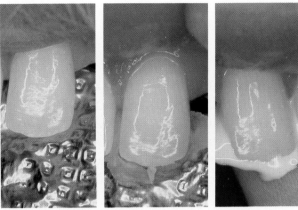

Figure 8-105 Foil simply held against the lingual surface produces little color change. With a composite material between the tooth and the foil, as in the center panel, considerably more "graying" is obvious. Opaque composite between the tooth and the foil eliminates the incisal discoloration (*right panel*).

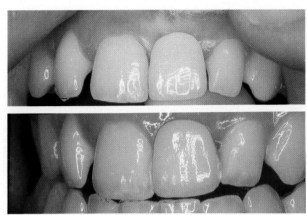

Figure 8-106 A bridge held against the lingual surfaces of the abutments produces no "shine-through". The bridge was cemented with a regular composite material without experimentation as to the effect of the composite application and the serious graying resulted.

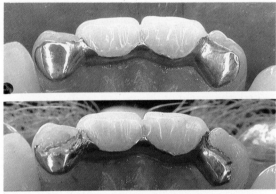

Figure 8-107 Extension of a metal framework close to the incisal is seen in the top panel. The lower panel shows reduction of this extension to correct the graying seen in Figure 8-108 (*top panel*). (The reduction was done subsequent to bonding—not a recommended procedure.)

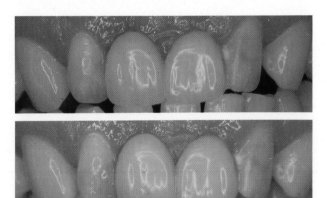

Figure 8-108 The before and after views show the significance of incisal extension and underscore the importance of determining this extension in the preliminary planning stages.

Clinical and Laboratory Techniques

Tooth Preparation

Enamel Modification. Following careful preplanning, as has been described, the clinical steps can proceed smoothly. Axial surface reduction can be initiated with a thin-tapered fissure diamond (700.9 VF, Two Striper[11]) and finished by means of a multifluted tungsten carbide bur (#9902[12]). For delicate reduction, the multifluted bur may be used for the entire procedure. The preparation of the anterior abutments can be facilitated by painting or spraying the involved surface with a disclosing type material (Occlude[13]). In this way the extension of the preparation can be more easily visualized (Figs. 8-109 and 8-110).

Existing Restorations. Existing restorations on abutment teeth may require special consideration. Large restorations that leave poorly supported enamel or esthetically compromised teeth make metal-bonded bridges impractical unless the restorations can be replaced by means of new techniques and materials (Chapters 1 and 2) which can solve many esthetic problems and actually provide internal support for undermined and weakened enamel walls (Figs. 8-111 and 8-112). Metal-bonded prostheses may be effectively luted to composite restorations after little preparation of the restoration at the time of bonding other than the cleansing, freshening action of the phosphoric acid during enamel etching. For this reason, and considering the effectiveness of some of the new posterior composite restorative materials, the replacement of posterior amalgams in abutment teeth may be considered an ideal approach (Figs. 8-113 to 8-115). When amalgam restorations are to be retained, the extent of the restoration dictates the type of mouth preparation to be employed. With a conservative class I restoration, an

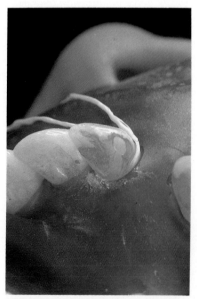

Figure 8–109 Proximal reduction through the disclosing solution enables the clinician to visualize the potential retention offered by the tooth modification.

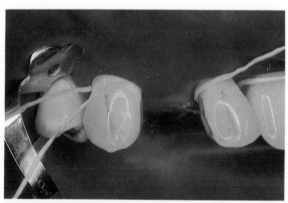

Figure 8–110 As viewed from the facial, the proximal extension within the area covered by the disclosing solution will not create an esthetic problem.

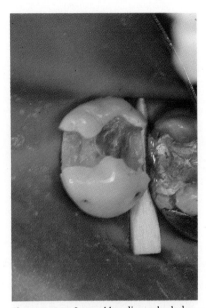

Figure 8–111 Internal bonding to both dentin and enamel surfaces allows the composite restorative material to "tie" weakened areas of this abutment together. Without this potential, the lingual wall of the tooth would not offer sufficient strength for the retentive surface of a cast-metal bonded bridge.

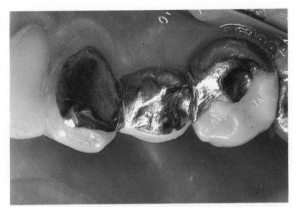

Figure 8–112 The composite restoration has been placed in the tooth as prepared in Figure 8-111, and a bridge has been bonded to the lingual and occlusal surfaces.

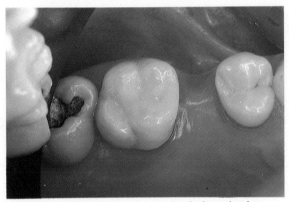

Figure 8–114 The composite restoration is shown in place.

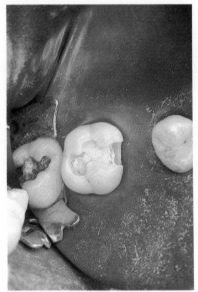

Figure 8–113 A class II amalgam has been removed in preparation for replacement with a posterior composite material.

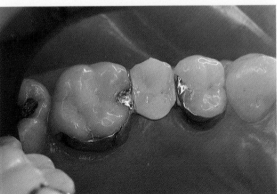

Figure 8–115 The cast-metal bonded bridge has now been bonded to both the enamel and the proximal and occlusal composite surfaces.

occlusal rest in the marginal ridge is not likely to alter the effectiveness of the restoration or to be compromised itself as an important part of the design of the prosthesis. When occlusion permits or requires, especially when a class II amalgam is not to be replaced, the metal framework can extend over varying amounts of the occlusal surface, and in such cases, the enamel may be slightly modified to produce a surface to which the casting may precisely seat (Figs. 8-112, 8-116, and 8-117). Another method that may be used with the class II amalgam involves preparing, in effect, a conservative proximal inlay within the amalgam extending out to the facial and lingual enamel surfaces, exposing this internal enamel for additional framework retention at the time of etching and bonding (Figs. 8-118 and 8-119).

Impression Procedures

Impression techniques are greatly simplified, primarily because gingival tissues are not involved. Any of the available elastic materials, with the exception of irreversible hydrocolloid, can produce the required impression. The stability of the polyvinyl siloxanes can be a real advantage if multiple casts are to be poured, as could be the case if a refractory die method of framework fabrication is used.

Shade Confirmation

At this appointment shades are taken to confirm the decisions made at a preliminary appointment.

Occlusal Records

Depending on the previous decisions regarding occlusion, records may be required to mount working models on a simple or a semiadjustable articulator with an appropriate facebow transfer. The latter is most desirable if an anterior prosthesis is to be fabricated with excursive function on the pontic(s) and/or the retainers. Whatever method and material are used in capturing jaw relationships, accuracy must be ensured to minimize adjustment on frameworks, already exceedingly thin and, as cast in base metal, difficult to adjust.

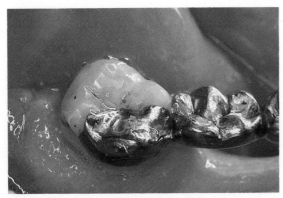

Figure 8–116 The framework design includes an extension over the mesial lingual cusp to secure additional retention and rigidity.

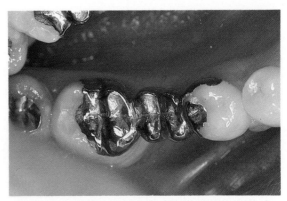

Figure 8–117 Where occlusion was absent on the mesial of the posterior abutment, the framework has been extended almost as a mesial onlay restoration.

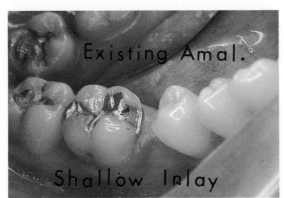

Figure 8–118 Note the removal of some of the proximal amalgam to create a shallow box preparation, exposing internal enamel surfaces on both the facial and lingual aspects of the box.

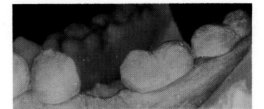

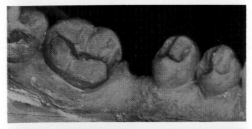

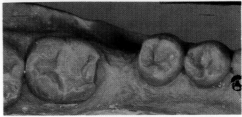

Figure 8–119 The top panel shows the reciprocating, almost parallel surfaces on the two abutment dies. The middle and lower panels show the preparation described in Figure 8-118 as it is reproduced in the working die.

Prosthesis Fabrication

Laboratory activity varies depending on the type of restoration prescribed. Most frameworks are fabricated from a pattern that is built up in resin or wax on master model dies and then removed, invested, and cast. The pattern thickness is carefully controlled so that it approximates the desired thickness of the final casting. A methymethacrylate pattern (Duralay Kit[8]) works best because of its greater strength, considering the delicacy of the patterns. In the case of perforated or etched metal retainers, the pattern material is added directly to the lubricated surface of the die. If the prosthesis is to be a perforated type, holes 1 mm in diameter, numbering 6 to 10 per retainer, are placed in the resin pattern and then countersunk for a tunnel effect on the external surface (Fig. 8-120). If a macrosurface retention design is to be fabricated, the pattern is prepared on the surface of the die by either molding a mesh pattern or applying beads or crystals to the retainer area as outlined on the die. The acrylic pattern material (in some cases wax, depending on particular manufacturer's instructions) is then added over the retention material and carefully extended out to the margins of the retainer (Figs. 8-121 to 8-124).

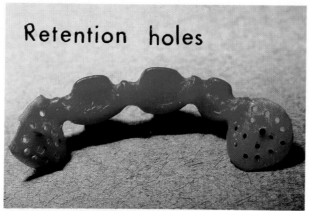

Figure 8-120   A combination Duralay-wax pattern removed from the dies. The retention perforations have been placed and the pattern is ready for investing.

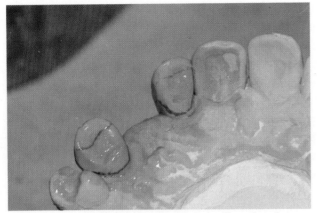

Figure 8–121 Adhesive-lubricant applied to the die surfaces in preparation for the application of salt crystals[6].

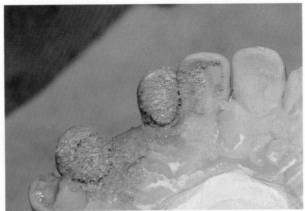

Figure 8–122 Crystals have been sprinkled on the dies and are shown adhering to the surface.

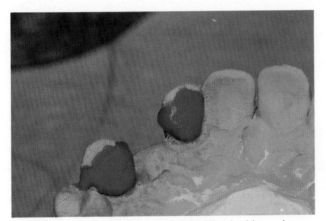

Figure 8–123 Methylmethacrylate (Duralay Kit[8]) in this case has been added as an external "skin" over the crystals, permitting them to be picked up from the surface of the dies.

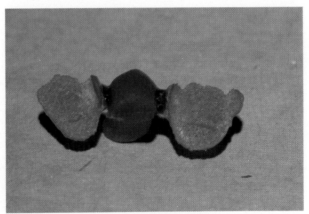

Figure 8–124 A view of the die surface of the porous retainer patterns after the crystals have been dissolved away.

The pontic framework is built up over an acrylic or a preformed pattern strut, attached first to one retainer and then to the other to avoid polymerization distortion. Pontic framework design depends on the pontic material prescribed (Figs. 8-125 to 8-129).

Some laboratories, particularly for large cases, prefer to use a refractory die technique. They either duplicate the master model in a manner similar to cast partial denture fabrication or use an investment die material, which permits the investing of the pattern and then casting of the metal framework directly on the master model dies (DVP Investment[16]).

A variety of metals are suitable, depending again on design. Base metal alloys are currently the most widely used, and although the laboratory undoubtedly has its favorite metal, the clinician who is prescribing an etched-metal prosthesis should confirm that the laboratory is using one of the base metals with the required etching potential (see Table 8-2). Investing and casting instructions are provided by the manufacturers and should be rigidly followed.

Following recovery of the casting and addition of the esthetic material, if required, the prosthesis is returned for trial seating and cementation, except in the case of etched-metal designs, which should be returned to the laboratory, following the try-in, for electrolytic etching.

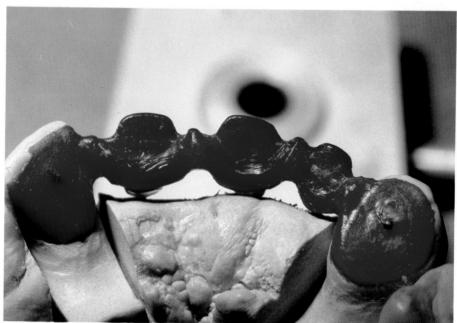

Figure 8-125 An acrylic strut has been attached to the retainers and porcelain pontic substructures built in the wax.

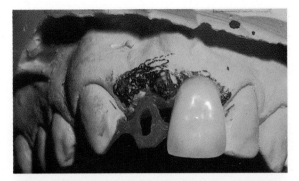

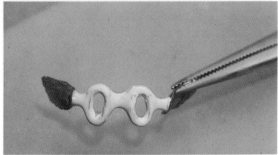

Figure 8–126 Acrylic (Duralay Kit[8]) loops fabricated between the retainers to provide retention for acrylic denture teeth or resin facings.[14] The left facing is being "fitted". The lower panel shows the two-pontic span with the loops cast and "opaqued".

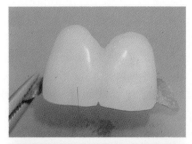

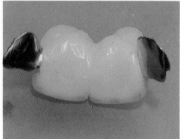

Figure 8–127 Labial and lingual views of the resin facings in place over the loops shown in the previous figures.

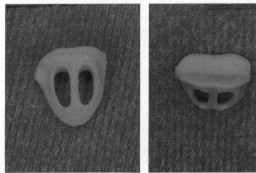

Figure 8–128 Examples of prefabricated pontic substructures. As these are cast and built up with porcelain or composite, a very strong framework is developed[15] (Shoher and Whiteman, 1983).

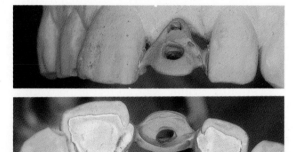

Figure 8–129 A pattern of the type shown in Figure 8-128 cast and ready for porcelain application. There is an obvious simplification in laboratory technique in the use of these patterns.

Electrolytic Etching

The survival of an etched restoration depends on the quality of its etch pattern. A clear understanding of the process and a diligent observance of the steps in the process are both essential.

The restoration must become one of the electrodes in the electrolytic bath. It is therefore secured with sticky wax to a stainless steel rod or copper wire (12- to 14-gauge) with at least two points of contact between the framework and the rod or wire. All areas of the restoration that are not to be etched are masked with sticky wax, as is any part of the rod or wire that will be in contact with the etching solution. Areas to be etched are then cleaned by air abrading with alumina (50 μ), and then the margins are reexamined and remasked if inadvertently exposed (Fig. 8-130). Since etching formulas (Table 8-2) require specific current densities, it is necessary to estimate the area to be etched in order to determine the total amount of current to be passed through the etching solution. This is readily done by comparing the prosthesis to a sample of known area (Fig. 8-131). Prior to location of the restoration in the etching solution, the existence of electrical contact between the retainers and the attached wire or rod is assessed by attempting to complete a circuit through the restoration. The restoration is mounted in the etching solution as the anode, the positive lead, while another stainless steel wire is attached as the cathode or negative lead. The electrodes are maneuvered in the clamp assembly so as to be approximately 2 cm apart when submerged in the etching solution. The etching apparatus is then activated in accordance with the appropriate etching formula and according to the instructions supplied with the etching equipment (Fig. 8-132). The current level may fluctuate initially, but should stabilize and, using an average three unit framework as an example, display readings within ± 20 ma of the required density. A noticeable color change occurs almost instantly so that after the first 30 seconds the prosthesis should appear black. Bubbles are in evidence on the cathode, and the solution around the prosthesis turns yellow. It is now suggested that stirring or ultrasonic agitation of the solution during etching is of no real importance to the success of the procedure (Del Castillo and Thompson, 1982).

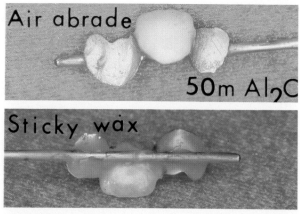

Figure 8-130 A three-unit bridge is shown attached to a stainless steel wire electrode; the surface to be etched is carefully abraded. The lower panel shows the outer surfaces of the bridge and the electrode totally masked with sticky wax.

TABLE 8–2   Etching Conditions

for Ni-Cr-Be Alloys

Rexillium III[19]	10% H_2SO_4	300 ma/cm² for 3 minutes
Bak-On NP[19]	10% H_2SO_4	300 ma/cm² for 3 minutes
Litecast B[19]	10% H_2SO_4	With methanol 9 parts to 1 200 ma/cm² for 6 minutes

for Ni-Cr Alloys

Biobond C & B[18]	0.5N HNO_3	250 ma/cm² for 5 minutes
NP[18]	0.1 HNO_3 + 2% glacial acetic acid	400 ma/cm² for 5 minutes (Pretreat with 5% NH_4OH Ultrasonic bath for 5 minutes)

From Simonsen R, Thompson V, Barrack G, 1983.

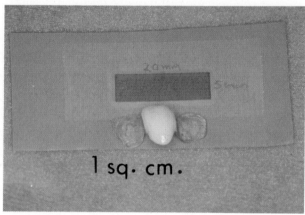

Figure 8–131   The surface area to be etched is being estimated by comparison with a 1-cm² piece of cardboard.

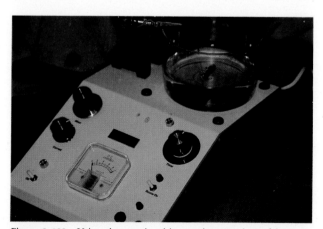

Figure 8–132   Using the metal etching equipment pictured here, one of several designs[17], samples to be etched are placed as one of two electrodes in the acid solution in the beaker shown at top and current is then passed through the solution with the instrument set at the predetermined milliamperage and time.

At the completion of the etching cycle, the restoration is removed from the solution, avoiding skin contact with the acid solution, rinsed with tap water, and then placed in an 18 percent hydrochloric acid solution. Fresh solution (approximately 150 ml) should be added for each cleaning cycle, and again the solution should not touch any exposed portion of the electrode. The acid container is placed in an ultrasonic cleaner for 10 minutes. The black surface coating (a debris layer) should quickly fall away from the surface of the restoration, and the cleaning should continue until a uniform gray surface appears. In fact, surface appearance varies with the alloy being etched. Ni-Cr alloys (Biobond C & B; NP[18]) are brighter and more metallic; Ni-Cr-Be alloys (Rexillium III; Bak-On NP; Litecast B[19]) are darker, sometimes with patches of brown or gray-black.

At this point, the surface of the restoration should be examined with stereoscopic magnification (at least 60 ×) to ensure that the etch pattern extends over at least 90 percent of the surface. If there is question as to the uniformity of the pattern, the restoration is re-etched for 60 to 90 seconds and then cleaned in hydrochloric acid as before.

Removal of the restoration from the electrode is a critical step. It must be accomplished without contamination of the etched surface with wax or even by skin contact. It is necessary to chill the sticky wax in ice cold water so that it can be fractured cleanly from the restoration. The restoration is immediately placed in an envelope to protect the etched surface until bonding is completed.

Credit must be given to the investigators at the University of Maryland for their work in the development of the metal-etching process. A number of etching units are now available, as well as suggested variations in etching techniques, but the original research effort expended by this team in the development and refinement of the formulas (see Table 8-2), along with the associated equipment and materials, has appropriately resulted in wide usage of these etching techniques, as described in the research literature and now in textbook form (Simonsen et al, 1983).

Prebonding Try-In

Careful inspection of the restoration for such details as marginal extension, internal blebs and bubbles, pontic contours, and occlusal contacts, preferably using magnification, can prevent the loss of valuable chairside time. As a precautionary measure, dental floss should be ligated or attached with sticky wax to the restoration before the framework is placed in the mouth.

An effective method of assessing the precision of the seating of the retainers, as well as the relationship of the pontic(s) to the soft tissues, involves the use of a wash viscosity polyvinyl siloxane impression material (Reprosil; President[20]) as a disclosing agent (Fig. 8-133). Adjustments are made, the impression material reapplied, and the prosthesis is reinserted until maximum seating is achieved. The restoration should manifest resistance to dislodgement except along its path of insertion. At this point, the occlusion on all areas of the prosthesis should be carefully analyzed and adjustments made if required. Because of the possible deleterious effects of heat transfer through the metal to the bonding composite in the event of occlusal adjustment after cementation, every effort should be made to refine the occlusion prior to bonding procedures.

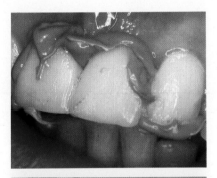

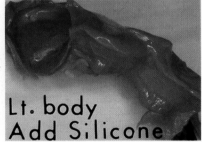

Figure 8-133   The fit of the bridge is being assessed using the low-viscosity impression material. High spots or positive defects on the internal surfaces can be readily visualized and removed.

The esthetic potential of the case is assessed and appropriate adjustments or modifications made (Figs. 8-134 to 8-137). If porcelain adjustments do not require the retexturing associated with reglazing (i.e., facial of the pontic surface as in Fig. 8-137), a clinically acceptable smoothness can be produced using available porcelain polishing wheels or pastes (Shofu Porcelain Polishing Kit; Insta-Glaze[21]). Resin facings may have their shade modified or be characterized by the addition of light-cured composite colorant materials. The appearance

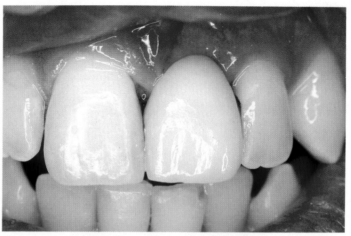

Figure 8–134   At prebonding try-in, the pontic (left central incisor) dimension and shape are unacceptable.

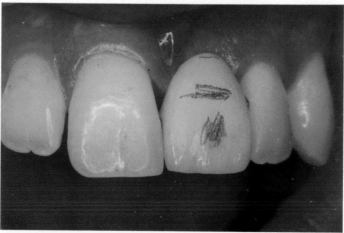

Figure 8–135   Areas where the porcelain requires modification are marked with pencil and removed.

of the finished restoration can be previewed by selecting a likely composite material, adding a drop of eugenol to the mix to inhibit polymerization, and then inserting the prosthesis. A solvent such as chloroform or acetone can be used to clean the framework following the "trial" cementation. Assuming fit, occlusion, and esthetics to be acceptable, the prosthesis may be cemented, unless of course it must still be electrolytically etched.

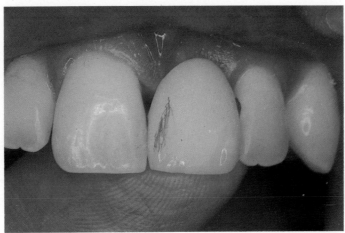

Figure 8–136 While reshaping is minimal, subtle change can result in substantial esthetic improvement.

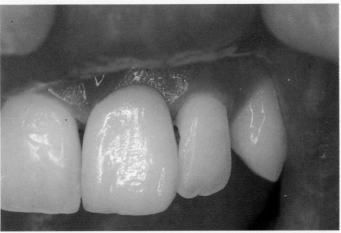

Figure 8–137 For a final modification, the prosthesis is returned to the laboratory for the addition of porcelain to reshape the mesial gingival area more in keeping with the shape of the adjacent central. The ground surfaces are glazed in the process.

Bonding Procedures

Many earlier cases have been successfully bonded by means of large-particle, macrofilled composite materials (Adaptic; Concise[1]). To obtain more intimate seating of the restorations, materials have now been developed with decreased filler-particle size and lowered viscosity (Comspan[22]), as well as with extended working times and opaque formulations (Comspan Opaque; Conclude; Retain; Resin Bonded Bridge Cement[10]). In preparation for bonding (Figs. 8-138 to 8-147), the teeth are isolated with a rubber dam, which is carefully inverted into the gingival sulcus so as not to encroach on the abutment surface. A prophylaxis with oil-free, nonfluoridated pumice is followed by copious water lavage. The abutments are etched for one minute using 37 percent phosphoric acid liquid or gel placed with light strokes of a sable-hair brush, or with a gel injected onto the tooth surface with a syringe, followed by a 30-second wash. If a gel etchant has been used, the water lavage should be increased to

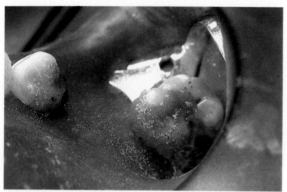

Figure 8-138 Rubber dam isolates the abutments; phosphoric acid gel has been applied to these areas of enamel to be covered by the retainers.

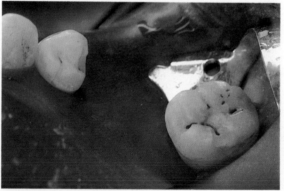

Figure 8-139 Following the rinse-dry cycle, the enamel appears opaque and frosted.

one minute, since many gels contain a glycerine base which is difficult to remove. The teeth must be examined for the efficacy of the etch. The enamel should demonstrate a white chalky surface. An inadequate etch may result from resistant (fluorosed) enamel, insufficient etching time, or moisture contamination. The mixing and application of the composite materials, followed by the seating of the prostheses, must be done strictly according to the manufacturer's directions; four-handed techniques greatly facilitate the procedures. Although variations are expected in the sequencing of the mixing and application of the composite materials, the critical nature of the procedure demands prior organization and even a "trial run" if the handling characteristics of the materials are unfamiliar to the operator and the assistant(s). Of absolute importance is the maintenance of the uncontaminated enamel surface following etching and following application of the low-viscosity resin. The composite resin materials, both filled and unfilled, must be applied to the abutments and to the prosthesis and then the prosthesis fully seated before *any* polymerization has occurred. (Some manufacturers suggest that working and setting times can be adjusted by varying the material ratios. Experimentation by the "office team" is required in advance of an actual bonding procedure if such adjustments are to be attempted.) A third critical point involves the application of the low-viscosity unfilled resin. It must not be pooled on either the abutment teeth or the metal framework. A quantity of this material triggers rapid polymerization, which would then seriously compromise the seating of the restoration. The clinician must stabilize the prosthesis and its abutments for the full polymerization cycle. The assistant should remove excess resin before it has hardened, particularly in difficult-to-reach embrasure and marginal areas. Care must be taken in post-cementation trimming, to avoid overheating the composite and the metal framework. A variety of instruments are effective in removing residual composite (# 7902; ET; Soflex Discs;[3] Carbide Finishing Knives[5]).

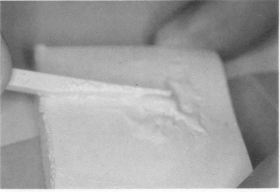

Figure 8-140 The composite "pastes" in this sequence were mixed first.

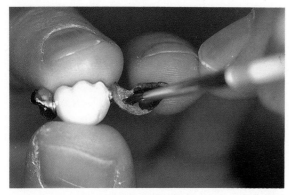

Figure 8-141 The unfilled resin was then mixed and applied to the teeth and the prosthesis. A well-etched retainer will appear to almost suck the free-flowing resin into its surface.

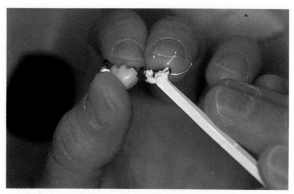

Figure 8-142 After the unfilled resin is thinned by blowing both the abutment teeth and the retainers with air, the composite is placed on the etched surfaces of the bridge retainers.

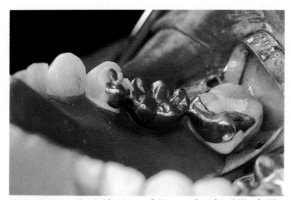

Figure 8-143 The bridge is carefully seated and stabilized. The excess composite, shown here immediately after insertion, is removed as much as possible before polymerization, without disturbing the bridge in any way.

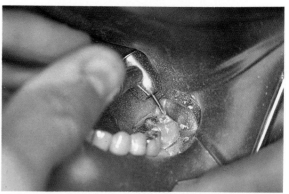

Figure 8-144 Finishing burs are used following polymerization to complete the removal of excess composite.

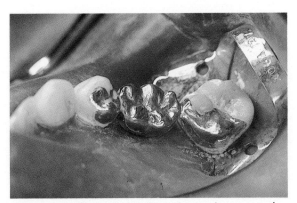

Figure 8-145 The bonded bridge is shown prior to removal of the rubber dam.

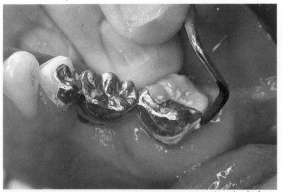

Figure 8-146 The enamel surfaces adjacent to the gingival margins are carefully inspected for residual composite.

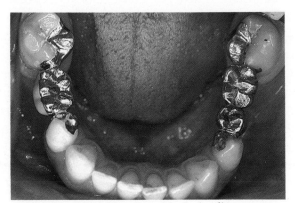

Figure 8-147 The bridge pictured in the bonding sequence joins a similar prosthesis inserted earlier in the contralateral quadrant. Both bridges continue to provide excellent service for the patient after approximately 1 year in the mouth.

Troubleshooting and Maintenance

Clinical experience with cast-metal bonded prostheses has identified a number of performance problems. These include partial or total "debonding" of the restoration, framework fracture, and pontic dislodgement or breakage.

Loss of Attachment

When there is total loss of attachment, a careful assessment of the prosthesis, the abutment teeth, and particularly the occlusion should be made to determine the cause of dislodgment. If dislodgment has occured because of trauma, retreatment will depend on the extent of the damage (Figs. 8-148 to 8-153).

When a "debond" occurs shortly after insertion without apparent trauma, inspection of the restoration and its abutments may reveal the composite to have fractured primarily at either the enamel or metal interface (Figs. 8-154 to 8-157). Careful assessment of the occlusal factors and then of the prosthesis may give evidence of (1) hyperocclusion on the pontics or retainers, (2) a lack of adequate framework design (check if bridge will move lingually when totally seated, indicating inadequate resistance form), (3) inadequate retention design (insufficient surface area and/or number of holes or inadequate etch, mesh, or bead pattern), or (4) faulty technique, permitting contamination (either metal or enamel surfaces). Depending on the conclusion, and a definite answer may not be possible ("debonding" could be a result of the combination of more than one or all of these factors), the prosthesis can frequently be considered for reinsertion, with appropriate steps taken to eliminate the probable causes of the previous trouble. Prostheses with apparently noncorrectible problems or oral environments evidently highly unfavorable, based on unsuccessful performance periods, require restoration remake or perhaps abandonment of the bonded prosthesis approach.

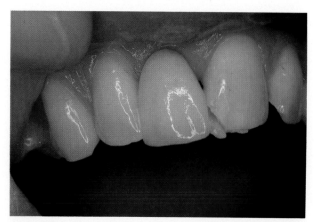

Figure 8-148 The metal-bonded bridge replacing the right central incisor has been loosened through patient "fall". The left central retainer has fractured away from the enamel except along the mesial incisal edge, which has fractured and remained attached to the framework.

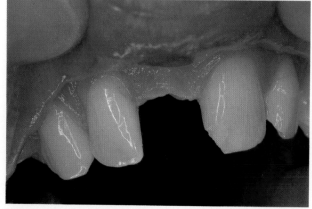

Figure 8-149 The right lateral retainer remained securely bonded, but was successfully tapped loose by means of a chisel at the incisal margin. The extent of the damage to the central is seen with the bridge removed.

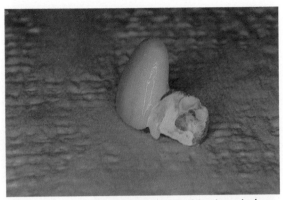

Figure 8–150 Note the composite retained by the etched metal surface along with the fractured incisal proximal enamel.

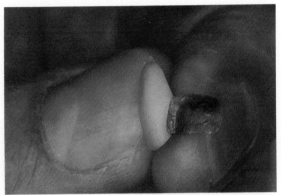

Figure 8–151 The retainer surfaces have had the composite burned off and have been re-etched.

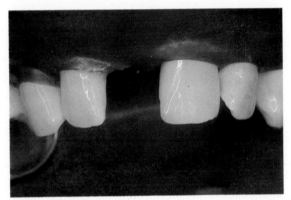

Figure 8–152 The fractured incisal corner has been repaired by use of a light-cured microfilled composite.

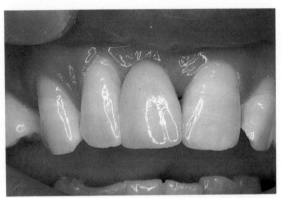

Figure 8-153 The bridge is shown successfully rebonded.

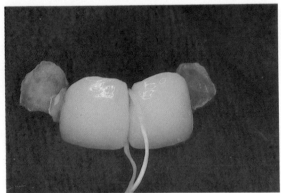

Figure 8–154 In this debonding of a perforated bridge, the composite has remained on the retainers. Enamel bonding technique may be suspected in this case.

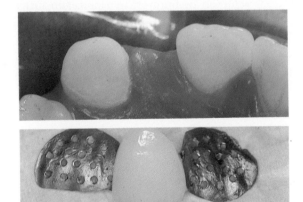

Figure 8-155 Another perforated debond, but this time failure has occurred at the metal-resin interface. Composite remains within the perforations. Stress encountered by the restoration evidently could not be "handled" by the composite-perforation retention mechanism.

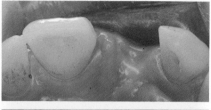

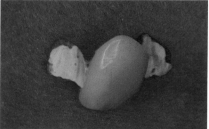

Figure 8–156 An etched metal bridge "debond" with the composite remaining on the retainer metal surface.

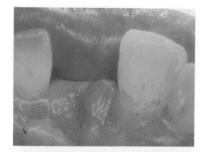

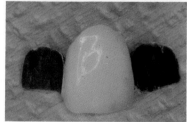

Figure 8–157 In this "debond" the composite has remained on the enamel surface. Contamination or inadequate metal etching should be considered a possible cause.

The same exercise faces the clinician when a prosthesis only partially "debonds", with the added problem of attempting its removal. The perforated prostheses are most readily removed in this situation by elimination of the composite from the holes and then use of an instrument to apply a shearing force at the framework enamel interface (Figs. 8-158 and 8-159). Although application of this type of force may dislodge retainers with the "sandwich" of composite, it may instead distort the framework or even tear enamel away from the underlying dentin (Fig. 8-160). Discretion then is required, and the restoration may have to be cut off and essentially destroyed (Figs. 8-161 and 8-162).

Following successful removal of a prosthesis and prior to rebonding, its retention mechanism must be reinstated. As previously pointed out, this is readily accomplished with the perforated design, less easily with a macrosurface design, and with difficulty in the case of the etched metal type. Removal of the composite from the etched surface has usually been achieved by burn-off in a porcelain furnace (700 °C for 10 to 15 minutes) followed by re-etching. Bridges with acrylic pontics which cannot be heated in this fashion have been treated by thorough sandblasting (alumina, 50 μ) and then etching; early results indicate this may be adequate (Gratton et al, 1984; Ullo et al, 1984). Rebonding procedures are identical to the steps followed in the original insertion.

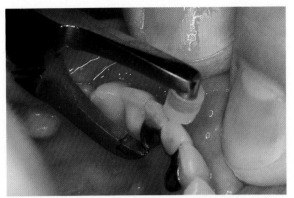

Figure 8-158 A lower etched metal bridge with one loose retainer. An orthodontic bond remover is being used in an effort to free the other retainer.

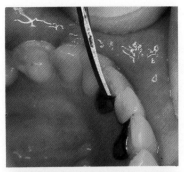

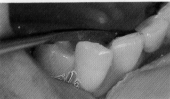

Figure 8–159 An alternative method of removal is being demonstrated on the same bridge. A chisel engaging the edge of the metal retainer is tapped sharply with a surgical mallet. The unpredictability of both of these methods is readily acknowledged, particularly with etched metal retainers.

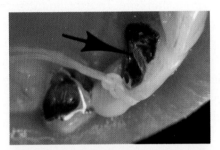

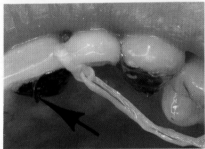

Figure 8-160 The "chisel" method in this case resulted in distortion and then tearing of the retainer before the composite finally fractured at the metal-enamel interface (*arrows*).

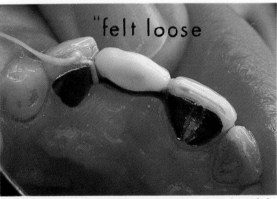

Figure 8-161 Another etched metal anterior bridge "debonded" on the lateral incisor. The bridge was ligated with floss and then efforts made to tap it loose.

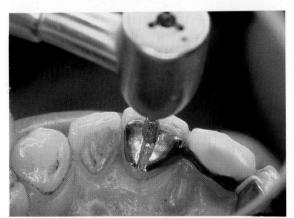

Figure 8-162 All efforts, short of force likely to damage the abutment tooth, were unsuccessful, and the retainer was "cut off", necessitating total remake of the bridge.

Framework Fracture

Framework fracture can be attributed to poor case selection, inadequate design, poor quality laboratory work, or a combination of these. Adherence to principles already discussed should prevent this type of problem, which obviously must be remedied by remake of the prosthesis or selection of a more conventional treatment form (Fig. 8-163).

Pontic Dislodgment and Fracture

Pontic loss or fracture can occur with trauma, from occlusal factors arising from inadequate integration of the pontics into the patient's occlusal scheme, particular habits of the patient, or failure of materials. Acrylic or resin pontics are much more easily repaired or replaced "in situ" (Figs. 8-164 to 8-167).

Porcelain pontics constitute a much more serious problem. To date, unquestionably, the best esthetic and functional results are to be obtained by refabricating the porcelain. Efforts to avoid this major "overhaul" by bonding composite materials to the residual porcelain and/or metal have not been entirely satisfactory (Figs. 8-168 to 8-170). This approach has been used for some time in the repair of porcelain fractures involving conventional bridges (Barreto, 1984), but results remain somewhat unpredictable. Newer techniques and materials for porcelain repair may provide improved esthetics and longevity.

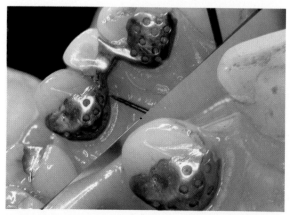

Figure 8-163 The explorer tip is placed at the site of a framework fracture. With the pontic and the incisor retainer removed, the failure is seen to have occurred along a then narrow connector area (*lower panel*).

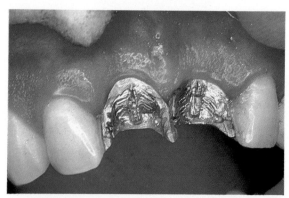

Figure 8-164 This patient presented, 6 months after insertion of the bridge, with loosening of the acrylic pontic facings.

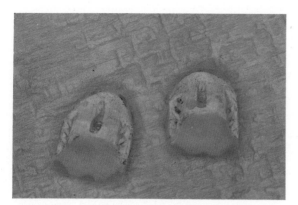

Figure 8-165 Most of the opaque masking resin has fractured from the metal surface, indicative of inadequate mechanical retention or metal contamination.

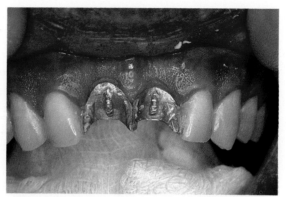

Figure 8-166 The framework retention was redefined prior to reattachment of the facings. Although not shown, increased mechanical retention was cut into the pontic facings.

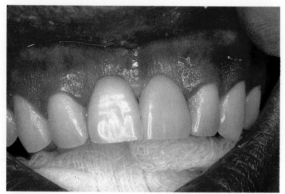

Figure 8-167 The pontics are shown after being reattached with an auto-curing composite resin. The increased strength of the composite resin is expected to provide a stronger attachment, although it is recognized that there will be no chemical union between the composite and the acrylic facings.

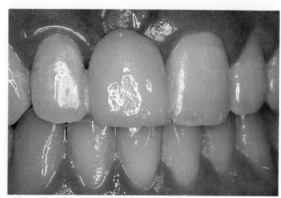

Figure 8-168 A porcelain pontic bonded by etched metal retainers to the right lateral and left central incisors (immediately post-insertion).

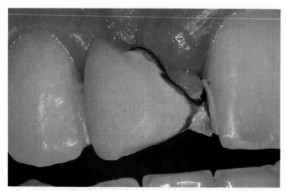

Figure 8-169 A traumatic fracture through the porcelain 3 months after insertion.

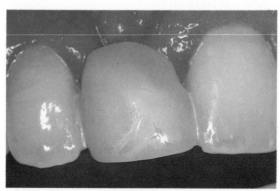

Figure 8-170 An attempted composite repair with less-than-hoped for results.

Clinical Variations

Many examples could be shown of cases that have required some modification of what could be considered the ''normal'' approach. While variations are almost as numerous as are individual clinical situations, one of these, the so-called ''combination case'' involving a conventional fixed unit attached through the framework to a metal-bonded retainer(s), is likely to be encountered with some frequency. Its practicality is greatly enhanced through the use of a semi-precision attachment in the conventional unit. When this attachment is used, the opposite ends of the prosthesis have some independence (important, as already discussed, from an occlusion-physiologic movement point of view), and inadvertent loosening of the bonded retainer does not require removal of a permanently cemented conventional crown (Figs. 8-171 and 8-172).

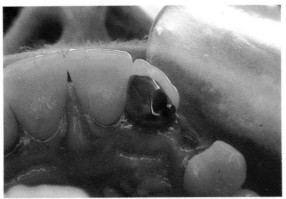

Figure 8-171 An example of a conventional full crown retainer over a post and core. The female segment of a semi-precision attachment has been placed in the distal to receive the male segment, which is part of a resin-bonded bridge from the virgin premolar. The attachment would of necessity be much smaller in a vital tooth.

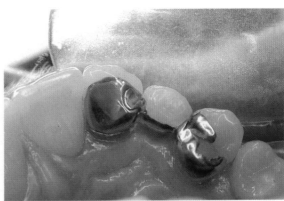

Figure 8-172 The distal segment of the bridge has been bonded to the premolar and coupled into the attachment in the mesial full crown retainer.

SUMMARY

The bonding of fixed prosthodontic restorations to natural enamel has opened a new horizon in restorative dentistry. Even though many questions remain to be answered, excellent service has and is being provided for large numbers of patients. As is common in clinical dentistry, certain design and technique considerations are critical to the use of these bonded prostheses. Attention to details of the techniques and materials now available should enable the practitioner to recommend these restorations even as we await the results of ongoing research.

The prospect of improved materials and refined techniques to produce better prostheses and even more predictable bonding to natural tooth structures (see Chapter 6) augurs well for the future of this ultraconservative approach.

References

Barreto MT. Failures in ceramometal fixed restorations. J Prosthet Dent 1984; 51:186.

Bergendal B, et al. Composite retained onlay bridges. Swed Dent J 1983; 7:217.

Buonocore NG. The Use of Adhesives in Dentistry. Springfield IL: Charles C. Thomas, 1975.

Del Castillo E, Thompson VP. Electrolytically etched non-precious alloys: Resin Bond and Laboratory Variables. Abstr Internat A Dent Res Program Abstr Papers 1982; 61:186.

Denehy GE, Howe DF. A conservative approach to the missing anterior tooth. Quintessence Int 1979; 7:1.

Eshleman JR, et al. Retentive Strengths of Acid Etched Fixed Prosthesis. Abstr Internat A Dental Res Program Abstr Papers 1981; 60:377.

Eshleman JR, Moon PC, Barnes RF. Clinical evaluation of cast metal resin bonded anterior fixed partial dentures. J Prosthet Dent 1984; 51:761.

Forbes JF, Horn JS. Characterization of bonding composites for two types of metal retainers. Abstr Internat A Dent Res Program Abstr Papers 1984; 63:320.

Gratton DR, et al. Unpublished data, 1984.

Gratton DR, Jordan RE, Teteruck WR. Resin bonded bridges: the state of the art. Ont Dentist 1983; 60:9.

Howe DF, Denehy GE. Anterior fixed partial dentures utilizing the acid-etch treatment and a cast metal framework. J Prosthet Dent 1977; 37:28.

Ibsen RL. Fixed prosthetics with a natural crown pontic using an adhesive composite. South Calif Dent A J 1973; 41:1000.

Jenkins CBG. Etch-retained anterior pontics: a four year study. Br Dent J 1978; 144:206.

Jordan RE, et al. Restoration of missing incisors by means of resin bonded techniques. Alpha Omegan 1981; 74:19.

Jordan RE, et al. Temporary fixed partial dentures fabricated by means of the acid etch resin technique: A report of 86 cases followed for up to three years. J Am Dent Assoc 1978; 96:994.

Jordan RE, Suzuki M, Gwinnett AJ. Conservative applications of acid etch resin techniques. Dent Clin North Am 1981; 25:307.

Kaiser DA. Fabricating a customized incisal guidetable. J Prosthet Dent 1981; 45:568.

Kochavi D, Stern N, Grajower R. A temporary space maintainer using acrylic resin teeth and a composite resin. J Prosthet Dent 1977; 37:522.

LaBarre EE, Ward HE. An alternative resin-bonded restoration. J Prosthet Dent 1984; 52:247.

Lambert PM, Moore DL, Elletson HH. In vitro retentive strength of fixed bridges constructed with acrylic pontics and an ultraviolet-light polymerized resin. J Am Dent Assoc 1976; 92:740.

Livaditis GJ. Cast-metal resin-bonded retainers for posterior teeth. J Am Dent Assoc 1980; 101:926.

Livaditis GJ. Personal Communication. February, 1981.

Livaditis GJ, Thompson VP. Etched castings: improved retentive mechanism for resin-bonded retainers. J Prosthet Dent 1982; 47:52.

McLaughlin G. Composite bonding of etched metal anterior splints. Comp Cont Ed Dent 1981; 2:279.

Moon PC. Resin-bonded bridge tensile bond strength utilizing porous patterns. Abstr Internat A Dent Res Program Abstr Papers 1984; 63:320.

Nykamp TL, Lorey RE. A comparison of the various mechanisms of etched-metal resin-bonded bridges. Abstr Internat Assoc Dent Res 1984; 63:331.

Portnoy L. Constructing a composite pontic in a single visit. Dent Surg 1973; 49:20.

Rochette AL. Attachment of a splint to enamel of lower anterior teeth. J Prosthet Dent 1973; 30:418.

Rochette AL. Adhésion par polymères et traitement de surface en odonto-stomatologie. Etrait Actualités, Odonto-stomatologiques 1972; 98:204.

Shoher I, Whiteman AE. Reinforced porcelain systems: a new concept in ceramometal restorations. J Prosthet Dent 1983; 50:489.

Simonsen RJ. Clinical Applications of the Acid-Etch Technique. Chicago: Quintessence, 1978; 71.

Simonsen RJ, Thompson V, Barrack G. Etched cast restorations: clinical and laboratory techniques. Chicago: Quintessence 1983; 15.

Sloan KM, Lorey RE, Myers GE. Evaluation of laboratory etching of cast metal resin bonded retainers. Abstr Internat Assoc Dent Res 1983; 62:220.

Stolpa JB. An adhesive technique for small anterior fixed partial dentures. J Prosthet Dent 1975; 340:513.

Sweeney EJ, Moore DL, Dooner JJ. Retentive strength of acid-etched anterior fixed partial dentures: An in vitro comparison of attachment techniques. J Am Dent Assoc 1980; 100:198.

Thompson VP, Livaditis GJ. Etched casting acid-etch composite bonded posterior bridges. Paediatr Dent 1982; 4:38.

Thompson VP, Del Castillo E, Livaditis GJ. Resin-bonded retainers. Part 1: Resin-bonded to electrolytically etched non-precious alloys. J Prosthet Dent 1983; 50:771.

Ullo C, Schlissel E, Gwinnett J. Etch cast retainers: surface preparation and rebonding strengths. Abstr Internat Assoc Dent Res 1984; 63:233.

Williams VD, Drennon DG, Silverstone LM. The effect of retainer design on the retention of filled resin in acid-etched fixed partial dentures. J Prosthet Dent 1982; 48:417.

Williams VD, et al. Acid-etch retained cast metal prostheses: a seven-year study. J Am Dent Assoc 1984; 108:629.

Product Information

Product	Manufacturer/Distributor	Purpose
1. Adaptic	Johnson and Johnson 20 Lake Drive, CN7060 East Windsor, NJ 08520	Composite materials for bonding all resin-bonded bridges
Concise	Dental Products/3M Company 3M Center 270–5N–02 St. Paul, MN 55144	
Prismafil	L. D. Caulk Co. P.O. Box 359 Milford, DE 19963	
Command Ultrafine	Kerr-Sybron Co. P.O. Box 455 Romulus, MI 48174	
2. Centrix Syringe	Centrix Inc. 480 Sniffens Lane Stamford, CT 06497	Composite syringe
3. #7902	Teledyne Densco Ltd. 3840 Forrest St. Denver, CO 80207	Multifluted carbide steel finishing bur
Esthetic Trimming Kit (ET)	Brasseler USA Inc. 800 King George Blvd. Savannah, GA 31419	Carbide steel and diamond finishing burs
Soflex Discs	Dental Products/3M Company 3M Center 270–5N–02 St. Paul, MN 55144	Aluminum oxide finishing discs
4. TMS Minikin	Whaledent International 236 Fifth Ave. New York, NY 10001	Self-threading pin
5. Carbide Finishing Knives 150:17/150:20	Brasseler USA Inc. 800 King George Blvd. Savannah, GA 31419	Carbide-tipped finishing instruments
6. Duralingual	Unitek Corp. 2724 South Reck Rd. Monrovia, CA 91016	Mesh pattern for macroretention
Micro Retention Beads	Vivadent USA Inc. P.O. Box 304 Tonawanda, NY 14150	Resin beads for macroretention
Cubic Salt Crystals	Moon, P.C. Medical College of Virginia, School of Dentistry Richmond, VA 23298	Dissolvable crystals for macroretention
Crystal Bond	Crystal Bond Products P.O. Box 179 Loma Linda, CA 92354	
7. WhipMix	WhipMix Corp. 361 Farmington Ave., Box 17183 Louisville, KY 40217	Semiadjustable articulator
8. Duralay Kit	Reliance Dental Mfg. Co. 5805 West 117 Place Worth, IL 60482	Methyl methacrylate pattern
9. MDS Truspot	MDS Products Inc. 1440 South State College Blvd. Anaheim, CA 92806	Thin articulating film
10. Comspan Opaque	L. D. Caulk Co. P.O. Box 359 Milford, DE 19963	Opaque composite luting materials

Product Information

Product	Manufacturer/Distributor	Purpose
Conclude	Dental Products/3M Company 3M Center 270–5N–02 St. Paul, MN 55144	
Retain	Pentron Corp. P.O. Box 771 Wallingford, CT 06492	
Resin Bonded Bridge Cement	Kerr-Sybron Co. P.O. Box 455 Romulus, MI 48174	Microparticle opaque composite
11. 700.9VF, Two Striper	ESPE-Premier Sales Corp. Romano Dr., P.O. Box 111 Norristown, PA 19401	Thin-tapered fissure diamond
12. #9902	Denco 260 Yorkland Blvd. Willowdale, Ontario M2J 1R7	Multifluted tungsten carbide bur
13. Occlude	Pascal Co. Inc. 2929 Northeast Northrup Way Bellevue, WA 98004	Disclosing material
14. Bioblend, Trubyte	Dentsply International 570 West College Ave. York, PA 17405	Acrylic denture teeth for aesthetic pontics
Isocette	Vivadent USA Inc. P.O. Box 304 Tonawanda, NY 14150	Resin facings for aesthetic pontics
15. Inzoma Patterns	Ivoclar/Vivadent Canada Inc. 1200 Aerowood Dr., Unit 23 Mississauga, Ontario L4W 2S7	Prefabricated pontic substructures
RPS Wax Structures	Williams Gold Co. 2978 Main St. Buffalo, NY 14214	
16. DVP Investment	WhipMix Corp. 361 Farmington Ave., Box 17183 Louisville, KY 40217	Investment die material
17. Time-Etch	Time Dental Laboratories 20 Strabain Cres. Baltimore, MD 21234	Metal etching equipment
Ultra-Etch	Tri-Dynamics Dental Inc. P.O. Box 787 East Brunswick, NJ 08816	
18. Biobond C & B	Dentsply International 570 West College Ave. York, PA 17405	Nickel-chrome alloys
NP	Howmedica Inc. 5101 South Keeler Ave. Chicago, IL 60632	
19. Rexillium III	Jeneric Industries P.O. Box 125, North Plains Ind. Rd. Wallingford, CT 06492	Nickel-chrome-berillium alloys
Bak-On NP	Johnson and Johnson 20 Lake Drive, CN7060 East Windsor, NJ 08520	
Litecast B	Williams Gold Co. 2978 Main St. Buffalo, NY 14214	

Product Information

Product	Manufacturer/Distributor	Purpose
20. Reprosil	L. D. Caulk Co. P.O. Box 359 Milford, DE 19963	Polyvinyl siloxane impression material
President	Coltene Inc. Feldwiesen Strasse 20, CH-49507 Altstatten, Switzerland	
21. Shofu Porcelain Polishing Kit	Shofu Dental Corp. 420 Bohannon Dr. Menlo Park, CA 94025	Porcelain polishing wheels
Insta-Glaze	George Taub Products & Fusion Co. Inc. 277 New York Ave. Jersey City, NJ 07307	Diamond paste for porcelain
22. Comspan	L. D. Caulk Co. P.O. Box 359 Milford, DE 19963	Small-particled, low-viscosity composite

9

RONALD E. JORDAN

RESIN-TO-RESIN BONDING

One of the unique clinical features of composite resin materials is that they are reliably bondable one to another by means of a simple but effective direct add-on clinical technique (Chan and Boyer, 1983; Miranda et al, 1984; Marshall et al, 1983). Recent research has shown that several parameters dictate the efficacy of the add-on result:

1. The *time* of repair: Repair bond strengths equal to that of the composite material itself may result after bonding to unprepared surfaces 30 minutes old (Boyer et al, 1978).
2. The *condition* of the surface: In attempting repairs on *aged* composite restorations, best results are obtained when the composite surface is lightly abraded, etched, and bonded before application of the new composite material (Murrey et al, 1983; Miranda et al, 1984; Meeker et al, 1983).
3. The chemistry of the composite substrate and adhesive: The closer the chemical similarity between substrate and adhesive, the better is the repair bond (Chan and Boyer, 1983).

MATERIALS

Because of their high degree of esthetic acceptability and color stability, the light-cured microfilled materials (Durafil;[1] Silux;[2] Visiodispers;[3] Certain[4]) are considered ideal for effecting resin-to-resin repairs. Such materials adhere well to conventional materials with a bond strength of approximately 75 percent of the tensile strengths of the resin materials (Chan and Boyer, 1983).

TECHNIQUE

Figure 9-1 shows the 4-year appearance of a class IV mesioincisal composite restoration. The surface is somewhat dull and nonreflective and demonstrates some degree of interproximal plaque accumulation. After proper isolation (Fig. 9-2), the composite surface is prepared with a thin, tapering, bullet-nosed diamond (201.3F[5]) (Fig. 9-3).

A 0.25- to 0.5-mm composite thickness is removed from the surface, and a chamfer finish line is established in the adjacent enamel (Fig. 9-4). A gel etchant (Scotchbond Etching Gel[6]) is now placed over the entire surface of the ground composite and the chamfered enamel (Fig. 9-5) and kept undisturbed for one minute.

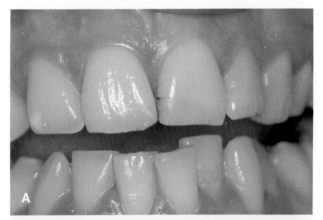

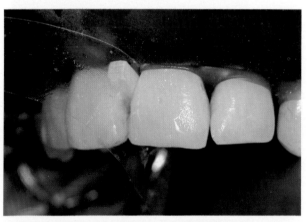

Figure 9-2   Rubber dam isolation of the field prior to rebonding.

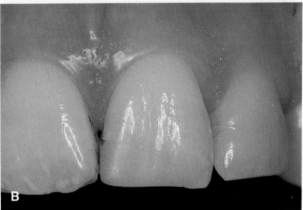

Figure 9–1   *A,* A 4-year mesioincisal composite restoration in the maxillary left central incisor. *B,* Close-up view.

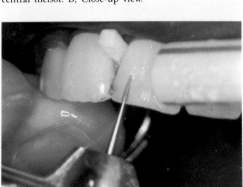

Figure 9-3   A tapering bullet-nosed diamond is used to prepare the composite surface.

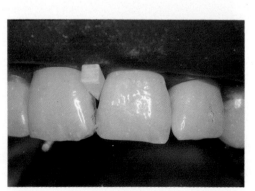

Figure 9-4   Prepared composite surface and enamel chamfer.

After a 45-second water lavage and careful air drying, the composite surface is thoroughly cleaned, and the etched enamel presents a white-opaque appearance (Fig. 9-6). A thin layer of bond resin (Scotchbond[7]) is placed over the composite enamel surface (Fig. 9-7) and gently blown with air (Fig. 9-8).

Microfilled composite (Silux[2]) is bulk-packed into position and a Teflon instrument (Felt No. 4 Instrument[8]) is used to grossly shape the anatomic form (Fig. 9-9). A fine, dry, sable brush is used to finally contour the restoration (Fig. 9-10). If care is taken to complete the contouring procedure without gross excess (Fig. 9-11), the need for gross finishing is minimal. The completed restoration is shown in Figure 9-12.

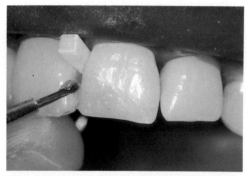

Figure 9-5 A gel etchant is placed over the composite and enamel surface.

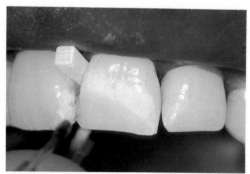

Figure 9-6 Appearance of the etched surface after washing and drying.

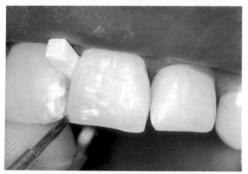

Figure 9-7 A layer of bond resin is applied to composite and enamel surfaces.

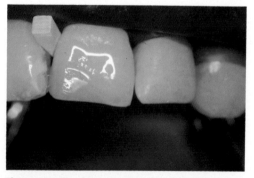

Figure 9-8 Bond resin surface after air blowing.

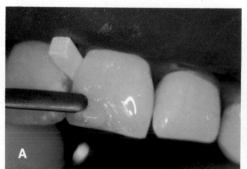
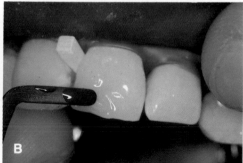

Figure 9–9 *A*, A Teflon instrument is used to "bulk pack" the composite material and, *B*, to preliminary shape the surface.

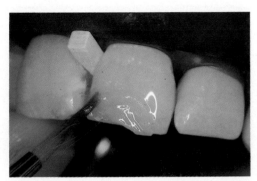

Figure 9-10 Final shaping of the composite is accomplished by means of a dry sable brush.

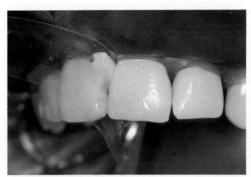

Figure 9-11 The add-on composite after contouring prior to light cure.

Although it is best to bond the adhesive composite to a composite substrate of similar basic chemistry, it is not always necessary for the clinician to know exactly what type of composite constitutes the substrate. Figure 9-13 shows a large discolored composite restoration in the maxillary right central incisor, the nature of which was unknown. After preparation etching and bonding, a light-cured microfilled composite material (Visiodispers[3]) was bonded to it, and the result at 2-year recall is shown in Figure 9-14. Microfilled materials are excellent adhesives when bonded to other microfilled restorations (Chan and Roger, 1983). Figure 9-15 shows a large, discolored, self-cured (Silar[9]) microfill restoration at 4-year recall. It was reveneered with its light-cured counterpart (Silux[2]), and the result is shown in Figure 9-16.

"Paint-on" light-cured microfilled materials (Rembrandt Natural[10]) are useful for resin-to-resin bonding techniques. Figure 9-17 shows two discolored and worn composite restorations reveneered with Rembrandt Natural[10] (Fig. 9-18).

Resin-to-resin bonding procedures are also useful when "stratification" or "sandwiching" is necessary. For example, Figure 9-19 shows a fractured maxillary left central incisor crown in a young patient. Protrusive and protrusive lateral occlusion are both heavy. To complicate matters further, the patient was undergoing orthodontic treatment involving direct bonded brackets. The coronal restoration was built up with a "heavy-filled" macrofilled composite material (Visiofil[11]), which was then overveneered (Fig. 9-20) with a microfilled material (Visiodispers[3]). The resultant "light on heavy" or "sandwich" restoration (Fig. 9-21) combines the best clinical features of the microfilled and macrofilled systems, i.e., polishability and fracture resistance, respectively.

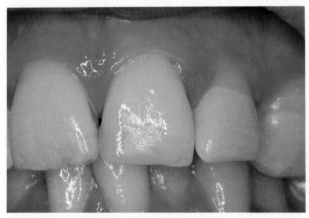

Figure 9-12 The completed restoration.

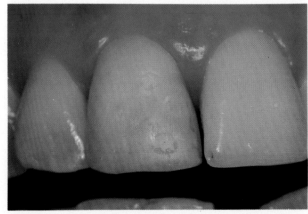

Figure 9-13 A large discolored composite restoration in the maxillary right central incisor.

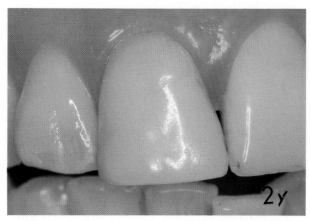

Figure 9–14   The incisor shown in Figure 9-13 after rebonding with microfilled composite at 2-year recall. Note the white color of the restoration which is characteristic of many light-cured microfilled composite materials at recall.

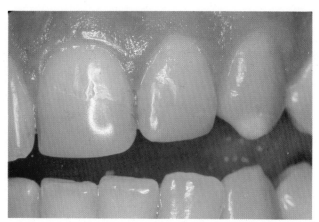

Figure 9–15   A discolored, self-cured microfilled composite restoration in the maxillary left central incisor.

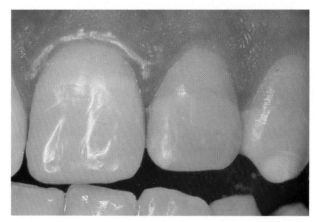

Figure 9–16   The incisor shown in Figure 9-15 after reveneering.

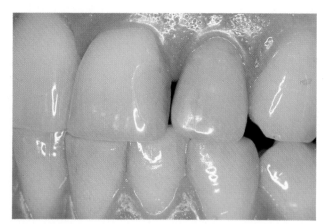

Figure 9–17   Discolored and worn composite restorations in the maxillary central and lateral incisors.

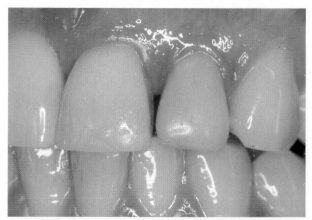

Figure 9–18   The restorations shown in Figure 9-17 after reveneering with a paint-on light-cured microfilled material (Rembrandt Natural[10]).

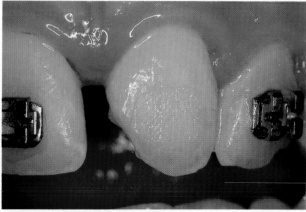

Figure 9–19   Fractured maxillary left central incisor.

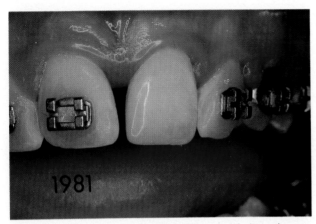

Figure 9-20 Build-up of the maxillary left central incisor using a macrofilled material veneered with a microfill.

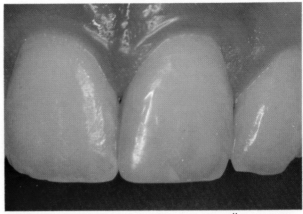

Figure 9-21 The sandwich restoration at 2-year recall.

The "light on heavy" or "sandwich" technique may be used with a wide variety of (heavy-filled or lightly filled composite) combinations:

Visiodispers[3] with Visiofil[11]
Durafil[1] with Estilux[12]
Prisma Fil[13] with Prisma Micro Fine[14]
Aurafil[15] with Certain[4]
P-30[16] with Silux[2]

Furthermore, it is not necessary to use the same manufacturer's products for the heavy-filled – lightly filled combinations; any of the heavy-filled materials listed may be used in combination with any of the lightly filled systems (Figs. 9-22 to 9-26).

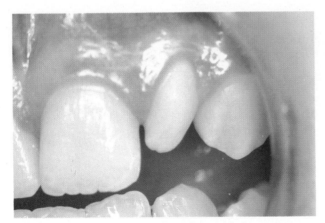

Figure 9-22 A peg-shaped maxillary left lateral incisor preoperatively.

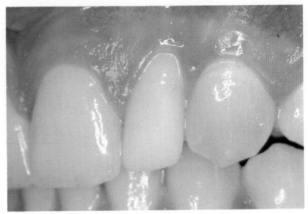

Figure 9-23 The peg lateral incisor crown restored with macrofilled composite (Prismafil[13]).

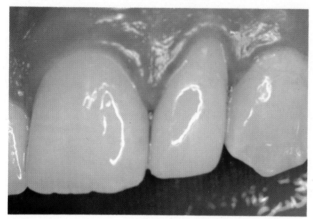

Figure 9-24 The same restoration after veneering with microfilled composite (Silux²).

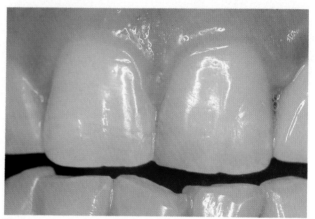

Figure 9-25 A rough, slightly discolored mesioincisal restoration (Miradapt¹⁸) in the maxillary left central incisor.

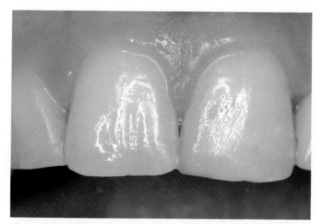

Figure 9-26 The restoration shown in Figure 9-25 after reveneering with a light cured hybrid material (Command Ultrafine¹⁹).

Another interesting application of the "light on heavy" technique relates to the use of a "filled glaze" resin material, Complus,[17] which is a clear paint-on Bis-GMA resin material, 50 percent by weight, filled with colloidal silica microfiller. The material is primarily indicated for "overcoating" semi-polishable and nonpolishable composite materials (Figs. 9-27 and 9-28), thereby giving them a smooth, lustrous surface. The abrasive wear resistance of such a material with time is not known.

Recently, similar materials of different shades (Comp-Guard[20]) have been introduced, enabling the operator to alter the shade of a preexistent composite restoration.

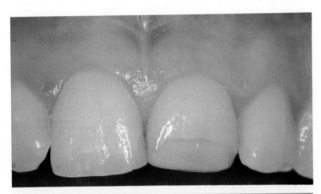

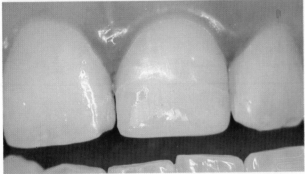

Figure 9–27 A discolored incisal restoration in the maxillary left central incisor preoperatively (*top*) and after replacement using a macrofilled material (*bottom*). The finished composite surface demonstrates a rough dull nonreflective surface.

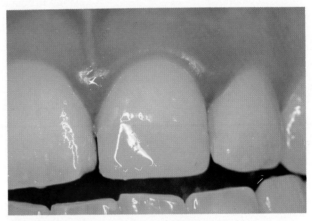

Figure 9–28 The restoration shown in Figure 9–27 after veneering with a filled glaze material (Complus[17]).

References

Boyer DB, Chan KC, Torney DL. The strength of multilayer and repaired composite resin. J Prosthet Dent 1978; 39:63.

Chan KC, Boyer DB. Repair of conventional and microfilled composite resins. J Prosthet Dent 1983; 50:345.

Marshall TD, Murrey AJ, Norling BK. Shear bond strengths of additions to composite resins. Personal Communication July, 1983.

Meeker HG, Hirsch SM, Kaim JM. Repairing voids at cavosurface-composite resin margins. J Prosthet Dent 1983; 50:636.

Miranda FS, Duncanson MG, Dilts WE. Interfacial bonding strengths of paired composite systems. J Prosthet Dent 1984; 51:29.

Murrey AJ, Marshall TD, Norling BK. Effect of resurfacing on additions to aged composite resins. Personal Communication July, 1983.

Product Information

Product	Manufacturer/Distributor	Purpose
1. Durafil	Kulzer Inc. 10015 Muirlands Blvd., Unit G Irvine, CA 92714	Light-cured, microfilled composite for add-on repair
2. Silux	Dental Products/3M Company 3M Center 270–5N–02 St. Paul, MN 55144	Light-cured, microfilled composite for add-on repair
3. Visiodispers	ESPE-Premier Sales Corp. Romano Dr., P.O. Box 111 Norristown, PA 19401	Light-cured, microfilled composite for add-on repair
4. Certain	Johnson and Johnson 20 Lake Drive, CN7060 East Windsor, NJ 08520	Light-cured, microfilled composite for add-on repair
5. 201.3F	ESPE-Premier Sales Corp. Romano Dr., P.O. Box 111 Norristown, PA 19401	Thin tapering diamond for preparing composite surface prior to repair
6. Scotchbond Etching Gel	Dental Products/3M Company 3M Center 270–5N–02 St. Paul, MN 55144	Viscous etching gel for application to composite enamel surfaces
7. Scotchbond	Dental Products/3M Company 3M Center 270–5N–02 St. Paul, MN 55144	Bonding agent
8. Felt No. 4 Instrument	American Dental Instrument Manufacturing Co. 2800 Reserve St., P.O. Box 4546 Missoula, MT 59801	Bulk-packing and initial shaping of composite material
9. Silar	Dental Products/3M Company 3M Center 270–5N–02 St. Paul, MN 55144	Self-cured microfill material
10. Rembrandt Natural	DenMat Inc. 3130 Skyway Dr., Unit 501 Santa Maria, CA 93456	Paint-on light-cured, microfilled material for resin-to-resin bonding
11. Visiofil	ESPE-Premier Sales Corp. Romano Dr., P.O. Box 111 Norristown, PA 19401	A light-cured, heavy-filled (80% by weight), macrofilled composite material
12. Estilux	Kulzer Inc. 10015 Muirlands Blvd., Unit G Irvine, CA 92714	Heavy-filled (76%), light-cured composite material
13. Prismafil	L. D. Caulk Co. P.O. Box 359 Milford, DE 19963	Heavy-filled (76%), light-cured composite material
14. Prisma Microfine	L. D. Caulk Co. P.O. Box 359 Milford, DE 19963	Lightly-filled (47%), microfilled composite material
15. Aurafil	Johnson and Johnson 20 Lake Drive, CN7060 East Windsor, NJ 08520	Heavy-filled (80%), light-cured, small-particle, macrofilled composite material
16. P–30	Dental Products/3M Company 3M Center 270–5N–02 St. Paul, MN 55144	Heavy-filled (87.5%), light-cured, hybrid composite material
17. Complus	Parkell Co. 155 Schmitt Blvd. Farmingdale, NY 11735	A clear, filled glaze resin used for smooth surfacing composite materials
18. Miradapt	Johnson and Johnson 20 Lake Drive, CN7060 East Windsor, NJ 08520	A heavy-filled (80%), self-cured, hybrid composite

Product Information

Product	Manufacturer/Distributor	Purpose
19. Command Ultrafine	Kerr-Sybron Co. P.O. Box 455 Romulus, MI 48174	A heavy-filled (76%), light-cured, hybrid material
20. Comp-Guard	DenMat Inc. 3130 Skyway Dr., Unit 501 Santa Maria, CA 93456	A shaded filled glaze material
21. Paste Laminate	DenMat Inc. 3130 Skyway Dr., Unit 501 Santa Maria, CA 93456	Light-cured, microfilled composite material

10

D A V I D J. J O R D A N

POTENTIAL DAMAGING
EFFECTS OF
LIGHT ON THE EYE

Light is radiant energy with electromagnetic properties and measurable wavelengths (Fig. 10-1). These extend from 0.001 Angstroms to 30,000 meters, yet the human eye perceives only those in the visible spectrum (380 nanometers to 780 nanometers) and interprets these wavelengths as color. When considering the damaging effects that light can have on the eye, one must take a closer look at the nonvisible range bordering the visible spectrum, i.e., ultraviolet rays (> 400 nm) and infrared rays (< 780 nm). The ultraviolet rays are invisible to the eye and can be subdivided into three groups: (1) UVC, which includes wavelengths below 286 nm and is effectively filtered out by the protective ozone layer surrounding the earth; without this protection, life on earth would be impossible, (2) UVB, which includes wavelengths between 286 nm and 320 nm and is responsible for sun tanning; and (3) UVA, which includes wavelengths between 320 nm and 400 nm.

The human cornea absorbs UV radiation below 300 nm (the lower portion of UVB), while the human lens absorbs UV radiation below 400 nm (UVA). The energy above 400 nm becomes the visible spectrum and is transmitted to the retina (Fig. 10-2).

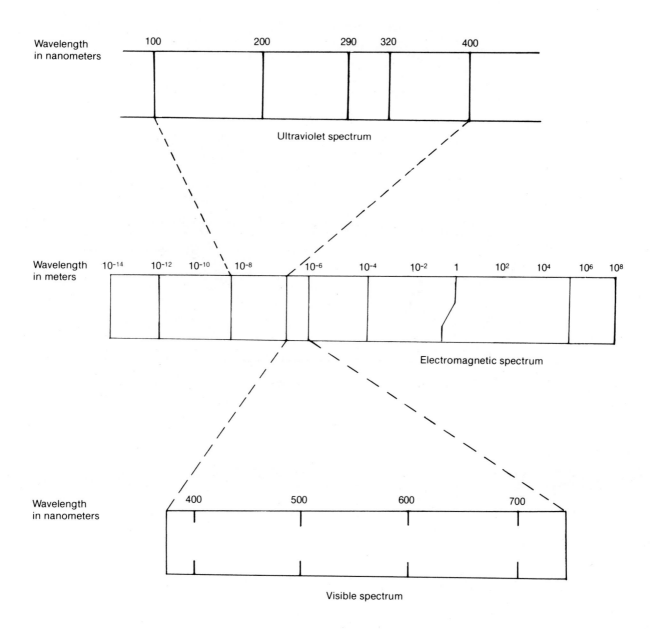

Figure 10-1 Electromagnetic spectrum showing the total spectrum in addition to expanded sections of the ultraviolet and visible light range. (Modified from Pitts DG. Threat of ultraviolet radiation to the eye—how to protect against it. J Am Optom Assoc 1981; 52:949–957.)

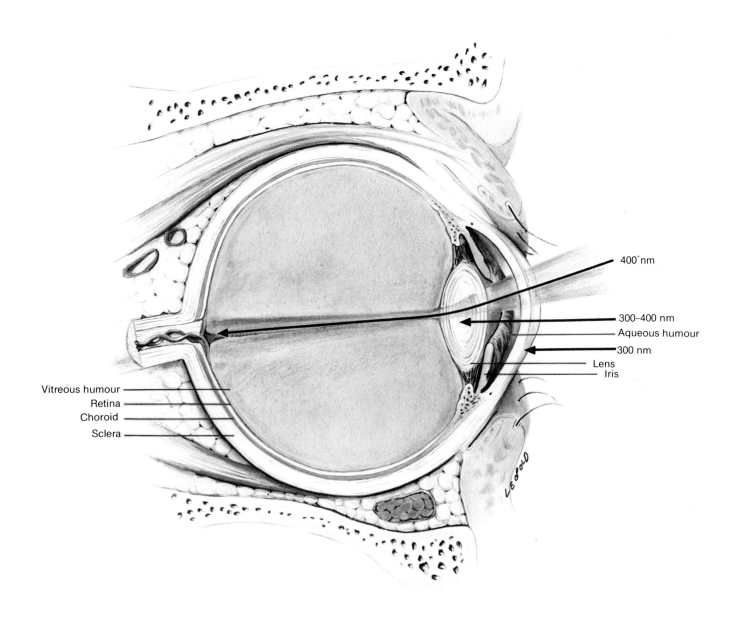

400⁺nm

300–400 nm
Aqueous humour
300 nm
Lens
Iris

Vitreous humour
Retina
Choroid
Sclera

Figure 10-2 The human eye is shown in cross section to illustrate the exposure of the eye to various wavelengths of the electromagnetic spectrum. The cornea absorbs those rays < 300 nm while the lens absorbs those rays between 300–400 nm. The retina is therefore exposed to light rays > 400 nm.

Various parts of the eye act as natural filters. The cornea is irradiated first and filters out whatever wavelengths of incident radiation it can (< 300 nm). The remainder of the light enters the aqueous, iris, lens, and vitreous. Each absorbs according to its spectral characteristics. The cornea and lens are the major filters, and an ever-diminishing amount of radiation penetrates to the retina. All the anterior structures of the eye are sensitive to injury from ultraviolet rays. However, the retina, which can also be injured by UV radiaiton, is only rarely exposed. On the other hand, visible and infrared rays reach the retina almost unattenuated and therefore may be hazardous (Sliney and Wolborsht, 1980). Direct observations of this latter form of radiation (as seen with molten glass, metal, arc lamps, infrared lamps) have been known to cause cataracts (Duke-Elder, 1972) as well as choroidal and retinal lesions (Sliney and Wolborsht, 1980; Lanum, 1978; Guerry et al, 1982).

Our visual perceptions are finely regulated by the amount, wavelength, and pattern of light that enter our eyes. In the past decade, after extensive research, our awareness has increased to the possible damaging effects light may have on the eye.

ANTERIOR SEGMENT (CORNEA AND LENS)

Cornea

Although ultraviolet rays are absorbed in the cornea and crystalline lens of the eye, excessive exposure can lead to cellular damage due to nuclear fragmentation of the cornea epithelium. Loss of cohesion between the epithelium and stroma also occurs. This type of injury occurs after unprotected exposure to a sun lamp or welder's arc (Moses, 1981) (photokeratitis, UV keratitis). Snow blindness (Sliney, 1983) and fibrovascular connective tissue overgrowths on the cornea (pterygium) (Grayson, 1979) are other UV exposure problems. These can be significantly reduced merely by taking adequate precautions and wearing a protective ultraviolet filter.

Lens

The lens serves as a natural filter, absorbing that part of the electromagnetic spectrum between 300 and 400 nm. This protective aspect of the lens increases from age 20 on as the gradually aging and yellowing lens absorbs a greater amount of UV light and short wavelength visible light (Guerry et al, 1982; Lerman, 1980, 1982). Removal of the lens would therefore put the retina at an increased risk of potentially damaging UV rays (Guerry et al, 1982; Ham et al, 1982).

During the past decade, there has been increasing evidence that sunlight and particularly long wavelength ultraviolet light in the range of 300 to 400 nm are positively associated with lens damage and cataract formation (Lerman, 1980; Zigman, 1971, 1977, 1983). Although only a small portion of the solar radiation normally enters the eye, continuous exposure of the lens to UV radiation in the 295-nm to 400-nm range may result in cumulative photochemical damage (Ham et al, 1982).

There appear to be two mechanisms whereby near-ultraviolet light (300 to 400 nm) may lead to cataractous change (Zigman, 1977, 1983). In one case, cytotoxic effects on lens epithelial cells can result from the formation of toxic photo products in the aqueous humor or in the cells themselves. This interferes with their growth, differentiation, and clarity. Another possible mechanism involves the elevation of molecules such as tryptophan (in free or in protein form) to excited states leading to altered protein interactions. This susceptibility of tryptophan to UV light results in abnormal lens proteins, which then begin to scatter (by aggregation) and absorb light (by pigmentation) rather than transmit it (Zigman, 1977, 1983).

There are natural protective agents within the lens and aqueous (glutathione, ascorbic acid), but they are not always present in high enough concentration to protect the lens from photo-oxidative damage (Zigman, 1983).

Several studies have been made of the incidence of cataract in areas where high intensity and long duration of sunlight occur (Lerman, 1980, 1982; Zigman 1971, 1977, 1983; Hollows and Morin, 1981). Recently, Hollows and Morin (1981) confirmed that the incidence of cataract observed among Australian aborigines was greater in areas of more intense UV radiation from sunlight than in areas with lower-level radiation. Cataracts also occurred at earlier ages. Although the impressively high numbers (over 100,000) might be attributed to the fact that aborigines use little protection against sunlight, other factors may be playing a role (e.g., genetics, type of cataract, nutritional status, use of drugs, other diseases). Although there appears to be a greater incidence of cataracts in areas where sunlight (UV radiation) duration is higher, the presence of sunlight does not in itself prove that exposure is the sole causative agent for cataracts (Zigman, 1971, 1983).

While sunlight is the greatest source of near-UV light (300 to 400 nm) exposure in man, artificial light sources such as those used for indoor lighting, occupational, or health-related activities also may expose humans to near-UV light. Variations in the quality and quantity of light energy emitted by these sources are enormous, as are the number of uses to which they are put. A short list includes fluorescent lamps, UV lamps for medical use (dermatologic treatments, sterilization), welding arcs, and near-UV lasers (Zigman, 1983). Ultraviolet radiation is used in the oral cavity in several different dental procedures. These include the photopolymerization of UV-sensitive methacrylates, illumination of teeth, as a light source in intraoral photography, operatory lights, and ceiling fixtures (Mills and Anderson, 1981).

Although the foregoing discussion indicates that ultraviolet radiation above 300 nm is capable of inducing a variety of changes within the human lens, clinical documentation of UV-induced cataracts is infrequent (Lerman, 1982; Crylin et al, 1980; Wojino et al, 1983).

The application of photopolymerization of plastic materials by UV light in dentistry began with the use of pit and fissure sealants in the early 1970s (Buonocore, 1970). These early materials contained photosensitizers (benzoin, methyl ether) with absorption peaks at 340 nm. Radiation sources, such as high-pressure mercury lamps (emitting 365 nm), were therefore required for successful polymerization (Cook, 1982; Pollack and Blitzer, 1982; Rock, 1974; Pollack and Lewis, 1981). One such instrument, the Caulk Nuva-Lite, was recalled in 1975 by the FDA for excessive leakage of UV radiation (Peterson et al, 1975; Birdsell et al, 1977). Lerman (1980) has reported three patients who developed lens opacities following documented exposure to UV radiation, 300 to 400 nm, for up to 200 hours during an 18-month period. Of the six people working in the dental office, only three used the Nuva-Lite (Lerman, 1980). None of the six had a positive history with respect to cataracts or any history of exposure to other known cataractogenic agents and drugs. All six used the same dental x-ray apparatus, which was subject to periodic checks and certified safe by a trained technician. Thus, ionizing radiation as the prime cataractogenic agent could be ruled out; furthermore, only three of the six patients developed lens opacities, and they were the ones who used the Nuva-Lite. Dr. Lerman demonstrated that each individual used the Nuva-Lite on several occasions beyond a calculated permissible exposure time.

Because of concern over possible UV damage to the eye with these curing units, alternative forms of light emitting higher wavelengths and in the visible spectrum have been designed. Pollack and Lewis (1984) and Cook (1982) describe several models used in the past few years and document the range of radiation emitted from each.

A number of dental curing lights are now available and, without question, have been an asset in resin restorations (Pollack and Blitzer, 1982; Pollack and Lewis, 1984). Their disadvantage, however, is the possibility of eye damage in the operator or assistant who looks at the light source (Pollack and Lewis, 1981; Pollack and Blitzer, 1982; Rock, 1974; Birdsell et al, 1977). The eye damage may involve the lens and/or the retina, depending on the wavelength of light emitted from the unit. Individual generators vary greatly in spectral distribution and radiation intensity (Council on Dental Materials, 1976, 1982). Although optimal curing light for most visible-light-curing resins has output in the spectrum of 450 to 470 nm, Pollack and Lewis (1984) have shown radiation from 400 to 500 nm in most generators, with different proportions of this spectrum being dominant in each generator. This portion of the visible spectrum is also potentially dangerous to the eye, particularly the retina (to be discussed), and caution is urged in the use of these units without the use of protective filters. A product monograph stating the range of electromagnetic radiation emitted, safety features, and the appropriate protective filters should be available in each case.

In summary, continuing research is under way to determine more quantitatively such properties as the absorption of near-UV light (300 to 400 nm) by the lens, the penetration of these wavelengths into the eye, the basic photochemical process leading to cytotoxic lens epithelial cell changes, direct effect of near-UV light on lens protein leading to aggregation, and epidemiology of cataracts relative to near-UV light or sunlight exposure (Zigman, 1977). The basic research completed so far implicates UV light (300 to 400 nm) in human cataractogenesis (Zigman, 1971, 1977, 1983; Lerman, 1980). For this reason, caution and eye protection are urged for those individuals who are repeatedly exposed to sources of near-ultraviolet radiation and blue light, i.e., dentists and dental assistants (Zigman, 1983; Ham et al, 1978). When one considers that continuous exposure of the lens to UV radiation between 295 to 400 nm may result in cumulative photochemical damage, the importance of lens filters cannot be overstressed (Lerman, 1982; Council on Dental Materials, 1982).

POSTERIOR SEGMENT (RETINA, CHOROID, RETINAL PIGMENT EPITHELIUM)

The ocular media in man, rhesus monkey, and rabbit transmit wavelengths between 400 and 1400 nm. Ham et al (1980) have described three types of radiation insult to the retina in this spectral range: (1) *mechanical disruption* of retinal structure resulting from high-powered shock waves engendered by short pulses of radiation and absorbed by the retinal pigment epithelium (RPE) and choroid, (2) *thermal insult* resulting from absorption of energy sufficient to raise the temperature in the retina, choroid, and RPE by 10 degrees Celsius above ambient, and (3) *actinic insult* from the photochemical effects of extended exposure to short wavelengths in the visible spectrum (400 to 550 nm) at power densities too low to produce temperatures of more than a few degrees Celsius above ambient. The important parameters determining the type of retinal insult are the power level, exposure duration, and wavelength (Ham et al, 1980). The power level entering the eye and exposure duration determine whether the damage is mechanical or thermal (Marshall, 1970). Both mechanical and thermal insult are potentiated by the shorter wavelengths down to approximately 500 nm, at which transmission through the ocular media begins to decrease rapidly (Ham et al, 1980).

When irradiance on the retina is reduced and exposure duration extended, a point is reached at which thermal effects become minimal or even completely negligible. At wavelengths above 550 to 600 nm and retinal temperatures only a few degrees Celsius above ambient, the retina remains undamaged even after extended exposures (Ham et al, 1979, 1980).

At wavelengths below 550 nm, the situation is felt to be quite different. Extended exposure produces actinic or photochemical effects at retina irradiances too low to produce thermal effects (Lanum, 1978; Ham et al, 1980; Friedman and Kuwabara, 1968). There is no sharp line of demarcation between thermal and actinic effects, and there is a point at which thermally enhanced photochemical effects most probably take place (Ham et al, 1980). The action spectrum for actinic effects in the retina increases at an expontential rate as the wavelength decreases toward 400 nm (Ham and Mueller, 1976). At wavelengths below approximately 450 nm, the lens start to absorb some of the electromagnetic rays, so that few photons in the far blue and violet end of the spectrum reach the retina. Whether the sensitivity of the retina continues to increase in the ultraviolet range is unknown, but obviously a hazard exists for patients whose lens is absent following cataract surgery (Ham et al, 1976, 1982).

The operating microscope used by the ophthalmologist as well as new dental curing lights and a host of other instruments emit some of their lights in the electromagnetic range between 400 and 500 nm (Pollack and Lewis, 1984; Cook, 1982; Calkins et al, 1980). Only in the past few years has it been realized that this portion of the unfiltered light may be having some untoward effect on the human retina. The aforementioned actinic effects are expressed at the shorter wavelengths in the visible spectrum (between 400 and 550 nm), where the retinal irradiance is too low to cause thermal damage (Ham et al, 1980). The photochemical reactions responsible for this type of retinal injury are not known, but they are believed to reside in the retinal pigment epithelium (Ham et al, 1980).

An interesting correlate can be seen when one studies the retinal damage induced by direct observation of the sun or an eclipse. Although a thermal etiology seems likely, there is now evidence that solar retinitis may in part be caused by the short wavelengths in the visible spectrum (400 to 500 nm), with some thermal enhancement from the longer wavelengths and near-infrared light (Peterson et al, 1975; Ham et al, 1976).

The sensitivity of the retina to blue light (blue peaks at 440 to 450 nm) may have more profound effects for man-made optical sources than for sunlight. The trend is toward ever brighter sources in the blue end of the spectrum; high-pressure mercury and xenon arc lamps, natural light sources, and dental curing lights are examples of these sources.

Many biologic factors of the organism and physical parameters of the inflicting light source influence photic injury to the retina. Thus, although exposure of the human retina to bright light may result in injury, several complicating factors (largely derived from animal work) must be considered (Lanum, 1978; Tso and Woodford, 1983). These include the susceptibility of different parts of the retina, dark adaptation of the retina, body temperature, pigmentation, age, species differences, motivational state, different wavelength, dose rate, continuous or intermittent light exposure, and whether or not the patient has had a cataract removed.

One also has to consider the possible cumulative effect that intermittent light exposure has on the retina (Lanum, 1978; Griess and Blankenstein, 1981; Sperling et al, 1980; Noell et al, 1966). Griess and Blankenstein (1981), working with rhesus monkeys, have recently shown that repeated subthreshold exposures to blue light (458 nm) produce cumulative retinal changes that are countered to some degree by a reparative process. Sperling and others (Sperling et al, 1972, 1980; Noell et al, 1966) have demonstrated that daily sessions of intermittent exposure to moderately intense, narrow-band blue light (463 nm) produces irreversible loss of blue sensitivity. Exposure to narrow-band green light produces loss of green sensitivity, which is recovered only after a number of days. Thus, blue light exposure eliminates the response of the blue-sensitive cones, whereas green light has only a temporary effect on the green-sensitive cones (Fig. 10-3). It appears that a selective absorption of energy by the photo pigments initiates a series of reactions which, if continued long enough, can permanently damage the photoreceptors (Lanum, 1978).

Histopathologic studies have not only demonstrated the damage produced by the blue end of the spectrum (Tso and Woodford, 1983; Anderson et al, 1972; Parver et al, 1983), but have also described reparative processes (Lanum, 1978; Tso and Woodford, 1983; Kuwabara and Gorn, 1968; Kuwabara, 1970). There seems to be a point beyond which recovery is impossible. Just how much damage must be sustained before it is irreversible is not entirely clear. The receptor cell bodies (rods and cones) must not be destroyed, and the less damage sustained by the RPE, the easier the recovery seems to be (Lanum, 1978).

In summary, light can cause retinal damage by mechanical, thermal, or photochemical (actinic) mechanisms. The nature and extent of light damage in primate retinas depend primarily on wavelength (color), exposure time, and power level (Ham et al, 1980). Mechanical and thermal injuries require an intense light exposure, whereas photochemical injury is caused by a prolonged exposure (primarily blue and near ultraviolet radiation) to levels that probably would be well tolerated if experienced only transiently (Mainster et al, 1983).

Since photochemical retinal damage exists in primates, does prolonged diagnostic or surgical light exposure cause retinal damage? This question has been the subject of much debate and no doubt will continue to be an important consideration. Animal studies have shown repeatedly that photochemical damage is much more pronounced for the short or blue wavelengths in the visible spectrum (Ham et al, 1976, 1980; Tso and Woodford, 1983; Griess and Blankenstein, 1981; Sperling et al, 1980; Marshall et al, 1971; Anderson et al,

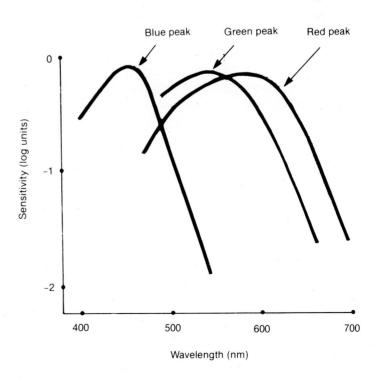

Figure 10-3 Measurement of cone pigments demonstrating three classes in the human retina with different but overlapping spectral sensitivities. Blue peak = 440 to 450 nm; green peak = 535 to 555 nm; red peak = 570 to 590 nm. (From Moses RA, ed. Adlers physiology of the eye. St. Louis: CV Mosby, 1981:548)

1972; Parver et al, 1983; Mainster et al, 1983). Light damage in the human retina, although not as extensive, is also present (Lanum, 1978). Solar retinitis and welding arc maculopathy probably are examples of photochemical injury (Ham et al, 1979; Naidoff et al, 1974). Furthermore, epidemiologic studies and clinical observation strongly suggest the association of light exposure history with macular injury and degeneration (Mainster et al, 1983; Schepens, 1980; Gladstone and Tasman, 1978; McDonald and Irvine, 1983; Sperduto et al, 1981; Marlor et al, 1973). Thus, there is a growing body of evidence to suggest the potential damaging effect of environmental and occupational light sources on the human retina. Adequate protective devices would obviously be of benefit, and until further conclusive evidence is obtained, their use should be stressed.

Ophthalmologists have become increasingly aware of the possible damage their lights may cause, and Mainster has suggested several methods to improve the safety of clinical light sources (Mainster, 1980). These can be applied to a number of areas where artificial light sources are in use. Suggestions include (1) using an interference filter to block wavelengths greater than 700 nm (infrared) as these rays add nothing to image quality, (2) filtering out wavelengths < 450 nm to eliminate the blue and near ultraviolet rays that are most hazardous, (3) using the minimum amount of light required when examining a patient and use of an occluder over the cornea with prolonged use of the operating microscope.

One other useful concept in the ophthalmic literature is that of maximal permissable exposure (MPE) or safe time (Calkins and Hockeimer, 1979, 1980). This is important since the ophthalmologist has to examine the eye regularly with light sources that are potentially damaging to the eye. Although the safety standards were originally developed for coherent light (laser) sources, they have recently begun to be adapted to incoherent light sources, such as those used in ophthalmic devices (Sperling, 1980). It is surprising to see how short some of the safe times are, and through personal experience, one realizes how often they are surpassed. Undoubtedly, many changes occur which are naturally repaired in healthy individuals; otherwise, we would all have been aware of light-induced damage by now (Calkins et al, 1980). The MPE is a useful concept and, with further research, may be developed for any light source that could have potentially damaging effects on the eyes of the patient or the operator. Pollack and Lewis (1981) have recently applied this concept to visible-light-curing units and have calculated the maximal permissible exposure time (for direct viewing) to be less than one second for some units. However, with filtered light reflected from a tooth, the safe viewing times goes up to over 30 minutes.

EYE PROTECTION

There are basically four separate types of hazards to the eye that must be evaluated for each light source (Sliney et al, 1980). These include (1) ultraviolet radiation from 200 to 400 nm, (2) thermal retinal injury hazard, (3) blue light photochemical retinal hazard, and (4) near infrared hazards to the retina and lens. We will concern ourselves with numbers 1 and 3.

To design any protective filter, it is first necessary to determine what light levels are safe and which wavelength region is most dangerous to the patient or operator.

Because there is sufficient evidence that near ultraviolet radiation has a role in human cataract development, most researchers in this field have suggested the use of protective lenses that filter out near UV radiation (300 to 400 nm) (Zigman, 1983).

Sunglasses are a common form of filter, but their use is often more for cosmetic purposes than for their filtering ability. Ideally, a sunglass should reduce visible radiation equally from the entire solar spectrum so that the spectral composition of radiation that normally reaches the eye is not altered. Furthermore, they should cut out the invisible radiation (infrared and ultraviolet). However, this is not always the case, and studies have shown the inefficiency of ordinary sunglasses in filtering out the UV rays (Segre et al, 1981; Anderson and Gebel, 1977). The use of lenses that reduce the visible spectrum more than the UV can cause two negative effects (Segre et al, 1981): (1) it gives a sense of protection leading to longer exposure and increased risk of high doses of UV rays, (2) it diminishes the intensity of transmitted light, thus causing dilation of the pupil and therefore allowing a greater quantity of radiation (including UV) to penetrate the eye.

With greater appreciation of the potential damaging effects caused by UV light, all the major optical product manufacturers have specifically designed lens filters to block near UV light from entering the eye. For several conditions of UV light exposure, special protective devices have been developed, such as the goggles worn by welders and the helmets worn by astronauts.

A relatively new feature is the production of a plastic lens with special chemical baked into it during formation, which then allows the reflection of all ultraviolet light below 400 nm and all infrared above 700 nm (Irex lenses[1]). These sunglasses are popular at present.

Adequate UV filters become increasingly important when one considers individuals at higher risk of potential damage. If, for example, a cataract is removed, one's retina becomes accessible to those potentially damaging rays normally filtered by the lens (300 to 400 nm). Ham et al (1982) have emphasized the importance of the UV protection provided by the natural human lens, and therefore such individuals would be ideal candidates for UV filtering lenses. Plastic lenses, such as the Orcolite[2] or UV 400,[3] have been designed to absorb near UV light and ensure complete protection from the ultraviolet spectrum to 400 nm. These generally permit 85 to 90 percent transmission of visible light, allowing patients to wear them with comfort indoors as well as outdoors and protect themselves from all sources of ambient UV radiation (e.g., fluorescent lamps, sunlight).

Those who experience occupational exposure to UV radiation (e.g., pilots, sailors, lifeguards, skiers) and those exposed to artificial light instrumentation also might benefit from filtering lenses. For example, light-curing units currently used in dentistry are known to transmit some ultraviolet (365 to 367 nm) and blue light (450 to 470 nm) (Cook, 1982; Pollack and Blitzer, 1982; Pollard and Lewis, 1984; Rock, 1974). This may be damaging to the clinician as he views the light reflected from the enamel, especially over time, when cumulative effects may be more important than isolated exposure (Lerman, 1982). Thus, an appropriate filter, such as the Liteshield 500[4], CPF 511[5], or Cure-Shield[8] would be useful to screen out rays below 500 nm or 511 nm respectively, thereby removing the blue and ultraviolet portion of the spectrum. Until more is known about intense light sources weighted in the blue end of the spectrum, caution is advised in limiting direct viewing of the light probe (UV or visible light units). The safe viewing time for some light-curing units has been calculated to be less than one second (unfiltered light) (Pollack and Lewis, 1981). Although light reflected off teeth is not, comparatively, as an intense exposure, familiarity with the unit's wavelength emission and adequate filtering devices are recommended.

Ultraviolet light filters are also useful for individuals who are undergoing phototherapy (psoralen-UVA therapy for psoriasis) and for those who are receiving photosensitivity drugs (sulfonamides, chlorthiazides, phenothiazines) (Lerman, 1982; McDonald and Irvine, 1983).

Protective filters, such as the CPF 527[6] or CPF 550[7] are available for patients with macular degeneration, albinism, retinitis pigmentosa, and other eye diseases to increase contrast, decrease photophobia, reduce glare, and decrease the number of potential damaging rays.

VISIBLE-LIGHT-CURING GENERATORS

There are many visible-light-curing generators on the market (Table 10-1). It has been reported that all light units cure all composite resin materials to a clinically acceptable depth (CRA Newsletter, 1982; Pollack and Lewis, 1984). For all practical purposes, the major differences in light units relate to convenience features, the most important of which are:

1. *The light-activator button.* Ideally it should be in a convenient location such as the handpiece head or a gun-type handle.
2. *Type of cord.* The cord in a light unit may be fiberoptic, fluid filled, or electrical. Fiberoptic cords may be hazardous since breakage of glass filaments in the bundles may occur over time of use, particularly if the cord is flexed or bent, thereby resulting in diminished cure. Fluid- or gel-filled cords tend to be stiff and unwieldy. Elimination of the fiberoptic cord in favor of a simple *electrical* cord results in a much more trustworthy instrument.
3. *End diameter of the light source.* Ideally, large diameters are used to eliminate the need to cure in several areas of the same restoration. Furthermore, light units that are available with several different-sized light tips are of distinct advantage.
4. *Portability.* The smaller lights, particularly those equipped with a handle for ease and safety in transporting between operatories, are preferred to large, bulky units.

The essential convenience features of the most commonly used lights are presented in Table 10-1.

TABLE 10–1   Visible-Light-Cure Units

Light	Manufac- urer	Light Activator Button	Timer	Type of Cord	Portability	End Diam. (mm)	Special Features
Command	Kerr-Sybron	On unit	Variable up to 30 sec	Fiberoptic	7.4 lbs + +	5.5 10	Delay switch, wide tip
Elipar	ESPE- Premier	Trigger— handpiece gun	20 sec; auto shut off	Electric	4.4 lbs +	8	Voltage regulator
Focus	Getz Teledyne	Trigger— handpiece gun	10, 20, 40 sec	Electric	3.1 lbs + +	8	
Heliomat	Vivadent	On hand- piece unit	Variable	Fiberoptic	10.5 lbs	5.5	Multifunctional
Initator	Solid State Systems	On unit	Variable	Fiberoptic	+	5	Time-delayed switch, multifunction tips
Insight II	Ritter/ Midwest Co.	On hand- piece head	Variable	Fiberoptic	6.3 lbs	6	Trans- illumination
Optilux	Demetron	Trigger— handpiece gun	10 sec; beeper	Electric	2.8 + +	7	5 tips of variable size available
Prismalite	L.D. Caulk	On hand- piece head	10 sec; beeper	Fiberoptic	17 lbs —	5.3	Voltage regulator; very quiet
Sunlight	Kinetic	On hand- piece head	10, 20, 40 sec	Fiberoptic	8.8 lbs +	7	
Translux	Kulzer Inc.	On unit	20 sec; beeper	Gel filled	9.9 lbs —	6	Plaque light attachment
Visar II	DenMat	On unit	15 sec; beeper	Fiberoptic	6.5 lbs + +	6 12	Light intensity control— curing or trans- illumination
Marathon	DenMat	On unit	15 sec; beeper	Fiberoptic	6.5 lbs +	8 12	
Visilux	3M	Trigger— handpiece gun	10 sec; beeper	Electric	2.8 lbs + +	7	5 tips of variable size

References

Anderson KV, Coyle FP, O'Steen WK. Retinal degeneration produced by low intensity colored light. Exp Neurol 1972; 35:233–238.

Anderson WJ, Gebel RKH. Ultraviolet windows in commercial sunglasses. Appl Optics 1977; 16:515–517.

Birdsell DC, Bannon PJ, Webb RB. Harmful effects of near ultraviolet radiation for polymerization of a sealant and a composite resin. J Am Dent Assoc 1977; 94:311–314.

Buonocore MG. Adhesive sealing of pits and fissures for caries prevention with use of ultraviolet light. J Am Dent Assoc 1970; 80:324–328.

Calkins JL, Hocheimer BF. Retinal exposure from ophthalmoscopes, slit lamps and overhead surgical lamps. An analysis of potential hazards. Invest Ophthalmol Vis Sci 1980; 19:1009–1015.

Calkins JL, Hocheimer BF. Retinal light exposure from operating microscopes. Arch Ophthalmol 1979; 97: 2363–2367.

Calkins JL, Hocheimer BF, D'Anna SA. Potential hazards from specific ophthalmic devices. Vision Res 1980; 20:1039–1953.

Cook WD. Spectral distribution of dental photopolymerization sources. J Dent Res 1982; 1436–1438.

Council on Dental Materials and Devices. Guidelines on the use of ultraviolet radiation in dentistry. J Am Dent Assoc 1976; 92:775–776.

Council on Dental Materials, Instruments and Equipment. Status Report: Dental visible light-curing units. J Am Dent Assoc 1982; 104:505.

Clinical Research Associates Newsletter. Vol. 6, Issue 5, May, 1982.

Crylin MN, Pedvis-Leftick A, Surgar J. Cataract formation in association with ultraviolet photosensitivity. Ann Ophthalmol 1980; 786–790.

Duke-Elder S, (ed). System of Ophthalmology. Vol XIV, Part 2. Injuries. St. Louis: CV Mosby, 1972:878–881.

Friedman E, Kuwabara T. The retinal pigment epithelium. The damaging effects of radiant energy. Arch Ophthalmol 1968; 80:265–280.

Gladstone GJ, Tasman W. Solar retinitis after minimal exposure. Arch Ophthalmol 1978; 96:1368–1369.

Grayson M. Diseases of the Cornea. St. Louis: CV Mosby, 1979:191, 274.

Griess GA, Blankenstein MF. Additivity and repair of actinic retinal lesions. Invest Ophthalmol Vis Sci 1981; 20:803–807.

Guerry et al. Find sun exposure causes photochemical eye damage. Ophthalmology Times, July 1, 1982.

Ham WT, Mueller HA. Retinal sensitivity to damage from short wavelength light. Nature 1976; 260:153–154.

Ham WT, Mueller HA, Ruffolo JJ, Clarke AM. Sensitivity of the retina to radiation damage as a function of wavelength. Photochem Photobiol 1979; 29:735–743.

Ham WT, Mueller HA, Ruffolo JJ, Guerry D, Guerry RK. Action spectrum for retinal injury from near-ultraviolet radiation in the aphakic monkey. Am J Ophthalmol 1982; 93:299–306.

Ham WT, Ruffolo JJ, Mueller HA, Clarke AM, Moon ME. Histologic analysis of photochemical lesions produced in rhesus retina by short wavelength light. Invest Ophthalmol Vis Sci 1978; 17:1029–1035.

Ham WT, Ruffolo JJ, Mueller HA, Guerry D. The nature of retinal radiation damage: dependence on wavelength, power level and exposure time. Vision Res 1980; 20:1105–1111.

Hollows F, Morin D. Cataract: The ultraviolet risk factor. Lancet 1981; 1:1249–1251.

Kuwabara T. Retinal recovery from exposure to light. Am J Ophthalmol 1970; 70:187–198.

Kuwabara T, Gorn RA. Retinal damage by visible light. Arch Ophthalmol 1968; 79:69–78.

Lanum J. The damaging effects of light on the retina. Empirical findings, theoretical and practical implications. Surv Ophthalmol 1978; 22:221–249.

Lerman S. Editorial: UV radiation photodamage to the occular lens: diagnosis and treatment. Ann Ophthalmol 1982; 14:411–413.

Lerman S. Human ultraviolet radiation cataract. Ophthalmic Res 1980; 12:303–314.

Lerman S. Radiant Energy and the Eye. New York: MacMillan, 1980.

Mainster MA, Ham WT, Delori FC. Potential retinal hazards: instrument and environmental light sources. Ophthalmology 1983; 90:927–932.

Marlor RL, Blais BR, Preston FR, Boyden DG. Foveomacular retinitis, an important problem in military medicine: epidemiology. Invest Ophthalmol Vis Sci 1973; 12:5–16.

Marshall JF, Turner BH, Teitelbaum P. Prolonged color blindness induced by intense spectral lights in rhesus monkeys. Science 1971; 174:520–525.

Marshall J. Thermal and mechanical mechanisms in laser damage to the retina. Invest Ophthalmol Vis Sci 1970; 9:97–115.

McDonald HR, Irvine AR. Light-induced maculopathy from the operating microscope in extracapsular cataract extraction and intraocular lens implantation. Ophthalmology 1983; 90:945–951.

Mills LF, Anderson F. Ultraviolet and microwave radiation in dentistry. General Dentistry 1981; 481–486.

Moses RA. Alder's Physiology of the Eye. St. Louis: CV Mosby 1981:58.

Naidoff MA, Noell WK, Walker VS, Kang BS, Berman S. Retinal damage by light in rats. Invest Ophthalmol Vis Sci 1974; 5:450–473.

Noell WK, Walker VS, Kang BS, Berman S. Retinal damage by light in rats. Inves Ophthalmol Vis Sci 1966; 5:450–473.

Parver LM, Auker CR, Fine BS. Observations on monkey eyes exposed to light from an operating microscope. Ophthalmology 1983; 90:964–972.

Peterson RW, Brostrom RG, Coakley JM, Ellingson OL. Measurement of the radiation emission from the Nuva-Lite dental appliance. DHEW Publ (FDA) No. 75-8031, April, 1975.

Pollack BF, Blitzer MH. The advantages of visible light curing resins. NY State Dent J 1982; 228–230.

Pollack BF, Lewis AL. Visible light resin-curing generators: a comparison. General Dentistry 1981; 488–493.

Pollack BF, Lewis AL. Visible light curing generators: an update. General Dentistry 1984; 193–197.

Rock WP. The use of ultraviolet radiation in dentistry. Br Dent J 1974; 455–458.

Schepens CL. Introduction to the problem. Visual Res 1980; 20:1037–1038.

Segre G, Pignalosa RB, Pappalardo G. The efficiency of ordinary sunglasses as a protection from ultraviolet radiation. Ophthalmic Res 1981; 13:180–187.

Sliney DH, Naidoff MA. Eye protective techniques for bright light. Ophthalmology 1983; 90:937–944.

Sliney DH. Retinal injury from a welding arc. Am J Ophthalmol 1974; 77:663–668.

Sliney DH, Wolborsht ML. Safety standards and measurement techniques for high intensity light sources. Visual Res 1980; 20:1133–1141.

Sperduto RD, Hiller R, Seigel D. Lens opacities and senile maculopathy. Arch Ophthalmol 1981; 99:1004–1008.

Sperling HG. Editorial: Are ophthalmologists exposing their patients to dangerous light levels? Invest Ophthalmol Vis Sci 1980; 19:989–990.

Sperling HG, Harwerth RS. Intense spectral light effects on spectral sensitivity. Optica Acta 1972; 19:395–398.

Sperling HG, Johnson C, Harwerth RS. Differential spectral photic damage to primate cones. Visual Res 1980; 20:1117–1125.

Tso MOM, Woodford BJ. Effect of photic injury on the retinal tissues. Ophthalmology 1983; 90:952–963.

Wojino T, Singer D, Schultz RO. Ultraviolet light, cataracts and spectacle wear. Ann Ophthalmol 1983; 729–731.

Wolborsht ML. Letter to the Editor. Invest Ophthalmol Vis Sci 1980; 19:1124.

Zigman S. Eye lens color: formation and function. Science 1971; 171:807–809.

Zigman S. Review Article: Near UV light and cataracts. Photochem Photobiol 1977; 26:437–441.

Zigman S. The role of sunlight in human cataract formation. Surv Ophthalmol 1983; 27:317–326.

Product Information

Product	Manufacturer/Distributor	Purpose
1. Irex Lenses	Imperial Optical Co. 21 Dundas Square Toronto, Ontario M5B 1B7	Reflect all ultraviolet light and infrared light
2. Orcolite 3. UV 400	Optical Radiation Corp. 1300 Optical Drive Azuza, CA 91702	Lenses absorb UV light up to 400 nanometers
4. Liteshield 500	Dioptics Professional Products 10015 Muirlands Parkway Ste. E. Irvine, CA 92714	Protects from all UV and visible light up to 500 nanometers
5. CPF 511	Corning Glass Works Houghton Park Corning, NY 14831	Screens all UV and visible light below 511 nanometers
6. CPF 527 7. CPF 550	Corning Glass Works Houghton Park Corning, NY 14831	Filters recommended for patients with macular degeneration, albinism, retinitis pigmentosa
8. Cure-Shield	ESPE-Premier Sales Corp. Romano Dr., P.O. Box 111 Norristown, PA 19401	For operator and assistant protection from all UV and visible light up to 500 nanometers
9. Nuva Lite	L. D. Caulk Co. P.O. Box 359 Milford, DE 19963	Ultraviolet-light curing instrument

11

A. JOHN GWINNETT
RONALD E. JORDAN

FISSURE SEALANTS

One of the most underutilized of the numerous applications of resin-enamel bonding is that of fissure sealant material for caries prevention in the young patient. General dentists apparently remain unconvinced that currently available research data more than justify their routine use. In addition, there is widespread controversy regarding sealant retention rates and relative cost-effectiveness. Furthermore, many practitioners are justifiably concerned about the long-term results of inadvertently sealing occlusal carious lesions. However, recent research has shown that the long-term retention rate of fissure sealants is reasonably high, and their cost-effectiveness is satisfactory provided a carefully controlled clinical technique is used in their placement (Mertz-Fairhurst et al, 1984). In addition, clinical research carried out at the University of Western Ontario for the past 8 years clearly indicates that there is no danger associated with the inadvertent placement of fissure sealant materials over occlusal carious lesions.

It is widely recognized that pits and fissures of teeth are the most susceptible sites for the onset and spread of caries (Backer-Dirks, 1961; Hennon et al, 1969; Lewis and Hargreaves, 1975). Systemic and topical fluoride applications appear to afford the least protection to occlusal sites where pits and fissures are most common (Graves and Burt, 1975). Although the occlusal surfaces represent little more than 10 percent of the surfaces at risk, they have been shown to exhibit almost 50 percent of the caries in the human dentition (Ripa, 1973). Paynter and Grainger (1962) indicated that the very presence of pits and fissures may be the single most important factor in precipitating caries in these sites. Black (1897) observed, however, that pits and fissures do not cause decay per se, but simply provide an opportunity and sanctuary for agents that are responsible for the disease. There exists a clear body of evidence to strongly suggest that caries is a multifactorial disease (Keyes and Jordan, 1963). Such factors are tooth anatomy, oral flora, and diet interacting over time. In the case of pits and fissures, these complex anatomic sites serve to encourage the accumulation and stagnation of microorganisms

(Galil and Gwinnett, 1975) (Fig. 11-1). They cannot be cleansed readily by the patient (Fig. 11-2) or dentist (Galil, 1975). Fermentable substrates ingested by the host accumulate in the pits and fissures where acidogenic microorganisms break them down into organic acids capable of demineralizing the tooth tissues. Given this understanding of the onset of occlusal caries, it is possible to formulate a caries preventive approach by eradicating the pits and fissures as a contributing host factor.

Methods aimed at eliminating pits and fissures have been investigated since the early 1920s. These have included their operative removal and placement of an amalgam restoration or the widening of the anatomic defect to ensure easier cleaning (Hyatt, 1923; Bodecker, 1929). Chemical agents and cements have been used to obtund pits and fissures, but with little clinical success (Miller, 1951; Ast et al, 1950). A significant breakthrough came almost 30 years ago when Buonocore (1955) developed a unique method of bonding plastic resin to tooth enamel.

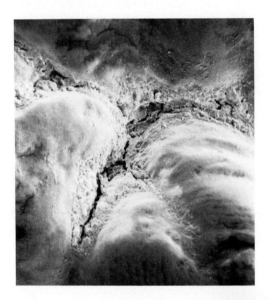

Figure 11-1 Scanning electron micrograph (20×) showing plaque in a molar fissure.

Figure 11-2 Many fissures and pits have a diameter significantly less than that of a toothbrush bristle (6 ×).

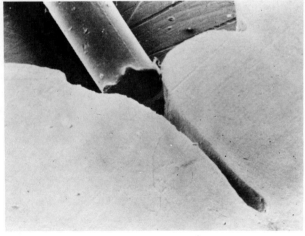

A review of the technical aspects of sealant placement allows us to understand the means by which it is retained as well as factors that may adversely affect its clinical performance. The mechanical cleansing of enamel is an important first step. The object is to remove plaque, *materia alba*, and calculus whose presence impedes the action and intent of the enamel conditioning agent. Miura et al (1973) demonstrated that maximal bond strengths were achieved between resin and enamel only when a thorough dental prophylaxis preceded enamel conditioning. The latter alone gave bond strengths approximately one-third less in value. Microscopic studies (Gwinnett, 1976) have shown that conditioning alone produces a non-uniform effect with islands of organic pellicle and organisms contaminating the conditioned surface (Fig. 11-3). A watery slurry of flour of pumice is usually recommended; a bristle brush or rubber cup is equally effective (Taylor and Gwinnett, 1973). A recent study showed no difference in clinical performance of sealants when a fluoridated toothpaste was substituted for pumice (Shey and Houpt, 1980). Further research is indicated.

Conventional mechanical cleaning methods leave significant residues in pits and fissures (Taylor and Gwinnett, 1973). There are no currently acceptable chemical methods to clean these sites. Debris, including microorganisms, remains sealed in pits and fissures, but is of little consequence or detriment to the host (Loesch, 1975; Going et al, 1978).

After careful tooth isolation from saliva and an inquisitive tongue (Fig. 11-4), a check should be made to ensure that the occlusal site is free of debris and is dry.

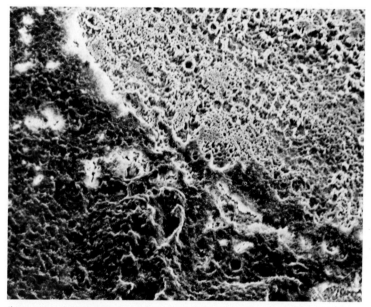

Figure 11-3 Scanning electron micrograph (500 ×) showing pellicle residue and microorganisms on enamel which had only been etched.

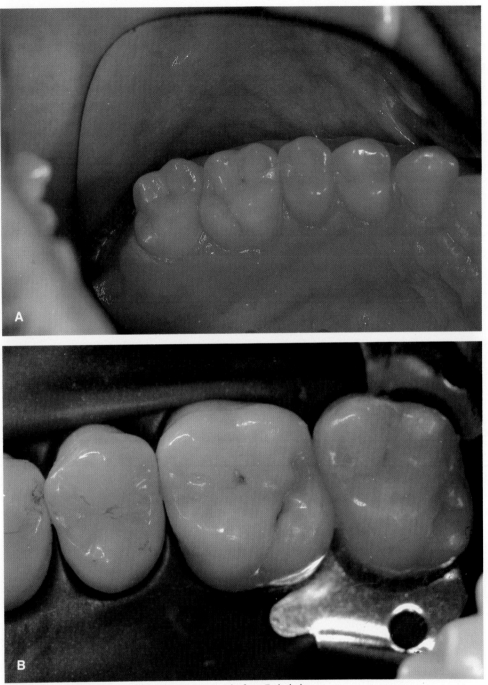

Figure 11-4 Maxillary left quadrant before, *A*, and after, *B*, isolation.

After proper isolation, the teeth to be sealed may be further cleansed by the application of 3% hydrogen peroxide on a cotton pledget (Fig. 11-5). A sharp explorer is then used to tease the peroxide liquid as far into the fissured defects as possible (Fig. 11-6). After a thorough water lavage, the occlusal surfaces are carefully dried. Drying should be accomplished by means of oil-free compressed air, preferably from a single syringe. Syringes that also deliver water may contribute moisture and should be checked by blowing air onto a mirror. Should moisture contamination be apparent, a commercially available warm air dryer (Handi-Dry[1]) should be used for thorough drying (Fig. 11-7).

The acid conditioning agent is now applied with a fine bristle brush, a cotton pledget, or a minisponge. The agent is available commercially in either solution or gel form. When using the solution, gentle agitation or dabbing is necessary to achieve the desired result. Rubbing the surface is to be avoided. If the gel is used (Fig. 11-8), it should be syringed into position and left undisturbed for the duration of its recommended application. Teasing the acid gel into the depths of the fissured defects, using a sharp explorer (Fig. 11-9) is recommended. The usual recommendation for solution and gel application is 60 seconds. However, recent research has suggested that shorter conditioning times may result in similar clinical performances of sealants (Stephen et al, 1982). Although several acids have been evaluated (Mullholland and deShazer, 1968; Brauer and Termini, 1972), phosphoric acid is currently the agent of choice. The concentration ranges upward of 30 percent. Chow and Brown (1973) showed that concentrations below 30 percent produced an insoluble reaction product on the enamel with the potential to reduce bond strength. It is interesting to note that the depth of the acid-conditioning effect increases as the concentration of phosphoric acid decreases (Gwinnett and Buonocore, 1965; Silverstone, 1975). One study reported higher bond strengths for sealants when a 30 percent concentration was used as compared with a 50 percent (Rock, 1974). A review of the literature, however, shows equivocation on this point with other studies reporting no differences (Retief, 1974; Williams et al, 1976). There does not appear to be any significant difference in clinical performance of sealants when these two concentrations are used. Concentrations in this same range have been shown to provide the most suitable architecture for bonding (Dennison and Craig, 1978). No differences in bond strengths have been found between acid gel and solution (Maijer, 1982).

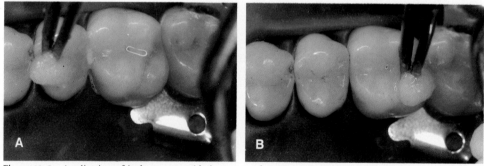

Figure 11-5   Application of hydrogen peroxide by means of a cotton pledget to, *A*, maxillary premolar and, *B*, maxillary first molar.

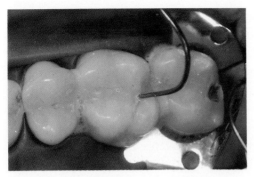

Figure 11-6 The use of a fine-tipped explorer to tease the hydrogen peroxide as deeply into the fissured defect as possible.

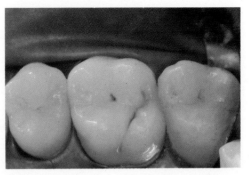

Figure 11-7 Appearance of the maxillary quadrant after thorough cleaning of occlusal surface.

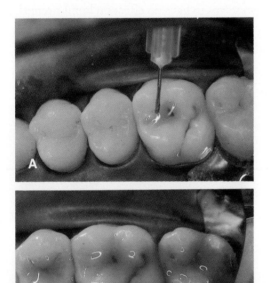

Figure 11-8 The gel etchant is syringed, *A*, to cover the enamel occlusal surfaces, *B*.

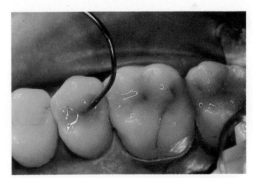

Figure 11-9 The gel etchant is worked as far into the fissured defect as possible by means of a sharp explorer.

Since enamel surfaces in vivo are contaminated physically and chemically complex, they have a relatively low surface energy not conducive to bonding. Acid conditioning removes old and fully reacted enamel and pellicle, increases the surface area, and enhances enamel porosity. As the enamel goes into solution, patterns reflecting the preferred dissolution of the microscopic rods develop (Figs. 11-10 to 11-12). Variations occur from site to site on the same tooth and from tooth to tooth owing to chemical and morphologic tissue variations (Gwinnett, 1971). The presence of prismless enamel, relatively common on newly erupted teeth (Ripa and Gwinnett, 1967), confers a morphologic difference in etching pattern (Fig. 11-13) and a smaller surface area for bonding (Gwinnett, 1973). However, this type of enamel does not appear to significantly affect the clinical performance of sealants (Hawes, 1973). Acid conditioning is confined to the inclined cuspal planes with regions below the fissural constriction being unaffected (Williams and von Fraunhofer, 1977).

After conditioning, the enamel is thoroughly rinsed with water (Fig. 11-14) and high-speed evacuation is used to capture the water and acid residue, which may taste unpleasant and cause an unwanted increase in salivary flow. Care should be taken to avoid splashing saliva onto the site. Wash times have been established at 10 to 15 seconds (Williams and von Fraunhofer, 1973) in which water composition seems to have no effect on bond strengths (Williams and von Fraunhofer, 1979). If gels are used, it is recommended that the wash time be doubled to at least 30 seconds to ensure removal of the gel and reaction products (Gwinnett, 1981).

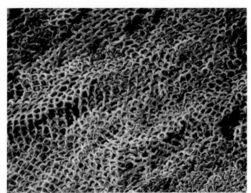 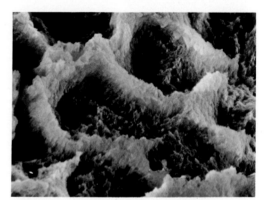

Figure 11-10 Scanning electron micrograph (1000 shows the typical surface morphology of etched enamel in which preferred dissolution of the rods is present.

Figure 11-11 Same as Figure 11-10. (5000×).

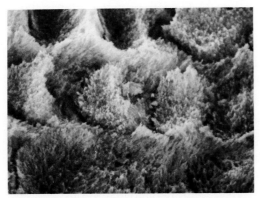

Figure 11-12 Same as Figure 11-10. (5000 ×).

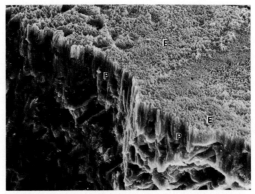

Figure 11-13 Conditioning of prismless enamel (P) confers porosity (E), but without disclosing a rod pattern (2000 ×).

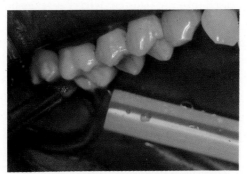

Figure 11-14 A 30-second period of water lavage is used to thoroughly clean the contaminant residues remaining after gel etching.

After washing, the site is thoroughly dried (Fig. 11-15) with oil-free compressed air. In the event that a rubber dam is not utilized, cotton rolls or absorbent pads should be carefully replaced, as necessary, to avoid contamination of the conditioned enamel with saliva. Fresh cotton rolls should be placed over existing ones before sliding the wet rolls from underneath. At this time, the surface energy of the enamel has been raised, and its integrity must be preserved until the sealant is in place and polymerized. Contamination with saliva (Fig. 11-16) physically alters the enamel surface and causes significant reduction in bond strength (Hormati et al, 1980). Should contamination occur, it is only necessary to recondition with phosphoric acid for 10 seconds in order to effectively remove the contaminant layer.

Enamel is a porous tissue in which intercommunicating pores and channels allow for the dynamic transport of fluid across the tissue. Acid conditioning enhances the size and volume of these spaces in the outer 20 to 30 micrometers of enamel (Gwinnett and Buonocore, 1965; Silverstone, 1975). The space created is large enough to accommodate the resin sealant molecules in monomer or liquid form, which readily penetrate the micropores. The resin sealants, filled and unfilled, are usually of the polymethacrylate type and are applied in a fluid, unpolymerized form. This is done with a brush (Fig. 11-17) or custom dispenser. The resin sealant should be teased into the fissured defects as far as possible by means of a sharp explorer (Fig. 11-18). Autopolymerized (Delton[2]) or light-cured (Prisma Shield[3]) sealants may be used. One of the advantages of visible-light-cured sealant materials is that they may be polymerized in a fraction of the time (30 to 40 seconds) required by self-cured sealants (90 seconds). The properties of the resin, achieved through careful formulation, penetrate 30 to 50 micrometers into the tissue and therein polymerize either chemically or by light activation. An examination of the interface between polymerized resin and enamel shows the former occupying space within the tissue (Gwinnett and Matsui, 1967) (Figs. 11-19 and 11-20). This mechanical entrapment of the resin by tag formation (Gwinnett and Buonocore, 1965) and its continuity with the bulk on the surface is the means by which the sealant is retained.

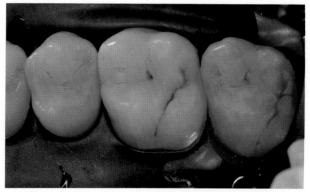

Figure 11-15 The enamel surface after acid etching, washing, and drying presents a white, frosty opaque appearance.

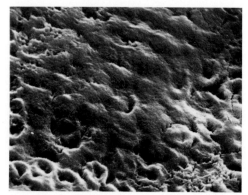

Figure 11-16 Scanning electron micrograph shows a contaminant of salivary protein on a conditioned enamel surface (2000 ×).

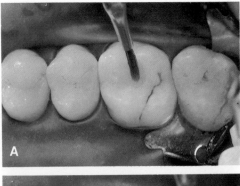

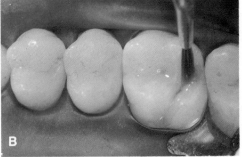

Figure 11–17 The sealant material is applied with the end of a fine-tipped brush, *A*, and carefully spread into the full extent of the fissured areas, *B*.

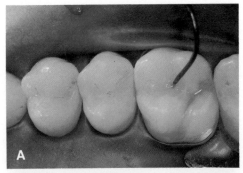

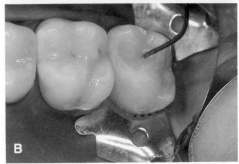

Figure 11–18 A fine-tipped explorer, *A*, is used to force the sealant material as far as possible into the depths of the fissured defects, *B*.

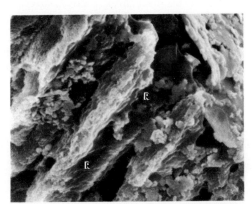

Figure 11–19 Scanning electron micrograph (2000 ×) shows the relationship between the resin (R) and conditioned enamel. Polymerized tags of resin have been disclosed by dissolution of the enamel.

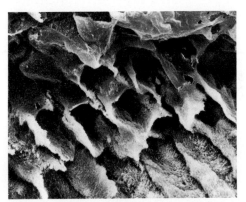

Figure 11-20 Same as Figure 11-19. (2000 ×).

The final step in the sealant procedure is to carefully examine the occlusal site for coverage by use of a good light and an explorer (Fig. 11-21). If isolation has been maintained, deficiencies can be remedied by simply adding fresh sealant. If the sealant is readily detached with an explorer, the procedure should be repeated from the beginning.

The results of controlled clinical trials have demonstrated the importance of sealants in caries prevention. As an adjunct to well-established methods such as fluoridation, sealants offer an exciting complement to facilitate reduction in caries attack rates of susceptible young individuals. Ripa (1973) has defined the cases in which sealants are indicated. These include recently erupted teeth with deep, narrow pits and fissures, a review of the general caries activity and the availability of other preventive procedures. Not all teeth of all patients require or are conducive to sealant application. Well-coalesced fissures are not at risk, nor are teeth that have been caries-free for 4 or more years. If many proximal lesions are present in an uncooperative patient, particularly where no preventive programs are available, sealants are not indicated.

Clinicians are understandably concerned over the possible consequences of inadvertently sealing active occlusal carious lesions since it is difficult, if not impossible, to reliably diagnose them in the incipient state. Recent research indicates that there is no need for real concern over this matter. In a long-term clinical investigation carried out at the University of Western Ontario, over 250 active occlusal carious lesions have been sealed and carefully followed for 7 to 8 years. Carious lesions that are sealed do not increase in size or extent over a long-term period provided the fissure sealant remains intact (Figs. 11-22 to 11-25). In fact, a certain degree of remineralization may well be associated with the hermetic seal (Figs. 11-26 and 11-27). Thus, if a clinician inadvertently seals an incipient occlusal carious lesion, arrest of the carious process occurs and remains for as long as the sealant is retained.

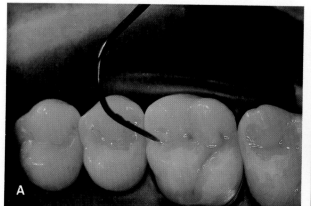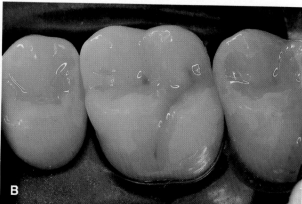

Figure 11-21 A sharp explorer is used, *A*, to ensure that the full extent of the fissured defects are properly sealed, *B*.

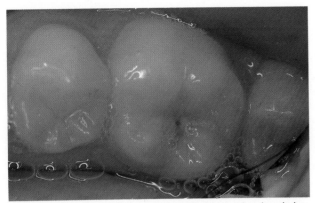

Figure 11–22 Clinical appearance of a typical occlusal carious lesion in the mandibular first molar, sealed in July, 1976.

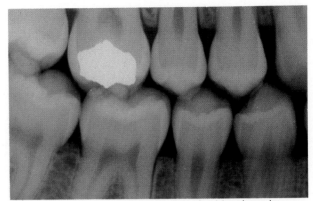

Figure 11–23 Bite-wing radiograph of the dentition shown in Figure 11-22, showing the extent of the carious lesion In the mandibular first molar approximately halfway between the dentin-enamel junction and the pulp.

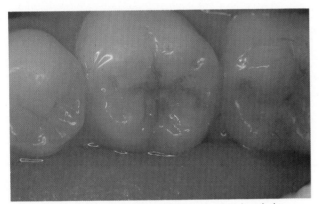

Figure 11–24 Clinical appearance of the occlusal carious lesion shown in Figures 11-22 and 11-23 in July, 1983 (7-year recall). The occlusal sealant is intact and there is no increase in size of the lesion.

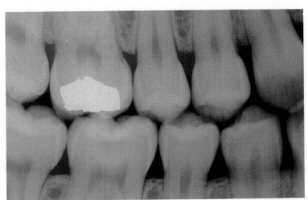

Figure 11–25 Bite-wing radiograph of the sealed mandibular first molar at 7-year recall (July, 1983). No increase in size of the lesion is apparent.

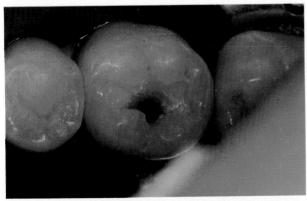

Figure 11–26 Occlusal view of the mandibular first molar shown in Figures 11-22 to 11-25, after the establishment of outline form for class I restoration. The carious dentin appears highly desiccated.

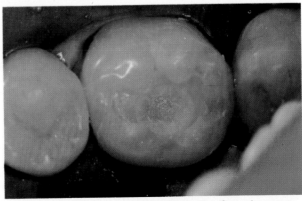

Figure 11–27 The same mandibular first molar after caries excavation. A layer of discolored but intact dentin is observed in the depths of the excavated lesion.

REFERENCES

Ast DB, Bushel A, Chase HD. Clinical study of caries prophylaxis with zinc chloride and potassium ferrocyanide. J Am Dent Assoc 1950; 41:437.

Backer-Dirks O. Longitudinal dental caries study in children 9–15 years of age. Arch Oral Biol 1961; 6:94.

Black GV. Descriptive Anatomy of the Human Teeth. Philadelphia: S.S. White Dental Manufacturing, 1897.

Bodecker CF. The eradication of enamel fissures. Dent Items Int 1929; 51:859.

Bowen RL. Dental filling material comprising vinyl silane treated fused silica and a binder consisting of the reaction product of bisphenol and glycidyl acrylate. U.S. Patent 3; 066, 122, 1962.

Brauer GM, Termini JD. Bonding of bovine enamel to restorative resin: Effect of pretreatment of enamel. J Dent Res 1972; 51:151.

Buonocore MG. Simple method of increasing the adhesion of acrylic filling materials to enamel surfaces. J Dent Res 1955; 34:849.

Chow LC, Brown WE. Phosphoric acid conditioning of teeth for fit and fissure sealants. J Dent Res 1973; 52:1158.

Dennison JB, Craig RG. Characterization of enamel surfaces prepared with commercial and experimental etchants. J Am Dent Assoc 1978; 97:799.

Galil KA. Scanning and transmission electron microscopic examination of occlusal plaque following tooth brushing. J Can Dent Assoc 1975; 41:499.

Galil KA Gwinnett AJ. Three-dimensional replicas of pits and fissures in human teeth. Scanning electron microscopy study. Arch Oral Biol 1975; 20:493.

Going RW, Loesch WJ, Grainger DA. The viability of microorganisms in carious lesions five years after covering with a fissure sealant. J Am Dent Assoc 1978; 97:455.

Graves RC, Burt BA. The pattern of the carious attack in children as a consideration in the use of fissure sealants. J Prev Dent 1975; 2:28.

Gwinnett AJ. Acid etch for composite resins. Dent Clin North Am 1981; 25:271.

Gwinnett AJ. Histologic changes in human enamel following treatment with acidic adhesive conditioning agents. Arch Oral Biol 1971; 16:731.

Gwinnett AJ. Human prismless enamel and its influence on sealant penetration. Arch Oral Biol 1973; 18:441.

Gwinnett AJ. Scientific basis for the sealant procedure. J Prev Dent 1976; 3:15–28.

Gwinnett AJ, Buonocore MG. Adhesives and caries prevention. A preliminary report. Br Dent J 1965; 119:77.

Gwinnett AJ, Buonocore MG. A scanning electron microscope study of pits and fissures conditioned for adhesive sealing. Arch Oral Biol 1972; 17:415.

Gwinnett AJ, Matsui A. A study of enamel adhesives: the physical relationship between enamel and adhesive. Arch Oral Biol 1967; 12:1615.

Hawes R. Clinical application of dental adhesives in primary teeth. Dental Adhesive Materials. Symp Proc US Department of Health, Education and Welfare, 1973:282.

Hennon DK, Stookey GK, Muhler JC. Prevalence and distribution of caries in pre-school children. J Am Dent Assoc 1969; 79:1405.

Hormati AJ, Fuller JL, Denehy GE. Effects of contamination and mechanical disturbance on the quality of acid etch enamel. J Am Dent Assoc 1980; 100:34.

Hyatt TP. Prophylactic odonototomy: the cutting into the tooth for prevention of disease. Dent Cosmos 1923; 65:234.

Jeronimus DJ, Till MJ, Sveen OB. Reduced viability of microorganisms under dental sealants. J Dent Child 1975; 42:275.

Keyes PH, Jordan HV. Factors influencing the initiation of dental caries. Mechanisms of Hard Tissue Destruction, American Assoc for Advancement of Science publication, 1963.

Lewis DW, Hargreaves JA. Epidemiology of dental caries in relation to pits and fissures. Br Dent J 1975; 138:345.

Loesch WJ. Bacterial studies related to sealants. Sealant Symposium, Am Assoc Dent Res, New York, NY, 1975.

Maijer R. Bonding systems in orthodontics. In: Biocompatibility of Dental Materials. Boca Raton: CRC Press, 1982:51.

Mertz-Fairhurst et al. A comparative clinical study of two pit and fissure sealants: 7-year results in Augusta, GA, J Am Dent Assoc 1984; 109:252.

Miller J. Clinical investigations in preventive dentistry. Br Dent J 1951; 91:92.

Miura F, Nakagawa K, Ishizaki A. Scanning electron microscopic studies on the direct bonding system. Bull Tokyo Dent Med Univ 1973; 20:245.

Mullholland RD, deShazer DO. The effect of acidic pretreatment solutions on the direct bonding of orthodontic brackets on enamel. Agle Orthodont 1968; 38:236.

Paynter KJ, Grainger RM. Relationship of morphology and size of teeth to caries. Int Dent J 1962; 12:147.

Retief DH. Failure at the dental adhesive-etched enamel interface. J Oral Rehabil 1974; 1:265.

Ripa LW. Occlusal sealing: rationale of the technique and historical review. JASPD 1973; 3:32.

Ripa LW, Gwinnett AJ. The prismless outer layer of deciduous and permanent teeth. Dent Radiol 1967; 40:38.

Rock WP. The effects of etching human enamel upon bond strengths with fissure sealant resins. Arch Oral Biol 1974; 19:873.

Shey Z, Houpt M. The clinical effectiveness of delton fissure sealant after forty-five months. Dent Res 1980; 59:428. (Abstract 642)

Silverstone LM. The acid etch technique. In vitro studies with special reference to the enamel surface and the enamel resin interface. In: Proceedings of the International Symposium on Acid Etch Technique. St. Paul: North Central Publishing 1975:13.

Stephen KW, Kirkwood M, Main C, Gillespie FC, Campbell D. Retention of a filled fissure sealant using reduced etched time. Br Dent J 1982; 153:232.

Taylor CV, Gwinnett AJ. A comparative study of the penetration of sealants into pits and fissures. J Am Dent Assoc 1973; 87:1181.

Williams B, von Fraunhofer JA. Possible factors in the adhesion of fissure sealants to enamel. J Oral Rehabil 1979; 6:345.

Williams B, von Fraunhofer JA. The influence of the time of etching and washing on the bond strength of fissure sealants applied to enamel. J Oral Rehabil 1977; 4:139.

Williams B, von Fraunhofer JA, Winter GB. Etching of enamel prior to application of fissure sealants. J Oral Rehabil 1976; 3:185.

Product Information

Product	Manufacturer/Distributor	Purpose
1. Handi-Dry	Lancer Pacific 6050 Avenida Encinas Carlsbad, CA 92008	For warm air drying enamel surfaces
2. Delton	Johnson and Johnson 20 Lake Drive, CN7060 East Windsor, NJ 08520	Self-cured sealant
3. Prisma Shield	L. D. Caulk Co. P.O. Box 359 Milford, DE 19963	Visible-light-cured sealant

INDEX

Page numbers followed by *t* indicate tables; those followed by *f* indicate figures.